THE USE OF THE CREATIVE THERAPIES WITH CHEMICAL DEPENDENCY ISSUES

THE USE OF THE CREATIVE THERAPIES WITH CHEMICAL DEPENDENCY ISSUES

Edited by

STEPHANIE L. BROOKE, Ph.D., NCC

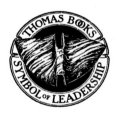

CHARLES C THOMAS • PUBLISHER, LTD.
Springfield • Illinois • U.S.A.

Published and Distributed Throughout the World by

CHARLES C THOMAS • PUBLISHER, LTD.
2600 South First Street
Springfield, Illinois 62794-9265

© 2009 by CHARLES C THOMAS • PUBLISHER, LTD.

ISBN 978-0-398-07861-4 (hard)
ISBN 978-0-398-07862-1 (paper)

Library of Congress Catalog Card Number: 2008049677

With THOMAS BOOKS *careful attention is given to all details of manufacturing
and design. It is the Publisher's desire to present books that are satisfactory as to their
physical qualities and artistic possibilities and appropriate for their particular use.*
THOMAS BOOKS *will be true to those laws of quality that assure a good name
and good will.*

*Printed in the United States of America
MM-R-3*

Library of Congress Cataloging in Publication Data

The use of the creative therapies with chemical dependency issues / edited by
Stephanie L. Brooke (with 16 other contributors)
    p. cm.
Includes biographical references and index.
ISBN 978-0-398-07861-4 (hard)–ISBN 078-0-398-07862-1 (pbk.)
1. Substance abuse–Treatment. 2. Arts–Therapeutic use. I. Brooke,
Stephanie L.
[DNLM: 1. Substance-Related Disorders–therapy. 2. Creativeness. 3.
Sensory Art Therapies–methods. WM 270 U848 2009]

RC564.U84 2009
616.89'165–dc22   2008049677

CONTRIBUTORS

I extend my deepest appreciation to the following contributors for sharing their expertise and experience regarding their work with chemical dependency issues. Each of these contributors was selected on the basis of his or her experience with respect to clinical issues, diversity in theoretical orientation, or treatment modality. As you read each chapter, it is my hope you will share in my appreciation for the insights contributed by the following individuals.

Mari Alschuler, LCSW, PTR

Sally Bailey, MFA, MSW, RDT/BCT

Brian L. Bethel, M.Ed., PCC/S LCDC III, RPTS

Corinna Brown, MA, MS, ADTR, CASAC, LCAT

Cosmin Gheorghe, MFT

Stephen Demanchick, Ph.D., LMHC

Meghan Dempsey, MS, ADTR, CMA, LCAT

D. Desjardins

Linda M. Dunne, MA, RDT

Katherin M. Fernandez, BA

Annie Heiderscheit, Ph.D., MT-BC, FAMI, NMT

Lisa D. Hinz, Ph.D., ATR

Ellen G. Horovitz, Ph.D., ATR-BC, LCAT

Shelley A. Perkoulidis, MA, MMH

Priyadarshini Senroy, MA DMT CCC

Stephanie Wise, MA, ATR-BC, LCAT

PREFACE

*T*he Use of the Creative Therapies with Chemical Dependency Issues is a comprehensive work that examines the use of art, play, music, dance/movement, drama, and poetry therapies with respect to treatment issues relating to substance abuse. The author's primary purpose is to examine treatment approaches which cover the broad spectrum of the creative art therapies. The collection of chapters is written by renowned, well-credentialed, and professional creative art therapists in the areas of art, play, music, dance/movement, drama, and poetry. In addition, some of the chapters are complimented with photographs of client artwork, diagrams, and tables. The reader is provided with a snapshot of how these various creative art therapies are used to treat males and females suffering from issues related to chemical dependency. This informative book will be of special interest to educators, students, and therapists as well as people struggling with substance abuse.

S.L.B.

CONTENTS

THE USE THE OF CREATIVE THERAPIES WITH CHEMICAL DEPENDENCY ISSUES

KNOWING

Feeling
My legs
Scrambling beneath me
Trying
Desperately
To balance my propelled upper body
Praying
That I won't hit the fireplace
That seems to be coming at me
Hoping
That I can walk away with some dignity
When it is finally over
Wondering
What my children
Must think
Knowing
That this is
All so wrong.

D. Desjardins (2004)

Chapter 1

INTRODUCTION–SUBSTANCE ABUSE ISSUES AROUND THE WORLD

Stephanie L. Brooke

For quite some time, I have had an interest in using the creative therapies–art, play, dance, music, drama, and poetry–for the treatment of a variety of issues including sexual abuse, eating disorders, and domestic violence. This work is dedicated to the use of these creative approaches to the treatment of alcohol and substance abuse. Given that most of the chapters in this book cover substance abuse issues within the United States and Canada, I wanted to provide the reader with a snapshot of chemical dependency issues around the globe. This chapter is by no means comprehensive but does cover the most recent research with respect to this issue. My hope is that the reader will share in my curiosity about how this pervasive problem affects other countries. Substance abuse creates a host of other issues affecting individuals, families, and society: Chemical dependency is associated with increases in violence, lower worker productivity, increased mental health problems, and sexually transmitted diseases such as HIV infection (Probst, Gold, & Cayborn, 2008). Substance use and abuse is on the rise, particularly with the use of methamphetamines. Just to give an example, worldwide production of illegal methamphetamine and amphetamine is estimated to be as high as 332 metric tons per year with 27 million recent users of which 2.7 million live in Europe, 4.3 million in the Americas, 16.7 million in Asia, 1.8 million in Africa, and 600 thousand in Oceania (Zabransky, 2007). This chapter will cite recent research on substance abuse in China, Japan, Africa, Russia, Greece, and Brazil.

3

Chemical Dependency Issues in China

In a study by Cheung and colleagues (2008), the sample included 1,749 participants with psychiatric diagnoses, of which there were 149 participants with substance use disorders as the primary diagnosis. Opioid was the major substance used by this group of participants (71%), with the remaining participants being addicted to alcohol (29%). For instance, in China and Hong Kong, opiod abuse was the most common drug-related problem. Given that these participants were recruited from the substance use treatment units at psychiatric hospitals and clinics, they were likely to be at the more severe end of the distribution of persons with chemical dependency problems in the Chinese community. Alcohol did not seem to be as much of a problem in this culture according to Cheung and colleagues (2008).

I also found a *CRDA 56th Report: Drug Statistics of the Central Registry of Drug Abuse,* by the Hong Kong SAR Government (2007). This report was very detailed and stated that drug abuse in the Chinese culture is more common among males than females. It reported that although males abused more than females, drug abuse among males was 6.8% lower in 2006 compared to 2005. The average age of male substance abusers was 35 in 2002, 37 in 2005, and then dropped to 36 in 2006. It concluded that female substance abusers were generally younger than their male counterparts with the average age of 27 in 2006.

According to Chen and Huang (2007), drug crime in China is on an overall rising trend. Major drug crime cases are becoming more common and the types of drugs being trafficked are more diverse. Further, the smuggling and trafficking of drugs into the country and the smuggling of precursor chemicals out of the country have formed a bidirectional cycle. They also reported a trend of internationalization with respect to the drug crimes in China. To counteract this problem, China has taken a number of measures against drugs including passing new laws and regulations against drugs, increasing the efforts to eradicate cultivation, establishing and expanding "drug-free communities" programs, and strengthening international cooperation in antidrug campaigns. The authors called for more scientific studies of drug problems within this culture (Chen & Huang, 2007).

Chemical Dependency Issues in Japan

McCurry (2005) provided an interesting historical overview to the alcohol abuse in Japan. Specifically, he looked at the drinking problem in Osaka, the world's second richest country. With the 1990 recession that hit Japan, many people lost their jobs and became homeless. McCurry reported that five of every 100 homeless people have a drinking problem with 2 percent being addicted to drugs. He describes the drug dealers as members of the local yakuza (mafia), who sell amphetamines and heroin through their car windows. Arrests are rare. Further, it was found that the prevalence of methamphetamine abuse since WWII is not known in Japan (Zabransky, 2007). Yet, the drug remains a matter of social concern and law enforcement priority. Indirect indicators suggest a recent sharp rise of its consumption (Zabransky, 2007).

Ahmad (2003) reported that amphetamines have been a problem for about six decades in Japan. Immediately after World War II, large quantities of intravenous methamphetamine stored for military use were made available to the general public. What ensued was methamphetamine use reaching epidemic proportions. "We are experiencing the third epidemic of methamphetamine abuse since World War II," says Kiyoshi Wada of the National Institute of Mental Health, Chiba-ken, Japan (as cited in Ahmad, 2003). During the past several years, crimes involving amphetamines have accounted for 90% of all drug-related crimes (Ahmad, 2003).

Chemical Dependency Issues in Africa

Reddy and colleagues (2007) compared prevalence rates and correlates of substance use among high school students in South Africa and the United States. The rates of alcohol and marijuana use were lower among South African students than among U.S. students, but rates of illicit hard drug use were higher. They found that being female was protective against tobacco, alcohol, and marijuana use in South Africa, whereas in the United States it was protective only against marijuana use. Black race/ethnicity was associated with lower rates of cigarette and alcohol use in both countries, yet the protective effect for alcohol use was stronger in South Africa (Reddy et al., 2007).

According to Obot (2007), a recent survey in central and southern Nigeria shows that 41.5% of male and 22% of female Nigerians consumed some form of alcoholic beverage. Compared to European countries, abstention rates are high in Nigeria, particularly among women. Yet, the country has one of the highest overall per capita consumption figures of recorded alcohol in Africa. Per capita, consumption of alcohol increased steadily throughout the 1970s and peaked at 8 liters in 1981, declined until about 1995 and increased slowly to an estimated 10 liters in 2001. Drinking begins early and surveys among youth show that high proportions report lifetime and current drinking (Obot, 2007).

Intravenous drug use is of great concern globally due to the transmission of HIV. The number of African countries experiencing intravenous drug use is reported to be growing (Dewing et al., 2006). Dewing and colleagues provide a thorough review of the available literature pertaining to intravenous drug use within six African countries: Egypt, Kenya, Mauritius, Nigeria, South Africa, and Tanzania. They report a contradiction in the prevailing view that intravenous drug use is extremely rare or non-existent in Africa. Intravenous drug users were shown to engage in high-risk sexual and injecting behaviors. According to UNODC (2004), approximately 0.2% of Africa's adult population uses heroin, a prevalence rate described as approaching the global average (as cited in Dewing et al., 2006). This is an in-depth article citing statistics of intravenous drug use.

Chemical Dependency Issues in Russia

In the 1990s, Russia experienced economic and political upheavals. Pridemore (2006) stated that Russian levels of alcohol consumption and suicide are among the highest in the world. Pridemore examined the cross-sectional association between heavy drinking and suicide mortality in Russia. A positive and significant association between alcohol and suicide was found. This study confirmed an association between heavy drinking and suicide in Russia, and when compared to findings from previous studies of other countries, it led to the thought that a nation's level of alcohol use may be as important as its drinking culture in the sensitivity of its suicide rates to alcohol consumption. Annual alcohol consumption in Russia is estimated to be nearly 15 liters per person as compared to average rates of about 10 and 7 liters per person in the Europe and the United States. The age standardized suicide rate in Russia in 2000 of about 38 per 100,000 persons and was reported to be second only to Lithuania and was two to three times higher than in Europe and the United States. In addition, Pridemore described three distinctive traits of Russian consumption: The preference for alcohol, binge drinking, and sociocultural tolerance for heavy drinking and concomitant behavior. Vodka represents about 75 percent of the alcohol consumed in the country and survey data showed that about one-third of Russian males admitted to binge-drinking vodka at least once per month (Pridemore, 2006).

Tompkins and colleagues (2007) were interested in the relationship between substance abuse and HIV transmission in Russia. Participants were an age-stratified, population-based random sample of men aged 25–54 years living in Izhevsk, Russia. Questionnaires ascertained about behavioral indicators of hazardous drinking derived from frequency of having a hangover, frequency of drinking alcohol, episodes in the last year of extended periods of drunkenness during which the participant withdraws from normal life (zapoi), consumption of alcoholic substances not intended to be drunk (surrogates), and socioeconomic position. Findings indicated that 79% of this sample drank alcohol and 8% drank surrogates at least sometimes in the past year; 25% drank alcohol and 4% drank surrogates at least weekly; and 10% had had an episode of zapoi in the past year. Education was strongly associated with indicators of hazardous drinking. Men with the lowest level of education compared to the highest level of education had an odds ratio of surrogate drinking of 7.7 (95% CI 3.2–18.5), of zapoi of 5.2 (2.3–11.8) and of frequent hangover of 3.7 (1.8–7.4). These indicators of hazardous drinking were also strongly associated with being unemployed. This research showed that the prevalence of these behaviors is high among working-age men in this Russian city. Further, these hazardous behaviors show a very clear socioeconomic pattern, with particularly high prevalence among those who have had the least education and are not in employment (Tompkins et al., 2007).

Chemical Dependency Issues in Greece

Greek society has grown increasingly concerned about the epidemic of drug misuse, particularly among young people (Arvanitidou et al., 2007). This study looked at the data on alcohol consumption among secondary education students and investigated the correlation to their health behaviors and parental socioeconomic status. A questionnaire was distributed to students from a representative sample of 15 schools from Thessaloniki, Greece. It was found previously that this city had the highest prevalence of drinking. A sample of 1,185 students (505 males, 680 females) participated in this study. It was found that 286 males (56.6%) and 329 females (48.4%) reported consuming alcohol. The average age of drinking was 13.2 years for boys and 13 years for girls. Alcohol drinking was positively associated with sociodemographic variables and negative health behaviors such as parental low level of education, lack of physical exercise, coffee consumption, and smoking. The authors concluded that although the results showed a decrease in alcohol use, being more pronounced in male students, the prevalence of frequent alcohol consumption is among the highest in Europe's countries. The authors suggested that changes like alcohol taxation and high alcohol prices, as well as a reduction in the amount of money available to people, influences the frequency of drinking (Arvanitidou et al., 2007).

In Greece, alcohol is considered to be an important part of culture with binge-drinking being largely avoided (Foster et al., 2007). Further, using other substances including illicit drugs is traditionally not encouraged. Foster and colleagues investigated prescription, over-the-counter and illicit drug use trends, and their link to mental health by synthesizing previous literature on chemical dependency issues. They examined a total of 184 articles, of which 23 were used. The review indicated that illicit drug use had increased threefold since 1984, with cannabis being the most frequently used drug by all age groups and both sexes. On the other hand, compared with other western nations, the use of opiates and cocaine is rare. They concluded that despite strong cultural disapproval, use is likely to continue to increase, especially since adolescents believe that access to such drugs is becoming easier (Foster et al., 2007).

Chemical Dependency Issue in Brazil

Pechansky and colleagues (2007) compared changes in AIDS awareness and risk behaviors among Brazilian cocaine users. The sample included 119 participants which were randomly assigned to either a standard or a standard plus "thought-mapping" intervention. The participants were re-interviewed two and eight weeks after intake using standardized data collection instruments. They found significant increases in AIDS awareness and condom use in the experimental group, as well as significant changes for sexual and drug-risk behaviors. On the other hand, they found that the experimental intervention was less successful in decreasing mean days of cocaine use when compared to the standard. They concluded that components of the experimental thought-mapping model might be useful in combination with other approaches (Pechansky et al., 2007).

Lima and colleagues (2007) wanted to examine differences in patterns of use in the context of gender. The authors looked at the patterns of alcohol consumption in a community sample from Sao Paulo City, Brazil. A survey was carried out with a representative urban sample, stratified by clusters. The GENACIS questionnaire was used in 1,473 face-to-face interviews. They found that for both genders heavy drinking (HD) was associated with having an HD partner and feeling less inhibited about sex when drinking. For men, HD was associated with a younger age and for women with drinking alone. A positive attitude towards drinking, sex, and having a partner who also was a heavy drinker were thus predictors of HD for both genders. Further, they found that younger men and women drinking alone were more at risk of heavy drinking. They sought to explain these differences from the biological point of view—women reach a higher blood alcohol concentration than men from the same amount of alcohol. From the sociocultural perspective, they stated that other aspects such as, for example, differences in social roles of men and women, have been described as factors associated with distinct patterns of alcohol use. They did mention the critique that it was possible that the rate was underestimated as a greater number of women were in the sample (Lima et al., 2007).

This presented a brief snapshot of research conducted on chemical dependency issues in other countries such as China, Japan, Africa, Russia, Greece, and Brazil. This book will examine creative therapy treatment approaches with the population of individuals classified as chemically dependent. The first section will focus on art therapy. The first art therapy chapter focuses on the use of this therapy with the Deaf and Hard of Hearing Population. The next chapter looks at the use of the open art studio method with a chemically dependent population in New York City. Chapter 3 discusses open studio art therapy in a Harm Reduction Center. Chapter 4 looks at the expressive therapies continuum as a framework for art therapy interventions in substance abuse treatment. In Chapter 5, the writer discusses the use of multifamily group art therapy with Australian adolescents. Chapter 6 is a quantitative study utilizing comic/cartoon drawings with clients at an inpatient treatment center and addressing ambivalence issues. In Chapter 7, the author discusses the use of play therapy with children. Chapter 8 discusses the use of play therapy, specifically filial therapy, to repair the relationship between a parent who is a substance abuser and the child. Chapter 9 provides an overview of music therapy in the treatment of substance abuse. Next, we move into dance/movement therapy as a means of decreasing anxiety and providing support for recovery. The next chapter looks at the use of the expressive arts therapy with a group of male offenders recovering from substance abuse in India. Chapter 12 looks at the use of dance/movement therapy with a person classified as dually diagnosed in a methadone treatment program. In Chapter 13, we move into drama therapy as a means of recovering identity and stimulating growth. Chapter 14 looks at the use of individual drama therapy in the treatment of alcohol-related issues. Chapter 15 discusses the use of existential drama therapy and addictive behaviors. Last but not least, Chapter 16 looks at the use of poetry therapy in the treatment of addictions. I thoroughly hope you enjoy this work!

References

Ahmad, K. (2003, May). Asia grapples with spreading amphetamine abuse. *The Lancet, 361*(9372), 1878.

Arvanitidou, M., Tirodimos, I., Kyriakidis, I., Tsinaslanidou, Z., & Seretopoulos, D. (2007). Decreasing prevalence of alcohol consumption among Greek adolescents. *The American Journal of Drug and Alcohol Abuse, 33*, 411–417.

CRDA 56th Report: Drug Statistics of the Central Registry of Drug Abuse, Hong Kong SAR Government. (2008). Retrieved July 24, 2008, from http://www.nd.gov.hk/text/stat/56_report.htm

Chen, Z. L., & Huang, K. C. (2007). Drug problems in China: Recent trends, countermeasures and challenges. *International Journal of Offender Therapy and Comparative Criminology, 51*, 98–109.

Cheung, F. M., Cheung, S. F., & Leung, F. (2008, June). Clinical utility of the Cross-Cultural (Chinese) Personality Assessment Inventory (CPAI-2) in the assessment of substance use disorders among Chinese men. *Psychological Assessment, 20*(2), 103–113.

Dewing, S., Plüddemann, A., Myers, B. J., & Parry, C. D. H. (2006, April). Review of injection drug use in six African countries: Egypt, Kenya, Mauritius, Nigeria, South Africa and Tanzania. *Drugs: Education, Prevention & Policy, 13*(2), 121–137.

Foster, J., Papadopoulous, C., Dadzie, L., & Jayasinghe, N. (2007, October). A review of the literature concerning illicit drugs, prescription drugs of abuse and their link to mental health in Greek communities. *Journal of Substance Use, 12*(5), 311–322.

Lima, M. C. P., Kerr-Corrêa, F., Tucci, A. M., Simao, M. O., Oliveira, J. B., Cavariani, M. B., & Fantazia, M. M. (2007). Gender differences in heavy alcohol use: A general population survey (The Genacis Project) of São Paulo City, Brazil. *Contemporary Drug Problems, 34*(3), 427–444.

McCurry, J. (2005, Jan-Feb). Drinking too much sake in Osaka. *The Lancet, 365* (9457), 375–377.

Obot, I. S. (2007, April). Nigeria: Alcohol and society today. *Addiction, 102*(4), 519–522.

Pechansky, F., von Diemen, L., Kessler, F., Leukefeld, C. G., Surratt, H. L., Inciardi, J. A., & Martin, S. S. (2007, September). Using thought mapping and structured stories to decrease HIV risk behaviors among cocaine injectors and crack smokers in the South of Brazil. *Revista Brasileira de Psiquiatria, 29*(3), No Pagination Specified.

Pridemore, W. A. (2006). An exploratory analysis of homocide victims, offenders, and events in Russia. *International Criminal Justice Review, 16*(1), 5–23.

Probst, T. M., Gold, D., & Caborn, J. (2008). A Preliminary Evaluation of SOLVE: Addressing Psychosocial Problems at Work. *Journal of Occupational Health Psychology, 13*(1), 32–42.

Reddy, P., Resnicow, K., Omardien, R., & Kamabaran, N. (2007). Prevalence and correlates of substance use among high school students in South Africa and the United States. *American Journal of Public Health, 97*(10), 0090036.

Tompkins, S., Saburova, L., Kiryanov, N., Andreev, E., McKee, M., Shkolnikov, V., & Leon, D. A. (2007). Prevalence and socio-economic distribution of hazardous patterns of alcohol drinking: Study of alcohol consumption in men aged 25–54 years in Izhevsk, Russia. *Addiction, 102,* 544–553.

Walley, A. Y., Krupitsy, E. M., Cheng, D. M., Raj, A., Edwards, E. M., Bridden, C., Egorova, E. Y., Zvartau, E. E., Woody, G. E., & Samet, J. H. (2008). Implications of cannabis use and heavy alcohol use on HIV drug risk behaviors in Russian heroin users. *AIDS and Behavior, 12*(4), 662–669.

Zabransky, T. (2007, Winter). Methamphetamine in the Czech Republic. *Journal of Drug Issues, 37*(1), 155.

Biography

Stephanie L. Brooke, Ph.D., NCC, teaches sociology and psychology for Excelsior College, University of Maryland, and Capella University. She also has written books on art therapy and edits books on the use of the creative therapies: *Tools of the Trade: A therapist's guide to art therapy assessments; Art therapy with sexual abuse survivors; The creative therapy manual; The use of the creative therapies with sexual abuse survivors; The creative therapies and eating disorders;* and *The creative therapies with domestic violence issues.* In October 2006, she was the chief consultant for the first Creative Art Therapy Conference in Tokyo, Japan. Dr. Brooke continues to write and publish in her field. Further, Dr. Brooke serves on the editorial boards of PSYCCritiques and the *International Journal of Teaching and Learning in Higher Education.* She is Vice Chairperson for ARIA (Awareness of Rape and Incest through Art). For more information about Dr. Brooke, please visit her web site: http://www.stephanielbrooke.com

Chapter 2

COMBATING SHAME AND PATHOGENIC BELIEF SYSTEMS: THEORETICAL AND ART THERAPY APPLICATIONS FOR CHEMICAL/ SUBSTANCE ABUSIVE DEAF CLIENTS

Ellen G. Horovitz

Introduction

Recovery programs for the chemically dependent individual presents numerous quandaries but when the patient is chemically dependent Deaf and/or hard-of-hearing, (herein referred to as HOH), obstacles may include: shame (lack of recognition or a problem within the community—hearing or Deaf); confidentiality issues; lack of substance abuse resources for Deaf/ HOH people; enabling from friends, family, and often professionals; and lack of funding for ongoing treatment and/or recovery.

To boot, there seems to be a dearth of treatment options for the Deaf/ HOH client that is not based in a hearing 12-Step management system. Therapeutic remedy is not readily apparent for this aforementioned population. Thus, bromidic results were culminated from a variety of theoretical underpinnings, all of which were informed by the common thread of shame and exploration of pathogenic belief systems.

Historical Review of the Chemical/ Substance Abusive Deaf Client

McCrone (1994) tabulated the following data regarding substance abuse amongst Deaf/ HOH people in the United States: 3505 Deaf heroin users, 31,915 Deaf cocaine users, 5101 Deaf crack users, and 97,745 Deaf marijuana users. (These figures were based on the 1992 U.S. Department of Justice

Reports of the overall illicit drug use in the United States and the assumption that Deaf people represent .5% of the general population (Guthmann & Blozis, 2001.) Additionally, the National Council on Alcoholism identified that approximately 600,000 people experience both alcoholism and hearing loss (Kearns, 1989). The widespread pathognomic perspective considers Deaf people to have an impairment that is in need of repair. Yet, the social minority viewpoint judges Deaf people to be members of a unique cultural and linguistic population (Horovitz, 2007; Lane, Hoffmeister, & Bahan, 1996; McCullogh, & Duchesneau, 2007). Historically, the American mental health system has woefully neglected to meet the needs of its Deaf clients (Pollard, 1994; Steinberg, Sullivan, & Loew, 1998).

Other than the McCrone report (1994), little data is available regarding the extent of substance and /or chemical abuse with the Deaf or HOH individual. Most research indicates that the Deaf and HOH person faces at least the same risk of alcoholism and drug abuse as hearing people (Horovitz, 2007; Lane, 1985; Moore, 1991). To date, approximately 123 specialized outpatient and 24 specialized inpatient mental health service programs for Deaf people exist in the United States (Kendall, 2002; Morton & Kendall, 2003). Yet, Deaf and HOH people have unique needs often not adequately tackled due to inadequate accessibility (Lane, 1985; McCullogh & Duchesneau, 2007; Pollard, 1994; Rendon 1992; Steinberg, Sullivan, & Loew, 1998; Whitehouse, Sherman & Kozlowski, 1991). The following barriers include:

1. *Recognition of the Problem*–Beyond the general lack of awareness of the problem of substance abuse in the Deaf community, this is compounded by a lack of appropriate education/ prevention curricula as well as limited access to educate Deaf people about alcohol and drugs through the mass media (Guthmann & Blozis, 2001; Whitehouse, Sherman & Kozlowski, 1991).

2. *Confidentiality and Shame*–Deaf individuals often fear that their treatment experience will become part of the Deaf "grapevine" and thus are reluctant to share their stories with others and/or seek treatment (Guthmann & Blozis, 2001).

3. *Lack of Resources*–Historically, chemical and substance abuse treatment services for the Deaf or HOH client have been limited. Further, there is a shortage of qualified professionals trained in the areas of substance abuse and Deafness (Guthmann & Blozis, 2001; Pollard, 1994; McCullogh & Duchesneau 2007; Whitehouse, Sherman & Kozlowski, 1991).

4. *Enabling*–Family members, friends, and even professionals (as will be evidenced in this case) often protect individuals who are labeled "disabled or handicapped," by hearing persons. Substance abuse exacer-

bates this problem often resulting in the Deaf or HOH person being unaccountable for his or her behavior (Guthmann & Blozis, 2001).

5. *Funding Difficulties*–Specialized programs with appropriately trained professionals and staff (interpreters, etc.) is costly and results in creating an additional barrier in and of itself (Guthmann & Blozis, 2001; Lane, 1985; McCullogh & Duchesneau 2007).

6. *Lack of Support in Recovery*–Detachment from "old friends" and relatively few Deaf role models result in a lack of support. Moreover, until recently, alcoholism or drug addiction was often viewed as morally inept (e.g., reprehensible) instead of a chronic disease, further contributing to shame and ostracism from the Deaf community (Guthmann & Blozis, 2001; McCullogh & Duchesneau, 2007; Rendon, 1992).

7. *Communication Barriers*–Traditional 12-Step treatment approaches often emphasize the use of reading/writing tasks and "talk therapy." HOH or Deaf people face additional problems including poor acoustical environments (environments predominately designed for a hearing population), inadequate lighting, inability to follow "group" conversations (especially if mixed in with hearing people), and lack of captioned or sign video-recorded material (Guthmann & Blozis, 2001; Larson & McAlpine, 1988; McCullogh & Duchesneau, 2007). Of exception is a unique program, the Minnesota Program (Minnesota Program for Deaf and Hard-of-Hearing Individuals) that uses methods based on the 12-Step model yet offers additional features such as asking clients to draw as a means of completing assignments and utilizing role-play and similar activities, which serve to activate the unique linguistic system of the Deaf (Horovitz, 2007).

Shame: Historical and Psychological Impact

Assessment is of utmost importance, not just in determining the sociohistory of the individual but also in appraising the Deaf/ HOH individual understanding of alcohol/ chemical dependency, and clinical jargon (McCullogh & Duchesneau, 2007). Often this information can be improperly interpreted especially when an interpreter is used who is not well-versed in mental health issues. This further complicates matters when working with a Deaf/HOH individual (Horovitz, 2007; McCullogh & Duchesneau, 2007). Regarding the use of art therapy with Deaf clients, McCullough & Duschesneau (2007) stated:

> As a unique assessment and treatment modality, art therapy has much to offer Deaf clients and the mental health professionals who work with them. Visual and tactile in nature, this particular type of therapy is especially well-suited for use

with Deaf people. The clinicians who can establish the most effective rapport with this population are those who possess an awareness and understanding of the diversity of Deaf people, their culture and language, as well as sensitivity to the historic patterns of oppression and paternalism they have endured within the American mental health system. Within this therapeutic framework, art therapy offers great potential for inspiring positive change. (p. 22)

Proper assessment of an individual's sociohistorical background is of utmost importance in ascertaining diagnostic appraisal, establishing a goal, and attaining best practice. Recent research points to the importance behind genogram-mapping of client issues. This visual map serves to underscore the pathogenic belief system, which informs a client's history and path to recovery (Horovitz, 2007; Horovitz-Darby, 1987; McGoldrick et al., 1999). Simultaneously, it offers the clinician a summation of all the historical and psychological aspects of a client and can include a timeline, DSM IV-TR diagnoses, IQ (if applicable and available from previous batteries), and most importantly a glimpse into transitional conflicts handed down from generation to generation (Horovitz, 2007). Transitional conflicts are keyed to the historical well that informs each client's pathogenic belief system. Without this compass, therapists might as well be navigating on an ocean sans a logistical map.

According to O'Connor and Weiss (1993), curtailing addiction and modifying pathogenic belief systems involves forming strong connections to other people. Without examining O'Connor and Weiss' application of "Control Mastery Theory" and/or looking at the literature on shame, "Psychology's Stepchild" (as suggested by Karen, 1992, p. 40), advancement is near impossible. While O'Connor and Weiss (1993) propose that addicted clients are motivated to recover from their addictive disease, their pathogenic beliefs (predated by their development and childhood experiences) curtail that possibility. But first, we will examine the core by-product of the pathogenic belief system, *shame.*

Shame appears to be the mother lode of the pathogenic belief system and psyche. Exploring treatment without its consideration is like kayaking without a paddle. Bad enough that you spin your wheels and go nowhere, you just might capsize, thus spiraling back into the arms of the all-comforting addiction. Shame has oft been confused with its sister, grief. But the twain is indeed different. A simple explanation will help: According to Karen (1992), guilt is about transgression, while shame is about the self. Guilt is the fearful remorse experienced when you steal from your mother's wallet, transgress with your neighbor's spouse, and say nothing when a co-worker is fired for your miscalculation. Relentless guilt torments until penance is completed. Until such time, life may actually feel suspended. While guilt is associated with behavior that has harmed others (transgression), shame is about not being good enough (self). Shame is more clearly associated with conformity and acceptability of character than it is about morality, integrity, and ethics. "To be ashamed is to expect rejection, not so much because of what one has done as because of what one is" (Karen, 1992, p. 47).

Guilt is more readily rectified through atonement, compensation, reparation, and apology, but sister shame? Well, that requires introspection and behavioral change. Not exactly a slice of cake. Even Freud readily admitted that shame (generally harboring in at the tender age of seventeen months) is more primitive than guilt; so why he focused so heavily on guilt is beyond most (Karen, 1992) including this writer. Freud's theory of psychoneuroses highlighted guilt as the anxious conflicts generated from the warring aspects of self (the rapacious id, the sensible ego, and the straitlaced superego). Shame, on the other hand, is associated with childhood failures and a defective self. Shame, however, can also occur at any time in one's life (incompetence, impotence, disease, job loss or the like); yet, is based in childhood messages often communicated (verbally or non-verbally) by parents or custodians.

Karen (1992) divided shame into several categories summarized below:

1. *Existential Shame*—Seeing yourself as you really are—that is too preoccupied (read: narcissistic) to notice that your child is failing or frightened to stand up for someone that you love. According to Karen, this type of shame lacks the "hopeless deformity" associated with childhood wounds (p. 58).
2. *Class Shame*—This can be a function of social power, class, skin color, serfdom, or slavery, class shame is a relentless pesky sense of inferiority. Class shame crosses the line from social pathology to individual pathology but breeds from a shared burden (with others) to a personal deficiency. And this gives rise to the next category.
3. *Narcissistic Shame*—Here the individual, suffering from class shame becomes singled out by the group. For example, a black child might be ridiculed for having darker skin or lighter skin, kinkier hair or straighter hair than his constituents. In modern-day society, it might be the obese woman who spills over into two airline seats instead of her appropriated one. This intractable humiliation contributes to shortcoming and deficiency that burrows into the very core of one's being.
4. *Situational Shame*—This is a passing experience that surfaces by way of rejection, humiliation, or violation of a social norm. Situational shame is akin to the Freudian moralistic superego—it keeps us bathing regularly, eating with utensils (civilized behavior), dressing suitably, and most importantly, functioning without relapse into aggressive and sexual

impulsivity. Situational shame can solidify into social disgrace or stigma, that human cesspool of waste. However, it is important to note that like a bad smell, it will eventually go away, unlike its cousin Narcissistic Shame, which never fully dissipates, but festers on as a negative self-regulator, which one is repeatedly trying to eradicate.

In medieval times, the self was protected from the pressures we experience today. The average town resident was untamed, unpredictable, and highly erratic. He murdered when incensed, vacillating between apology, guilt, and sorrow, and was chock full of physical and psychological quirks: he ate from common food bowls with his hands, defecated openly, fornicated and mourned with great passion; yet, remained rather indifferent about other's opinions or whimsical ideas of maladjustment.

According to Karen (1992, p. 61):

> Given our anxiety about our flaws, our uncertainty about the legitimacy of our feelings, and our lack of mutual trust, our modern psyches would seem especially fertile ground for narcissistic shame . . . traditional, hierarchical, religious society has given way to a world shaped by the freedoms, insecurities, and loneliness of modernity . . . guilt, class shame, situational shame, and the fear of authority have in varying degrees grown less powerful. They are no longer the chief forces around which inner controls are organized. Narcissistic shame has taken up the slack.

Narcissistic shame is just one causative factor in a litany of psychiatric conditions. Like bacteria, it breeds into the psyche inflaming its structure. At the very least, narcissistic shame creates a resistance to exploration, stopping a therapist dead in his tracks. Without working through this arena, deeper areas of conflict and addictive mentality will resurface. In the words of Karen (1992, p. 65), "Repressed shame must be experienced if we are to come to terms with the good, the bad, and the unique of what we are."

Control Mastery Theory

Differing opinions have evolved about the value of individual psychotherapy with drug-dependent or alcoholic clients (McLellan et al., 1988; Winick, 1991; Zweben, 1986, 1989). O'Connor and Weiss (1993) proposed that addicted clients are not gratified by their symptoms but instead suffer from their addiction and harbor unconscious plans for recovery. However, healing involves overcoming the direct psychological and neurological effects of addiction and mastering the problems that predate its use. Here is where revisiting the genogram comes in. O'Connor and Weiss' (1993) theory springs from revisiting childhood history and reviewing the connection with the abusive and/or neglectful parental situations. Clients from such family systems blame themselves for their parents' maladaptive behavior and/or imitate this conduct out of a misinformed sense of loyalty. Like Karen's (1992) theory on shame, O'Connor and Weiss (1993) propose that the deprivation, which these clients experience is justified by their defectiveness. Clients of this ilk simultaneously fear and need healthy attachments. Encouraging attachment to people in recovery programs—friends, mentors, sponsors—"may be crucial to the recovery process . . . and may help clients to modify the pathogenic belief that they do not deserve connections and thus may provide curative experiences" (O'Connor & Weiss, 1993, p. 288).

Indeed, O'Connor and Weiss (1993) stipulate that the attachment to an individual therapist may permit the client to begin attachments in the recovery program. Conversely, if the client was abused, neglected, and/or rejected, he might test his right to a dependent relationship thus fostering excessive dependency and resulting in the feared rejection. Since most therapists perceive dependency as maladaptive, they frustrate this by responding with neutrality. However, if O'Connor and Weiss' (1993) control mastery theory is employed, the aforementioned behavior is viewed as a "useful form of testing to disconfirm the pathogenic belief that warns them against the attachment to others" (p. 288).

The format of control mastery theory encourages an open-meeting structure, where clients can come and go as they like. This endears the client to perceive the 12-Step program as acceptable to want to belong, desire dependence while maintaining distance. Thus, the control mastery theory provides addicted and recovering clients with a therapeutic relationship in which they disconfirm their pathogenic beliefs while working towards abstinence, accept manageable parameters of dependency, and break the lifelong struggle of isolation.

Characteristics of Chemical Dependency

According to Guthmann and Sandberg (1998) and Schaefer (1996), there are four characteristics of chemical dependency:

1. *Primary Disease*—Chemical dependency is a primary disease that can give rise to other disorders, emotional, physical, cognitive, behavioral, etcetera. The chemical dependency must be treated first in order to alter the side effects that may follow such as depression, unemployment or the like.
2. *Progressive Disease*—Chemical dependency left untreated will get worse.
3. *Chronic Disease*—There is no cure except abstinence and a recovered lifestyle adjustment.

4. *Fatal Disease*–Left untreated, the user is prone to increased falls (accidents), suicide, and/or premature death. While this research may be daunting, 7 out of 10 chemically dependent people who accept treatment and use the knowledge and tools find sobriety (Schaefer, 1996).

Patterns of alcohol and chemical abuse fall into four broad categories: (a) use, (b) misuse, (c) abuse, and (d) dependency (addiction). Additionally, chemical abuse and alcoholic dependency may include several of the following items: loss of control, use to extreme intoxication, blackouts, preoccupation and multidrug use, use throughout the day, binge use, solitary use, financial repercussions/ losses, protecting supply, changing friends, tremors, and so forth (Guthmann & Sandberg, 1998).

Even Darwin (1913) explored this topic when he introduced the classic publication, *The Expression of the Emotions in Man and Animals.* Here, Darwin proposed three chief principles: (a) the first principle was that serviceable actions become habitual in association with certain states of the mind, and are performed whether or not they are of service, (b) the second principle was force of habit such as inheritance which contributed to habitual movements in humans, and (c) the third principle was reflex actions, the passage of the aforementioned habits into reflex actions. Since that groundbreaking work, psychology has concluded that "emotion is a complex web of physiological response, overt behavior, facial expression, and cognition" (Karen 1992, p. 47).

Shame and Sexual Abuse

While not necessarily connected to addiction, the cases herein were further complicated by sexual abuse. So a minute dip into the art therapy literature is required. Johnson (1990) discussed creative therapies and addiction in the art of transforming shame akin to the "toxic shame" that Bradshaw (1988) addressed in his trade and stock opus, *Healing the Shame that Binds You.* In Johnson's treatise, she used art qualitatively as a shamanistic healing agent to undo the wellspring of shame associated with addiction. Here, art was employed as the healer invoking group ritual, imagery, and restoration of inner demons.

In contrast, Brooke (1995) surveyed the quantitative aspects of utilizing art therapy with sexual abuse survivors. Due to the recurring problem of sexual abuse in our culture, there is an increased likelihood that addiction counselors will encounter people who have been victimized by this type of abuse. The purpose of the study conducted was to determine if art therapy with sexual abuse survivors would significantly improve self-esteem. The study consisted of two groups of sexually abused women of similar ethnicity and social class: (a) one group (the control group) did not receive group art therapy treatment; (b) the other group (the experimental group) received group art therapy treatment. Both groups were given the same pre and post assessment questionnaire. There was a statistically significant positive rise in self-esteem for women in the experimental group.

Her focus was on cognitive relabeling of the experience and developing self-esteem. An important aspect of this study is that it provided a method for understanding the impact of sexual abuse. Brooke like others (Jackson et al, 1990; Mayer, 1983; Kosof, 1985) concluded that sexual abuse is characterized by selflessness, somatic complaints, emotional constriction, low self-image, internalized guilt and shame, and often results in internalized sexual identity issues and substance abuse.

Brooke (1995) concluded via utilization of self-inventory (pre art and post art activity), investigation of dependent variables (such as locus of control) and working with expressive art materials that art can indeed improve self-esteem. In one very interesting exercise, Brooke devised a brilliant strategy of using a round mirror in the center of the paper, looking at the self, and using collage or drawings to surround the mirror and depict the self. This could easily be translated into a formative, corrective experience for surveying addiction as transformer of self.

Cohen-Liebmann (2003) found the following advantages of using art with those who may have been sexually abused:

- Art may gain access to the unexpected thoughts, feelings, and reactions of the victim.
- The pressure on the victim to verbalize is removed.
- Art is a less stressful and threatening way to assess the victim of sexual abuse.
- The artwork can be a recollective tool in the courtroom.

Diagnostic indicators of sexual abuse have been the focus of many research studies; it has been hypothesized that the drawings of sexually abused children (victims) will be significantly different to those of non-abused children (Brooke, 1997). Indeed, the graphic indicators found in the drawings varied according to the practitioner; however, some indicators were identified in several studies, suggesting a general consensus (although not a significant one). The composite list of 27 indicators is a compilation of the common indicators seen in the art of sexually abused children (Cohen-Liebmann, 2003).

The composite list of indicators:

1. Accentuated arms and legs

2. Artistic regression
3. Avoidance of sexuality
4. Bodies without lower halves
5. Circles
6. Compartmentalization
7. Detailing
8. Disorganization of body parts
9. Distortions
10. Elaboration
11. Encapsulation
12. Erasures
13. Genitalia
14. Heads without bodies
15. Heart-shaped imagery
16. Heavy and uneven pressure or varied lines
17. Heightened awareness of sexuality
18. Omissions
19. Phallic-like imagery
20. Position or placement of figures
21. Sexual connotation
22. Shadings
23. Small figures
24. Transparencies
25. Use of a complimentary color scheme
26. Weather
27. Wedges

Cohen-Liebmann (2003) found that genitalia was the most commonly identified indicator; recognized in 7 of the 16 studies. Indicators should not be used as sole and definitive diagnostic decision as to whether or not someone has been abused, but the information gleaned can alert the clinician to the possibility of such abuse. Presently it is the responsibility of the art therapist involved in legal proceedings to provide evidence of the probative value of the use of children's drawing in sexual abuse litigation.

Case: Diane, Adult Deaf Female

What was most unclear when I received the referral for this case was that the therapist referring the patient was in fact her lover. When I took the referral and exchanged information with the referring clinician, what was NOT clear was that Jane (the clinician) was indeed involved with Diane (the patient). Even at the first meeting, both Jane and Diane showed for the appointment; I was unsure why Jane accompanied Diane but primarily chalked it up to her need to make sure that I was (a) comfortable with the issues of working with the Deaf, and (b) was able to understand Diane's communication system. (There are numerous styles of sign language communication.)

Although I met with Jane and Diane for only a total of 13 sessions, I did not receive the background information on Diane until the tenth meeting. (This was because a previous therapist did not respond to my request for release of information.)

Nevertheless, halfway through the initial intake, it became abundantly clear to me that Jane was not just "accompanying" but "with" Diane in the literal sense. Normally, that breach alone might have sent some powerful triggers to even the most incipient therapist but I was used to working with unusual, albeit non-traditional cases. Internally, I questioned Jane's ethics, (e.g., forging a relationship with her past client); yet, it did not prevent me from treating her lover (Diane), nor Jane, in the capacity of couple's work. But after that primary intake, I suggested that Diane return the following week by herself. Below is an abbreviated timeline and genogram offering a snapshot of Diane's history. (The only information that I knew of Jane was that she was a well-respected clinician in the Deaf community and was close with her family of origin.)

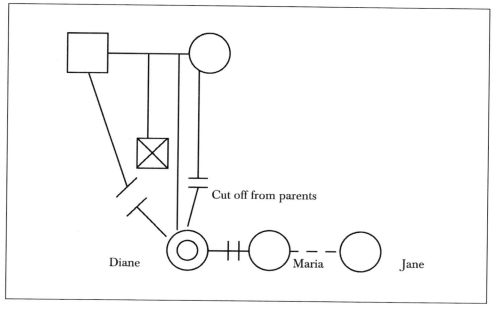

Figure 2.1. Diane's genogram.

Diane's Timeline

- Diane born Deaf—90 decibel loss in both ears, no one learned sign language.
- Relied on speech-reading and oral communication to communicate with her family.
- Educated at a residential school for the Deaf.
- Age 4.5–14—Sexually abused by an MR older Deaf boy every day after she exited the bus. Other neighborhood boys took turns abusing her daily. Diane told no one. This information was revealed during Session 8.
- Age 14—Brother struck by lightening and dies in sailboat. Diane was in the boat and witnessed the accident. Diane's mother begins alcoholic behavior.
- Age 20—Diane's first suicide attempt. Diane was rejected by a woman lover; she beat herself in the face until unconscious and overdosed on alcohol.
- Age 21—Diane's mother attempts suicide (details unclear). (But the alcoholic behavior and suicidal ideation of both Diane and her mother suggests a folie à deux.)
- Age 27—moves in with Maria—Relationship was very rocky; nevertheless they exchanged "vows" with each other and were "married" by a local minister (although this was not a legal union). Diane again overdosed on alcohol and pills and told Maria. Diane was taken to the hospital where she had her stomach pumped. She was hospitalized for a short stay.
- Age 28—Diane's mother attempts second suicide attempt (details unclear).
- At onset of Art Therapy, Diane was taking 150mg daily of Desipramine for her depression.
- Diane often stopped medication when she felt better.

Diane's history was mired with red flags: A family that refused communicating with her in her native language (American Sign Language), stormy relationships with past lovers; alcohol and substance abuse addiction, self-injurious behavior; suicidal ideation and depression (commingled with her mother's alcoholic and suicidal ideation); trauma regarding the loss of her brother (age 14); and then in the 8th session, Diane revealed a horrid story of being sexually abused daily by neighborhood boys (ages 4.5–14). Clearly this was a woman with a boatload of problems.

After the first meeting, I felt it would be best to see Diane individually and then in due course add Jane to the mix (thus mirroring the theoretical construct of O'Connor & Weiss, 1993). But, it was apparent from the get-go, that

Jane was wearing two hats: Clinician and lover. Her ability to function clinically (from the onset of her treatment with Diane) was compromised by her desire to be with Diane, when she was her patient. As a result, Jane's relationship with me was a mixture of professional jealousy blended with a genuine desire to help Diane with her issues.

Apparent during that first meeting was that (a) Jane was overprotective of Diane and feared losing her to her previous lover; (b) Diane had never resolved her lost relationship with Maria (her ex-spouse), was still harboring fantasies about a reconciliation; and (c) Jane had much difficulty separating herself as a professional therapist, removing her clinical hat, and getting in touch with her own feelings.

By the third session, Jane was able to admit the difficulty in separating her clinical self from the relationship, confessed being jealous of me (due to Diane's alliance with me during the session), and Diane declared that between sessions, she strongly resisted continuing treatment. All of these signs I perceived as both constructive and appropriate to treatment. It was not long before Diane acted on impulse: She slept with Maria. The result was beyond disastrous: not only did this drive a wedge between Diane and Jane's already tenuous relationship, it also caused Maria to verbally and physically threaten Jane and Diane. In an emergency phone call to me in the middle of the night, Diane reported that Maria had threatened her. I urged Diane and Jane to contact the police before Maria arrived. (Maria had apparently made similar threats in the past while wielding a knife.) These new threats led to increased depression for Diane and she cancelled the next appointment.

By session five, Diane verbalized her feelings of rejection by both Maria and Jane (thus affirming the theoretical need for control mastery theory as espoused by O'Connor & Weiss, 1993): She cried openly about her unresolved relationship with Maria and admitted suicidal ideation. As Diane was alone for this session, I engaged her with the art materials. She drew a picture of a campfire complete with four and one-half triangular-shaped fires. In sign language, triangles are the visual equivalent of vaginas and so I became suspicious based on several rationales: (a) according to Shoemaker (1977) the first art piece articulated by a client generally tells the whole story (and I had witnessed this to be quite accurate), (b) Spring (1985) had reported triangular shapes occurring in the work of her sexually abused clients, and (c) Diane appeared sullen and very guarded immediately following the completion of the artwork. Suffice it to say, my antenna was up. While I questioned her about four and a half and whether anything had happened to her at that age, she seemed surprised when I asked but averted any questions and /or meaning ascribed to the artwork. By session eight, she revealed the true meaning behind the work when she confessed the sexual abuse she had sustained from age four and one-half through the age of fourteen.

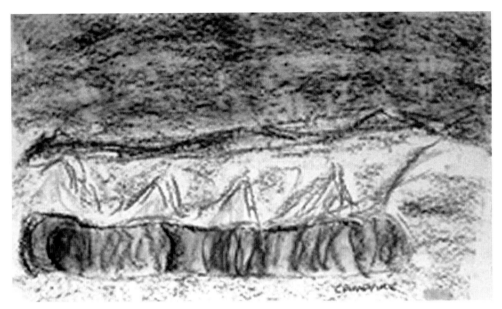

Figure 2.2. Campfire.

By the next session, Jane informed me that she had received a job offer from another city. They made a decision to leave, thus requiring Diane to sell her house and forfeit a job she had maintained successfully for eight years. Diane naively purported that this would solve their problems; yet, admitted that there might be "kinks" in their relationship. Jane's decision to uproot from the area also enabled Diane (as discussed by Guthmann & Blozis, 2001). Diane upheld that she and Maria could continue their "friendship." Naturally, Jane objected; she knew that the delicate balance that Diane hoped to achieve was unattainable.

As termination became closer, Jane and Diane bonded more closely with me. This is not unusual in treatment (Guthmann & Blozis, 2001). In fact, Diane and Jane felt the need to meet with me twice weekly (in preparation for their departure). This created a pseudorealistic relationship, thus allowing Diane to divulge information that she had never shared with her previous therapists. As well this mirrors the stance of clients who are shamed and need to distance as outlined in the above research of Karen (1992) and O'Connor and Weiss (1993). (Indeed, it has always been my experience that patients divulge information more readily during the termination process. Perhaps this is due to the knowledge that therapy will be ending and the sharing of information becomes safeguarded from analysis precisely because continued therapy is no longer a possibility.)

As noted above, during the eighth session, Diane revealed that she had been sexually abused between the ages of four and one-half and fourteen years of age. This confirmed my suspicion of the "campfire" artwork (Figure 2.2) and I interpreted that directly to Diane; the result was that both Diane and Jane began to talk about their sexual relationship and its complexities. Apparently, Diane was used to a sadomasochistic relationship with Maria and Jane desired a gentler, loving relationship than Diane could offer. Thus the remainder of the session revolved around my coaxing them in alternative strategies in order to satisfy sexual relations for both and discussing the aspects of the pathogenic belief systems that had compromised Diane's ability to interact in a healthy, non-dependent manner (Guthmann & Blozis, 2001; Karen, 1992; O'Connor & Weiss, 1993).

In another session, Diane spoke openly about her unease regarding sexual relations and expressed shame about her bodily image. I connected her childhood sexual abuse (O'Connor & Weiss, 1993) and encouraged her to act this out using psychodrama techniques. This cut through her issues and she sobbed. I suggested using clay art materials in the next session. The result was Brian, the abuser.

Interesting was his portrayal without a body, suggesting Diane's denial of bodily association and need to decathect from the experience. The image sported an overly aggressive smile, suggesting concomitant victimization and

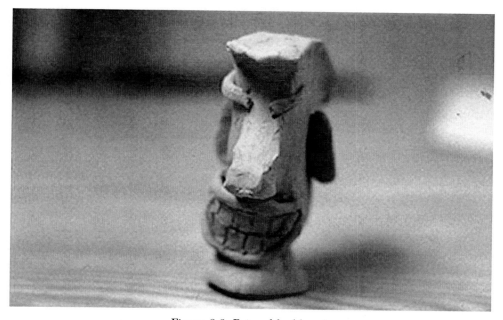

Figure 2.3. Brian, blockhead.

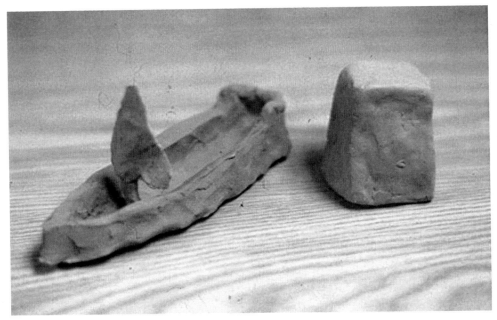

Figure 2.4. Jane's work: Sailboat and block.

identification with the aggressor. During this same session, I assigned Jane with the same task. She depicted Brian as a block because she felt "blocked because (she) didn't know him" and she then created herself as a sailboat. (On a deeper level, this "block" may have also represented her challenge relating to Diane as well as the pathogenic belief system which disabled Diane from functioning in a healthy, sexual relationship.)

The sailboat seemed an obvious stand-in for Jane's concomitant nurturance issues and desire to escape therapeutic confrontation (e.g., moving to a new town) and thus avoid therapeutic resolve of both her and Diane's problems. Diane also asked me to work on something regarding Brian while Jane asked me to incorporate Diane's relationship with Maria. My work resulted in my depicting Diane as a bird and the scissor at her neck as Brian, destroying her voice and ability to sing. The chain at the bird's tail was my rendition of Maria, but I severed a link at the end suggesting that Diane had the strength to terminate this unhealthy relationship.

I then asked Diane to create a sculpture symbolizing me. (I requested this because she had difficulty expressing her anger with me for bringing these issues to a head (no pun intended) and was clearly struggling with the therapeutic transference relationship as Karen (1992) and O'Conner and Weiss (1993) predicted. Figure 2.6, which she named "Falcor, the luck dragon" was described as "very sweet." I was unfamiliar with this character. They relayed

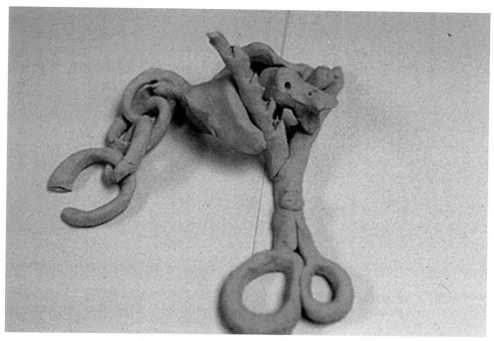

Figure 2.5. My work–"Broken Song."

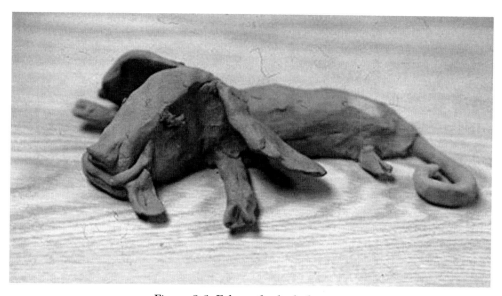

Figure 2.6. Falcor, the luck dragon.

the tale behind *The Neverending Story.*

When I told Diane she could do whatever she wanted with the Brian figure, she hesitated. I pointed out her inability to get angry. With some encouragement, she made another model of a man only this time she vehemently squashed it with her hands and purposefully threw it into the trash. I then encouraged her to create a sculpture representing her current relationship with Jane. She created a broken heart to depict her relationship with Maria and then a larger heart in which she placed smaller hearts to represent the new found relationship with Jane. (Again these symbols have been associated with sexual abuse (Brooke; 1997; Spring, 1985.)

Later that evening, I rented the videotape of *The Neverending Story* since I thought it would help me understand the role in which Diane had cast me. After I watched the video, it became clear that the luck dragon was indeed the protagonist and savior in this story and that Diane was bestowing omnipotent powers onto me. Thus, I knew that I had to address this in the next session.

In our last session, Jane and Diane arrived bearing gifts so I would "never forget them." I addressed the protagonist issue and their obvious feelings of loss as I transferred them to a colleague in their new town. I suggested that they create a sculpture regarding what they would do "without the luck dragon."

Figure 2.7 is this final project: They described that the heart-shaped piece contained eyes to symbolize their new outlook on their relationship, the ear reflected improved communication, a hand in the universal sign for "I love you," a cat to represent their love for their animals, and a lump of clay to echo their feelings about art therapy.

I created a Superwoman insignia plaque with a fissure running through it (Figure 2.8) to illuminate my limitations as their therapist and implored them to relinquish the false role in which they had cast me. I suggested that they transfer those feelings onto their new therapist, who was a pioneer in the field of Family Therapy, addiction, and worked with the Deaf. While the new therapist was male, both concurred that his gender made no difference. I reminded them that they would not be leaving their problems behind with the move and that they should seek treatment as soon as possible.

I opened their gifts after they left. The first was the book, *The Neverending Story.* The other gift was a beautiful Sierra Wilderness calendar and I recalled Jane's words, ". . . something for you to look at every day so that you will never forget us." Little did they know how prophetic their statement was.

Aftermath

While I had hoped that they would connect with their new therapist, they

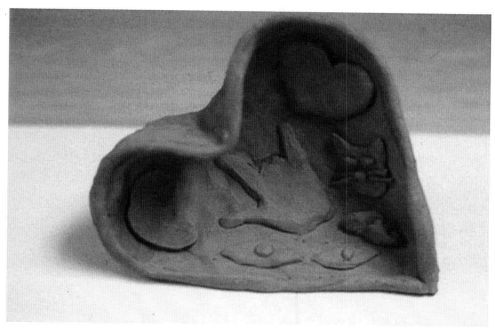

Figure 2.7. Termination piece.

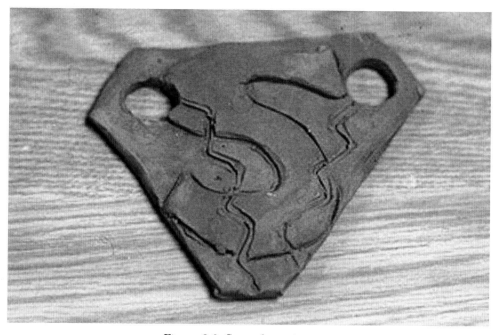

Figure 2.8. Supertherapist, not.

resisted for several weeks. As matters began to deteriorate, they finally connected with the new therapist; nonetheless, Jane left me messages continually pleading for me to call. Trying to get them to connect with their new therapist seemed futile. On one occasion, Jane actually reached me by phone and protested that the new therapist was doing "nothing" for them. I reminded her that she needed to give him a chance and that hanging onto me negated that possibility. With their signed consent, I telephoned the new therapist and apprised him of the situation. Yet, the calls continued. In retrospect, I probably should have continued in "phone therapy" for some duration to get them over the "hump." But I resisted, hoping they would connect with their new therapist.

One day, Jane called and left a message on my machine: she had been badly beaten. She shamefully skipped work and avoided sessions with the new therapist. Around this time, she drove back into town and asked to see me. Her jaw was swollen, her demeanor depressed and she was understandably angry. While I again tried to redirect her to her current therapist, she only sang my praises. What I failed to recognize was that like my "supertherapist" plaque, I had been triangulated. Several weeks later, Jane called again and reported on my machine that she had been avoiding treatment, altercations were increasing, and the battering was continuing. I began to feel guilty (as suggested by Karen, 1992). I called her back and pointed out how unhealthy the relationship was and urged her to take care of herself, seek treatment and move out.

Naturally, Jane avoided this suggestion. Several weeks later, she called to say she had temporarily moved in with some friends. I felt relieved since I did not hear from her for several months.

Then I received a message from Jane and when I returned her call, she was not present, so I left her a voicemail. This time, she did not call back. Somehow, I felt at peace, sensing that she was all right. Several months later, I was preparing a presentation on this case and so I contacted Jane.

Jane and I spent over an hour conversing about what had transpired. About the time of our last contact, Diane required a brief hopitalization. Predictably, there was a short-lived reconciliation. Battering continued but fortunately for Jane, her friends were aware of the situation. According to Jane, at one point she had been beaten unconscious. Frightened by what she had done, Diane telephoned Jane's friends who revived her and moved her out that evening. Since that point, Jane attended church religiously, became involved in other triangular relationships and entertained the idea of seeking therapy to resolve her issues. Diane had returned to town and was attempting to live out her fantasy—she had moved back in with Maria.

Concluding Remarks about the Case

I contacted Jane months later and a detailed written response of her reaction to this case was previously reported (Horovitz-Darby, 1992). Many of Jane's comments unnerved me. I was not aware that she was confused about my sexual orientation. Yet, in hindsight, I understood. It is true that one has to "like" one's patients as Boscolo (1987) puts it, if that is missing then one cannot become "passionately involved" and "co-create." If there is an aversion to a client, obviously the work cannot be done and the client should be referred out. Yet, I was unaware that my "concern" was mistaken for genuine attraction.

After much supervision and deliberation on this case, I concluded that "analytic neutrality" is a mythological position of which I am clearly incapable. And that is because alas I am human. In working with pathogenic belief systems, addiction, chemical and substance abuse, this is nearly impossible since it requires inordinate skills on the part of the therapist. In the words of the great Jay Haley (1988, p. 88):

> *Be passive.*
> *Be inactive.*
> *Be reflective.*
> *Be silent.*
> *Beware.*

Given the need to ascertain the pathogenic belief system of the chemical substance abusive client (Deaf or hearing), perhaps the above adage should be inscribed above every therapist's doorway. It is on mine and remains as a reminder to always be on the outlook, to ascribe to further research, and to steel oneself with continual supervision. Working with the chemically abusive client (Deaf or hearing) requires continual introspection not just of the pathogenic belief systems that clients bring to the table but also those that lie dormant in the legs that therapists bring to the stand.

Clearly, therapists need to revisit their own belief systems in relation to the pathogenic responses of their clients. This is inherent in charting a course for recovery with this population. Working towards eradication of shame, be it existential, class, situational, or narcissistic is inherent in recovery and mastery of primary, progressive, chronic or fatal aspects of addiction as disease (Guthmann & Sandberg, 1998; Schaefer, 1996). In this case, while Diane returned to the unhealthy arms of Maria, her addiction was finally mastered as she moved towards recovery and a dependency that was for her, manageable. While this case might not be viewed as successful to some, two years later Diane was drug free, had abstained from alcohol and was still engaged in a relationship with Maria. And Jane? She was free to reflect on her transgressions (with her past patient, Diane) and work towards reparation, penance, and a much-needed dose of self-regulation and supervision. And perhaps that is enough. While clearly, more could have been done, one can only work within the confines that people can handle. In this instance, I can only hope. In the words of Emily Dickenson: "Hope" is the thing with feathers—That perches in the soul—And sings the tune without the words—And never stops—at all. . ." (Franklin, 1951).

Appendix—Terms

Alcohol and chemical abuse—(a) use; (b) misuse; (c) abuse; and (d) dependency (addiction). The disease can progress from primary, progressive, chronic and if left untreated fatal. Control Mastery Theory provides addicted and recovering clients with a therapeutic relationship in which they disconfirm their pathogenic beliefs while working towards abstinence, accept manageable parameters of dependency, and break the lifelong struggle of isolation.

Deaf people—are primarily visually-oriented people. Deaf people can be descended from families with six or more generations of Deaf relatives or they may be the only Deaf member of their family. They may be native users of American Sign Language (ASL), or if they come from hearing families, they may have learned to sign when they entered school or college, or even afterwards. Everyone in the family may sign, making communication a non-issue; or there may be no signing family members at all, resulting in the Deaf person experiencing a sense of isolation. Deaf people may have been born Deaf or they may have become Deaf later in life. Some Deaf people may opt to use hearing aids or cochlear implants; others choose not to use amplification devices. (The word Deaf is often capitalized to show respect to this unique culture.) Sometimes Deaf people are also referred to as Hard-of-Hearing (HOH) but Deaf people discriminate between these terms depending on their auditory decibel loss.

Enabling—(of Deaf or HOH individuals)—Family members, friends, and even professions (as was evidenced in this case) often protect individuals who are labeled "disabled or handicapped," by hearing persons.

Genogram—is a pathogenic belief system, which informs a client's history and pat to recover. Simultaneously, it offers the clinician a summation of all the historical and psychological aspects of a client and can include a timeline, DSM IV-TR diagnoses, IQ (if applicable and available from previous batteries), and most importantly, a glimpse into transitional conflicts handed down from generation to generation.

Guilt is about transgression (for example: the fearful remorse experienced when you steal from your mother's wallet, transgress with your neighbor's spouse, and say nothing when a co-worker is fired for your miscalculation).

Minnesota Program for Deaf and Hard-of-Hearing Individuals—uses methods based on the 12-step model yet offers additional features such as asking clients to draw as a means of completing assignments and utilizing role-play and similar activities, which serve to activate the unique linguistic system of the Deaf.

MR—mentally retarded

Phone therapy—working with the client over the telephone (or in modern times, using SKYPE, IChat, Sightspeed or a similar software program that allows for communication over the telephone or Internet).

Sexual abuse characteristics—categorized by selflessness, somatic complaints, emotional constriction, low self-image, internalized guilt and shame, and often results in internalized sexual identity issues and substance abuse.

Shame is about the self (i.e., about not being good enough (self). Shame is more clearly associated with conformity and acceptability of character than it is about morality, integrity, and ethics). Shame can be categorized into several categories: existential, class, narcissistic or situational and:

- *Existential Shame*—Seeing yourself as you really are - that is too preoccupied (read: narcissistic) to notice others
- *Class Shame*—This can be a function of social power, class, skin color, serfdom, or slavery.
- *Narcissistic Shame*—Here the individual, suffering from class shame becomes singled out by the group. (e.g., In modern day society, it might be the obese woman who spills over into two airline seats instead of her appropriated one—becomes a negative self-regulator.)
- *Situational Shame*—This is a passing experience that surfaces by way of rejection, humiliation, or violation of a social norm—it keeps us bathing regularly, eating with utensils (civilized behavior), dressing suitably, and most importantly, functioning without relapse into aggressive and sexual impulsivity. Situational shame can eventually go away, unlike its cousin Narcissistic Shame, which never fully dissipates, but festers on as a negative self-regulator, which one is repeatedly trying to eradicate.

References

Boscolo, L. (1987, April 7–8). *The Milan Group.* (sponsored by the Family Therapy Workshops, Rochester, NY.)

Bradshaw, J. (1988). *Healing the shame that binds you.* Deerfield Beach, FL: Health Communications.

Brooke, S. L. (1995). Art therapy: An approach to working with sexual abuse survivors. *Arts in Psychotherapy, 22*(5), 447–466.

Brooke, S. L. (1997). *Healing through art: Art therapy with sexual abuse survivors.* Springfield, IL:

Charles C Thomas Publishers.

Cohen-Liebmann, M. S. (2003). Drawings in forensic investigations of child sexual abuse. In C. Malchiodi (Ed.), *Handbook of Art Therapy* (pp. 167–180). New York: Guilford Press.

Darwin, C. (1913). *The expression of the emotion in man and animals.* New York: D. Appleton & Co.

Franklin, R. W. (Ed.) (1951). *The poems of Emily Dickinson.* Cambridge, MA: Harvard College: Presidents and fellows of Harvard College.

Guthmann, D., & Sandberg, K. (1998). Assessing substance abuse problems in Deaf and hard of hearing individuals. *American Annals of the Deaf, 143*(1), 14–21.

Guthmann, D., & Blozis, S. A. (2001; July).Unique issues faced by Deaf individuals entering substance abuse treatment and following discharge. *American Annals of the Deaf, 146*(3), 294–304.

Haley, J. (1988). *The power tactics of Jesus Christ and other essays.* New York: W. W. Norton & Company.

Hammer, E. F. (1980). *The clinical application of projective drawings.* Springfield, IL: Charles C Thomas.

Horovitz, E. G. (2007). *Visually speaking: Art therapy and the Deaf.* Springfield, IL: Charles C Thomas.

Horovitz-Darby, E. G. (1987; October). Diagnosis and assessment: Impact on art therapy. *Journal of Art Therapy,* 127–137.

Horovitz-Darby, E. G. (1988). *Art therapy assessment of a minimally language skilled deaf child.* Proceedings from the 1988 University of California's Center on Deafness Conference: Mental Health Assessment of Deaf Clients: Special Conditions, Little Rock, Arkansas: ADARA.

Horovitz-Darby, E. G. (1992). Countertransference: Implications in treatment and post treatment. *Arts in Psychotherapy, 19,* 379–389.

Jackson, J. L., Calhoun, K. S., Amick, A. E., Maddever, H. M., & Habif, V. L. (1990). Young adult women who report intrafamilial sexual abuse: Sexual adjustment. *Archives of Sexual Behavior, 19*(3), 211–221.

Johnson, L. (1990). Creative therapies in the treatment of addictions: The art of transforming shame. *The Arts in Psychotherapy, 17,* 299–308.

Karen, R. (1992; February). Shame. *Atlantic Monthly,* 40–70.

Kearns, G. (1989). A community of underserved alcoholics. *Alcohol Research Health and World, 14,* 27.

Kendall, C. J. (2002). Unpublished predissertation. *Psychiatric hospitals and residential facilities in the United States specifically serving Deaf adults with mental illnesses.* Gallaudet University.

Kosof, A. (1985). *Incest: Families in crisis.* New York: Franklin Watts.

Lane, H., Hoffmeister, R., & Bahan, B. (1996). *A journey into the Deaf world.* DawnSignPress: San Diego, CA.

Lane, K. E. (1985; April). Substance abuse among the Deaf population: An overview of current strategies, programs, and barriers to recovery. *Journal of American Deafness and Rehabilitation Association, 22*(4), 79–85.

Larson, E. W., & McAlpine, D. E. (1988). Treating the hearing-impaired in a standard chemical dependence unit. *Journal of Studies on Alcohol, 49*(4), 381–383.

Liebmann, M. S. (2003). Drawings in forensic investigations of child sexual abuse. In C. Malchiodi (Ed.), *Handbook of art therapy* (pp. 167–180). New York: Guilford Press.

Lowenfeld, V., & Brittain, W. L. (1975). *Creative and mental growth* (6th edition). New York, NY: Macmillan.

Mayer, A. (1983). *Incest: A treatment manual for therapy with victims, spouses and offenders.* Holmes

Beach, Fl: Learning Publications.

McCrone, W. (1994). A two year report card on Title 1 of the Americans with Disabilities Act: Implications for rehabilitation counseling with Deaf people. *Journal of the American Deafness and Rehabilitation Association, 28,* 1–20.

McCullogh, C. A., & Duchesneau, S. M. (2007). Mental health and Deaf people. in E. G. Horovitz (Ed.), *Visually speaking: Art therapy and the Deaf* (pp. 7–23). Springfield, IL: Charles C Thomas.

McLellan, A. T., Luborsky, L., Woody, G. E., & O'Brien, C. P. (1988). Is the counselor in 'active ingredient' in substance abuse treatment? *Journal of Mental and Nervous Diseases, 176,* 423–430.

McGoldrick, M., Gerson, R., & Shellenberger, S. (1999). *Genograms, assessment and intervention.* New York: Norton.

Moore, D. (1991). Substance misuse: A review. *The International Journal of Addictions, 26*(1), 65–90.

Morton, D., & Kendall, C. J. (2003). *Mental health services for Deaf people: A resource directory,* 2003 edition. Washington, DC: Gallaudet.

O'Connor, L. E., & Weiss, J. W. (1993; Oct–Dec). Individual psychotherapy for addicted clients: an application of control mastery theory. *Journal of Psychoactive Drugs, 25*(4), 283–291.

Oster, D. G., & Gould, P. C. (2004). *Using drawings in assessment and therapy* (2nd ed.). New York & Britain: Brunner-Routledge.

Pollard, R. Q. (1994). Public mental health services and diagnostic trends regarding individuals who are Deaf or hard of hearing. *Rehabilitation Psychology, 39*(3), 147–160.

Rendon, M. E. (1992). Deaf culture and alcohol and substance abuse. *Journal of Substance Abuse Treatment, 9,* 113–110.

Schaefer, D. (1996). *Choices and consequences: What to do when a teenager uses alcohol/drugs.* Minneapolis, MN: Johnson Institute.

Shoemaker, R. H. (1977) Published in *The Dynamics of Creativity,* Proceedings of the Eighth Annual Conference of the American Art Therapy Association, by AATA Publications, Comm. Baltimore.

Spring, D. (1985). Symbolic language of sexually abused, chemically dependent women. *American Journal of Art Therapy, 24,* 13–20.

Steinberg, A. G., Sullivan, V. J., & Loew, R. C. (1998). Cultural and linguistic barriers to mental health service access: The Deaf consumer's perspective. *American Journal of Psychiatry, 155*(7), 982–984.

Winick, C. (1991). The counselor in drug treatment. *International Journal of the Addictions, 25,* 1479–1502.

Whitehouse, A., Sherman, R., & Kozlowski, K. (1991). The needs of Deaf substance abusers in Illinois. *American Journal of Drug and Alcohol Abuse, 17*(1), 103–113.

Zweben, J. E. (1986). Recovery-oriented psychotherapy. *Journal of Substance Abuse Treatment, 3,* 255–262.

Zweben, J. E. (1989). Recovery-oriented psychotherapy: Patient resistance and therapist dilemma. *Journal of Substance Abuse Treatment, 6,* 123–132.

Biography

Ellen G. Horovitz, Ph.D., LCAT, ATR-BC is Chair of the Creative Arts Therapy Department, Professor / Director of Graduate Art Therapy and the Art Therapy Clinic at

Nazareth College of Rochester, New York. She has had over thirty years of experience with myriad patient populations and specializes in family art therapy with the deaf. Dr. Horovitz currently is in private practice. Dr. Horovitz is the author of numerous articles, book chapters and the following books: *Spiritual Art Therapy: An Alternate Path; A Leap of Faith: The Call to Art; Art Therapy As Witness: A Sacred Guide;* and *Visually Speaking: Art Therapy and the Deaf.* As well, Dr. Horovitz has directed and produced ten films available in DVD format. (Dr. Horovitz's films are available through www.arttxfilms.com) Dr. Horovitz is past President Elect of the American Art Therapy Association (AATA). For additional information contact: Dr. Ellen G. Horovitz, ATR-BC/Director of Graduate Art Therapy/Nazareth College/4245 East Avenue/ Rochester, N.Y. 14618/ E-mail: ehorovi4@naz.edu ehorovi4@naz.edu

Chapter 3

EXTENDING A HAND: OPEN STUDIO ART THERAPY IN A HARM REDUCTION CENTER

STEPHANIE WISE

Introduction

Among the most marginalized people in contemporary society are persons who suffer from chemical dependency and poverty. Drug users and the homeless have few options available to enable development of healthy interpersonal experiences based upon mutuality and creativity. In the opinion of this author, utilizing art therapy in an open studio context facilitated some interpersonal bridge building across the abyss of social isolation which often appears to accompany addictive behaviors. This personal sense of connection to others possibly helps offset some of the negative impact of loneliness which may exacerbate the continuation of unhealthy lifestyle behaviors.

Offering hope and connection in place of despair and loneliness, the Open Art Studio Model of Art Therapy was implemented for the past two years at the Lower East Side Harm Reduction Center (LESHRC/The Center) located in New York City. The partnership between harm reduction and open art therapy studio models is synchronistic in that both therapeutic modalities encourage personal agency and empowerment.

Harm reduction theory supports the philosophy of helping people help themselves to develop safer behaviors while they are still actively involved with chemical addiction. While the generally accepted ideal within our society sets goals for the client to ultimately leave their drug addiction behind, the pragmatic intent of harm reduction at first glance might appear less lofty—it is to reduce the drug-using behavioral harms to the self and others as much as possible while the addict remains an active user. Proverbially speaking, this is where the rubber meets the road. It is a model without judgment, acknowledging the influences of poverty, class, racism, social isolation, past trauma, sex-based discrimination, and other social inequities. These influences are considered vulnerabilities. Harm reduction does not ignore the damage caused by chemical addiction but instead addresses the relationship of the person to the drug-using behaviors and the aims, as much as possible, to increase the likelihood of "safer choices" as a means to reducing harms.

The Open Art Studio in many ways parallels the values of Harm Reduction. The studio is a safe, open space where participants are able to become as deeply involved in the art process as they wish. They can come and go at will as the group is open-ended. The art therapist serves more as a facilitator/therapist, encouraging the creative experience, group process, and personal expression while at the same time lending a creative hand when indicated. Importantly, open studio is a place where healthy interpersonal connections can be developed. Through art making, activities, and social response and reflection upon the artwork occurs, engagement with others and renewed playfulness incorporating imagination are encouraged.

There is an immense social disconnect for persons actively addicted. Loneliness, frustration, and shame often prohibit the natural flow of positive interpersonal experiencing. By providing a safe therapeutic studio space, with simple art supplies, music, and camaraderie, the beginnings of relational exchange may begin to occur—elements of hope and possibility through creative activity offered a supportive environment to explore concepts of safer behaviors in the face of serious addiction. This model of working with chemically dependent persons draws upon our skills as therapists to lend a therapeutic hand to those who are often considered invisible in our society.

Harm Reduction

Those supporting the concept of harm reduction tend to define the model in general terms. It is considered more as a pragmatic way of thinking and approaching the problems of addiction rather than as an intra-psychic theoretical formula for working with clients. The Harm Reduction Coalition defines this model as a, "perspective and set of practical strategies to reduce the negative consequences of drug use, incorporating a spectrum of strategies from safer use to abstinence" (The Harm Reduction Coalition, www.harm-reduction.org/section.php?id=62).

According to Tatarsky (2002), "Harm reduction rejects the presumption that abstinence is the best or only acceptable goal for all problem drug and alcohol users. Harm reduction sees substance use varying on a continuum of harmful consequences to the user and the community" (p. 2). Another component within the harm reduction model is the respectful attitude which is fostered for the client. This occurs most readily because the intention of the moral model language is changed. Marlatt (1998) stated the following:

> The shift is from speaking of "drug abuse" to speaking of the "harmful use of drugs" or from labeling someone a "drug abuser" to calling him or her a "consumer" who experiences harmful or helpful consequence. The word consumer seems particularly apt, because people consume both substances and services; drug users also represent a significant economic consumer group (if we consider the high purchase costs of both licit and illicit substances from tobacco to heroin). (p. 58)

Psychologist, Patt Denning (2000), writes about harm reduction psychotherapy, expressing the concerns about the harm that therapists may do to their clients if chemical dependency treatment ignores the "biopsychosocial phenomenon" (p.7), which lays the groundwork for creating, "forces acting on him or her to create the conditions necessary for a serious and persistent problem" (p.7). Thus, the arena for public debate on best practices in managing the challenges of addictions necessitates including the whole cloth of society so the harms and the people are no longer invisible. The "buy in" requires that we see the problem as "ours" not just "theirs."

Harm Reduction Simplified

Most definitions of the harm reduction model come down to the following principles:

1. Focus is on harms associated with drug use and other risk taking behaviors.
2. It is in favor of any positive change as defined by the person making the change.
3. There is a continuum of drug use from non-problematic to extremely problematic.
4. Any reduction in drug-related harm is a step in the right direction
5. Direction and control of treatment remains with the client.
6. Compassionate pragmatism replaces moral idealism. (Marlatt, 1998, p. 56)

It was within this model that the open studio art therapy program was provided.

Open Studio Art Therapy

It is likely that for every art therapist, there is a personal and immediate internal concept that comes to mind when asked, "What does the studio mean to you? How would you define it?" The concept of studio is charged with meaning. Moon (2002) offers much to ponder on this topic when referencing the thoughts of other art therapists: "Kramer (1994) . . . the healthy studio environment is a place where there is "space for improvisation, openness to the unexpected, acceptance of the eccentric" (p. 92). Allen (1995b) identifies the primary attribute of a studio setting to be energy, while McKniff (1995) describes the studio as an "ecology of mutual influences" (p. 181) and Henley (1995a), believes the effective studio provides both inspiration and sanctuary" (as cited in Moon, 2002, p. 72).

There are many styles and challenges in running open studios. Impediments to envisaging the creation of the studio may thwart accomplishing the task of actualizing the space. Moon (2002) goes on to state: "Because it does not seem possible to achieve in many environments assumptions are made that the studio model of art therapy may be impossible due to limitations of setting or the lack of resources to transform the setting. The ability to imagine the ideal studio setting becomes a roadblock rather than point of access towards making that ideal as real as possible" (p. 69). The transformation of the room into a studio often necessitates a leap of faith that we believe in this space as studio and thus it becomes one.

Such was the case at the Lower East Side Harm Reduction Center. The collaborative process of studio-making necessitated participants pushing tables together, cleaning them off, placing enough chairs around, and declaring, "This is the studio." The collective imagination and efforts of staff and participants converted a rather cluttered and dull space into the art-making environment.

Most open art therapy studios, even in their variety of theoretical stances, share some commonalities. The first is that a high level of safety must be present. Safety is the foundation from which all relationships, creativity, and healing develop. There is a necessary attitude of intentionality in the definitive creation of the studio environment (Moon, 2002). The studio needs to be regarded and understood as such. Whether the studio is in the hospital, prison, women's shelter, school, or any other location, the environment, atmosphere, or milieu must sustain the creative forces that will be unleashed.

The open studio can also be viewed as a "model for social action" (Block, Harris & Laing, 2005). The Open Studio Project began in 1991 and was located in Chicago, IL. These three art therapists developed a working studio environment where clients and therapists created side by side making art and writing. The initial goal was personal transformation. By 2000, they took their work into their own communities with the intent of reaching recognized people as "being in transition" (p. 37). People were encouraged to take responsibility for their own actions and make their own choices about safety and privacy.

Dan Hocoy in Kaplan (2007) describes art therapy and social action as linked through the "versatility and power of the image" (p. 22), which brings the discussion right back to the here and now. A sense of self agency is reinforced metaphorically through the act of creative expression. The participants make the art which is most relevant to them and the art speaks.

Finally, Malchiodi (2002) eloquently states: "What is important is to trust ourselves to take the risk of self-expression. In doing so, we immediately begin a journey of exploration that brings with it, inevitable surprises. Along the way, we may even find the answers to a problem or question that has baffled us for months. . . . Moments of astonishment or wonder are common to the arts. . ." (p. 192). The open studio is filled with the unexpected. The participants coming session to session always vary. The art-making process and images that come forth are unplanned and open-themed. The state of mind and physical health may change week to week for any particular person. Different needs emerge and differing modes of expression are embraced. The art therapist in this environment is continually called upon to be flexible and willing to flow with the mood of the studio.

The Lower East Side Harm Reduction Center (LESHRC/The Center)

The Lower East Side Harm Reduction Center is a community-based non-profit organization whose mission is to reduce the spread of HIV and Hepatitis C among New York City's injection drug users. Over the past 16 years, LESHRC has grown from a grassroots volunteer collective to a multiservice provider that responds to the many needs of its target population.

Approximately every other week, for two years, I would go to The Center which is located in the lower part of Manhattan where Chinatown and the old Jewish sections of the city are quickly becoming part of a changing neighborhood. There is a certain smell on the streets of fish vendors and produce being delivered in bulk. The sidewalks are always filled with people rushing about. It is noisy. People seem to be moving at even a faster clip than on the average city street. Things are happening. It is easy to miss the entrance to the Center. There is no large sign of welcome. The front of the building looks much as all the others on this block. It is a place where something is going on inside but no clues are given from the street.

Upon arrival, my routine was always much the same. From the entrance into the building it was a straight shot directly in to the studio. Well before I got there, I had it in my mind that the room where I would be working was already a studio. Usually there were a handful of participants sitting around eating lunch or watching television. Some participants were asleep–perhaps from sheer exhaustion due to homelessness or medications, methadone, depression, and so forth. It is a very exhausting life that necessitates vigilance at all times. Participants were robbed constantly. They had to manage governmental bureaucracy often. They may have been separated from their loved ones and social supports. Often the only relief they received was time in the Center.

The Center is often the central hub of their lives. Participants receive medical Hepatitis C information, mental health counseling, housing, and substance use counseling. Kinesiology, chiropractic, Reiki, acupuncture as well as arts and crafts are also available. Social workers help with a myriad of issues such as housing, food stamps, and other vital resources. Legal referrals are available.

In the studio area there is a microwave oven, tea and coffeemaker, chairs, heat, and a place to just "be." To simply stop and take a rest and have people to talk with is an enormous benefit of being in the Center. There are bathroom facilities.

Fours year ago, the Executive Director, David Rosenthal and I applied for a Johnson and Johnson, Society for Arts in Healthcare grant which we received. For the duration of the grant, I ran a women's art therapy group with the help of a student intern, Eiko Kijima, from New York University. When the grant was completed, David, who is a firm believer in the efficacy of the expressive therapies, asked me if I would run an open art therapy studio to continue to have this modality present in the Center. Thus, the open art therapy studio began.

The Population

The participants come from all walks of life. I met people in every field imaginable from veterans, teachers and artists to blue collar workers, beauticians, telephone operators, and gang members. There is also a sizeable percentage of the homeless mentally ill with nowhere to go and few resources. Almost all races, religions, ethnic groups, and gender/sexual orientations are represented in some time or other at the center.

The Sessions

Each session lasted 1 and a half hours. I always tried to bring fresh art supplies so the participants would experience, on some level, that they were valued by me. All participants at the center were always welcomed to the group and people could come and go as they pleased. We did establish a few rudimentary rules. No eating or drinking was permitted on the art tables. A few times, when this rule was not observed, drinks accidently were spilled, endangering both the artworks and the serenity of the participants. Music was allowed but it had to be low enough that the studio still felt quiet.

I would distribute the art supplies across the four tables. We had drawing materials, paints, and collage. Some participants would complain about having to give up their place for "art time" but on the whole, people were very receptive to having the opportunity to be creative and take what supplies they wanted to use.

Over time, I would begin to see the "regulars," those participants who came time and time again. They might not always make art. Sometimes, if a participant had received medication s/he might not be able to remain awake for the session. Other times, that same participant would be actively engaged, talking, and alert. The studio was a place of energy.

Participants

There are some very talented artists at LESHRC. Henrique, a deliberate, quiet and somewhat aloof African American man, would come to session and inspect the quality of all the black lead pencils. He appeared to be a loner, unwilling to engage in light conversation. He could be critical of my pencil sharpening skills and take me to task if the erasers were a bit worn at the edges. This actually became a source of our opening dialogues when greeting for a session. Over time, we developed humor on the topic of my trying harder to make the points on his pencils more to his liking.

Henrique had been a professional cartoonist as a young man. Once he started talking about drawing, he was unstoppable. His sentences would flow without pause and there was an almost musical quality to the sound of his words. He had a wealth of knowledge about animation, rendering, and illustration. Other participants were so impressed by his technical skill that they freely complimented his artistic abilities. Henrique became much more engaged with other people during the time he was participating in art-making. The participants expressed positive regard for Henrique when responding to his artwork.

Janie presented as quite shy and frightened. A petite Caucasian woman, she vehemently denied having any artistic ability whatsoever. She would come to session dressed in multiple layers of clothing, dragging one or two overstuffed bags alongside her. Even when the weather was warm she would be bundled up. She told me she had to keep her "stuff" near her because people were always robbing her.

As we met over the weeks and months, she shared her life story with me. She and her life partner had lived in a modest one-bedroom apartment. They were both animal lovers and they rescued dogs and cats at every opportunity. Their apartment was teeming with animal life. Janie indicated they really took in too many animals and often sacrificed having enough

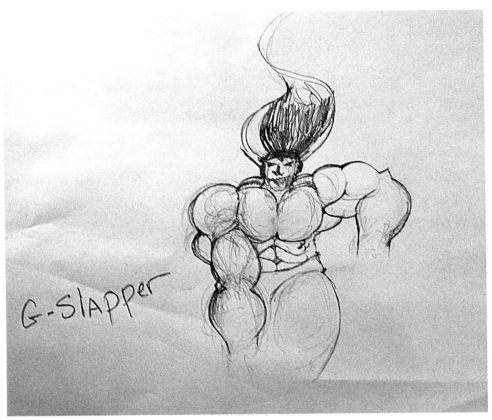

Figure 3.1. G-slapper.

food for themselves so they could keep their pets well-nourished.

Sadly, Janie's partner died leaving her bereft and unable to support her home and the animals. Her animals were confiscated and Janie became homeless. She never told me when she started her drug use. She has shared with me that the deep longing and loneliness make life so very difficult and depression is always with her. Many times she has expressed her goal of one day having a simple one-bedroom apartment and a few pets again.

In spite of her small stature, which she identified as a handicap on the street because she believed her size rendered her more vulnerable to being assaulted, Janie had powerful revenge fantasies. She would speak at length about how she would, "beat the crap" out of the next person who tried to steal her property. Her artwork was always contained, tight and compact. She worked cautiously and with great care. Much the way Janie physically presented, her drawings contained a quiet certitude which belied the tension roiling just under the surface.

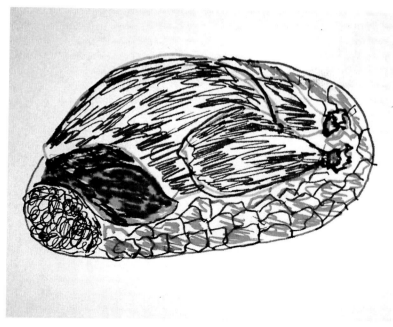

Figure 3.2. Turkey.

She made this drawing at Thanksgiving time. The participants responded to her "Turkey" with a group conversation around the meaning of Thanksgiving as well as reflections on holidays of the past. There was a bittersweet quality to these holiday conversations. A number of the participants expressed gratitude for "being alive" or "having friends" or "one more day" as well as sadness and loss. Others avoided the topic. Some participants were anticipating sharing their holiday meal at the Center.

There are many veterans at the LESHRC. The male vets who were present during most of the art therapy sessions tended to hover around the edges of the studio experience in pairs. Their relationships seemed private and particular. These "buddies" appeared powerful and mysterious, a brotherhood perhaps forged from the commonalities of difficult lives lived both on the battlefield and the embattled streets with the hardships of addiction and homelessness ever present. Generally very measured and polite, the men often nodded out in group and I would find myself watching attentively as images and lines would begin to be drawn just to stop mid-stroke.

One vet, who also identified as having been an artist before he went into combat, drew meticulous renderings of boats and war machinery. Every session that he attended he worked with steady intensity, always choosing ballpoint pen and plain paper as his medium. One crisp fall day he came in and

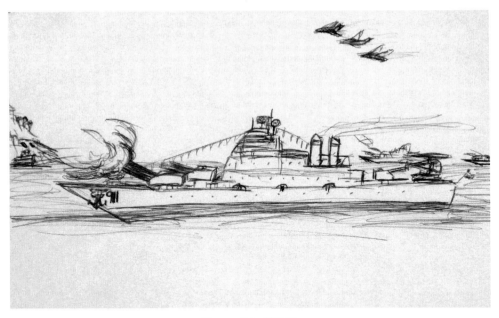

Figure 3.3. PT911.

made a drawing of a patrol boat entitled "PT911" (Figure 3.3). He told me he had lived on the streets near the tip of Manhattan when 9/11 happened and that the weather this day reminded him of the day of the day of the attack. Along with the name of the boat, "9/11" emblazoned on the bow, the two smoke stacks clearly replicate the destroyed Twin Towers. As he reflected upon his feeling about 9/11, the other participants joined in the discussion, connecting their individual experiences with one and other.

For many of the veterans, more often than not, the drawings they made ended in disconnected imagery and unfinished compositions. Introducing collage helped. The collage work often appeared to stimulate and coalesce the heart of the veterans' inner experiences much more successfully. Political commentary merged with personal sentiment in the selection and placement of images and words. There appeared to be less drifting off during the sessions when the men worked with scissors and glue as they removed pictures from magazines and reconstructed them into meaningful works of art (see Figure 3.4), During collage making, they were more actively engaged in conversation with other members of the Center. The art table became a source of interpersonal exchange.

There were many images acknowledging the devastating impact of unsafe sex, drugs, and gang behaviors (see Figure 3.5) on the lives of the participants. These drawings often included religious symbols and references to 12-

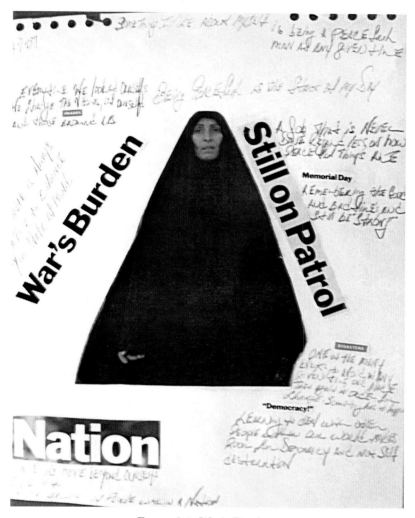

Figure 3.4. War's Burden.

Step slogans. Participants who had some "sobriety" would tend to make more art centered around recovery themes and there were times when showing their artwork to the group would stimulate discussions about how to take medications, to seek safer ways to live on the streets, to take care of possessions, and so forth.

Many participants had feelings of being overwhelmed by life (see Figure 3.6). This common theme sometimes stimulated conversations about fear and concerns about the future. In these moments, more optimistic participants tended to offer solace to the others. These were experiences of deep

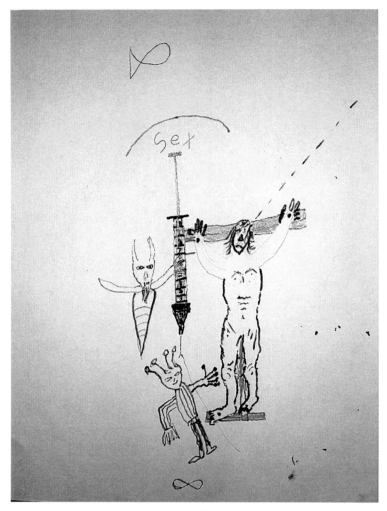

Figure 3.5. My Way.

connection within the studio. Sometimes, humor developed relieving some of the tension. I learned that this is a population with a good ability to find the humor in rather dire circumstances. I also discovered that even within this terribly disenfranchised group of people, where chaos abounded in everyday life, it was possible to find the lighter side to the pressures of stress, especially when we worked together and had a sense of belonging.

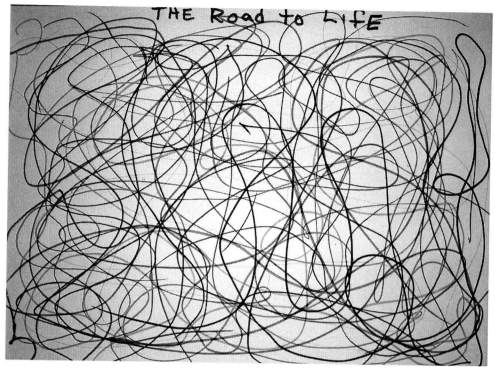

Figure 3.6. The Road to Life.

Discussion

The open art therapy studio at the Lower East Side Harm Reduction Center offered participants the safe opportunity to relax and explore through creative activity. Through sharing the art making experience and reflecting upon the artwork, individuals appeared to find a measure of acceptance and patience with each other. Commonalities developed which were broader than identities based solely upon addiction and homelessness status. Activating imagination became a vehicle for permitting metaphor to speak and the artists to be seen. There was much understanding expressed verbally between participants during the sessions.

The openness of the studio allowed people to come and go as they pleased. Some participants could tolerate being in the studio only a very few minutes. Others would stay the entire session, asking when the next gathering would be happening. It was a noisy, active, living space enriched, in particular, by a wall-sized mural made by a former long time participant, Mary, who had recently died. Mary's image stood as a tree of life, with people growing out of branches intertwined and reaching out towards one another.

The metaphor that we are all, in deep and meaningful ways, lending each other a hand as interconnected persons remains inescapable.

Appendix–Terms

Art therapy–a therapeutic profession which combines the process of creative visual expression with psychological and spiritual healing.

Harm reduction–practical, empathic, and non-judgmental approach to managing the adverse impact of harmful behaviors which often accompany chemically dependent persons.

References

Block, D., Harris, T., & Laing, S. (2005). Open studio process as a model of social action: A program for at-risk youth. *Art Therapy: Journal of the American Art Therapy Association, 22*(1), 32–38.

Denning, P. (2004). What is harm reduction? In P. Denning (Ed.), *Practicing harm reduction psychotherapy: An alternative approach to addictions* (p. 7). New York: Guilford.

Hocoy, D. (2007). Art therapy as a tool for social change: A conceptual model. In F. Kaplan (Ed.), *Art therapy and social/action* (p. 22). London: Kingsley.

Malchiodi, C. (2002). *The soul's palette: Drawing on art's transformative powers* (p. 192). Boston: Shambhala.

Marlatt, G. A. (2002). Harm reduction around the world: A brief history. In G. A. Marlatt (Ed.), *Harm reduction: Pragmatic strategies for managing high-risk behaviors* (pp. 41–68). New York: Guilford.

Moon, C. (2002). *Studio art therapy: Cultivating the artist identity in the art therapist* (pp. 69–72). London: Kingsley.

Tatarsky, A. (2007). Introduction. In A. Tatarsky (Ed.), *Harm reduction psychotherapy: A new treatment for drug and alcohol problems* (p. 2). Maryland: Aronson.

The Harm Reduction Coalition. Retrieved February 11, 2008 from www.harmreduction.org/section.php?id=62

Biography

Stephanie Wise, M.A., ATR- BC, LCAT is a Diplomat of the American Academy of Experts in Traumatic Stress, Board Certified in Professional Counseling and an Editorial Advisory Board member of the American Psychotherapy Association. Stephanie received her BFA from The Cooper Union and her Master's Degree from the Graduate Art Therapy Program at New York University. She earned her certificate from the International Trauma Studies Program/International University for Mental Health and Human Rights, New York University and Copenhagen University. She has worked in the field of Harm Reduction at both Project Hospitality and The Lower East Side Harm Reduction Center for many years. Stephanie is currently Clinical Assistant Professor in the Art Therapy Program at Marywood University in Scranton, PA. She is a Core Leadership Clinician for the ArtReach Foundation and maintains a small private practice.

Chapter 4

ORDER OUT OF CHAOS: THE EXPRESSIVE THERAPIES CONTINUUM AS A FRAMEWORK FOR ART THERAPY INTERVENTIONS IN SUBSTANCE ABUSE TREATMENT

Lisa D. Hinz

Clinicians, researchers, and writers in the field of art therapy have attempted to integrate the goals and methods of art therapy into substance abuse treatment programs for at least 30 years (Forrest, 1975; Head, 1975; Moore, 1983; Virshup, 1985). Early on, Head (1975) reported many advantages of art therapy as an adjunctive treatment with addicted individuals such as: adding structure to group therapy, providing a voice for non-verbal patients, objectifying conflicts making them easier to disclose and discuss, affording some kinesthetic activity, and stimulating affect. In an early review of the literature, Moore (1983) expanded upon the advantages of art therapy especially as a gently confrontive method of allowing emotionally avoidant persons access to feelings, and as a means of increasing mastery and control.

Friedman and Glickman (1986) in analyzing substance abuse treatment programs for adolescents found that the inclusion of art therapy was one important component of successful programs. However, despite early endorsements as to the importance and efficacy of art therapy in substance abuse treatment, art therapists have been slow to take up the challenge of its definition and implementation in this arena. A small number of more recent studies have demonstrated the efficacy of art therapy in the training of staff members (Adelman & Castricone, 1986; Biley, 2006), in the assessment of substance abuse disorders (Dickman, Dunn & Wolf, 1996; Francis, Kaiser & Deaver, 2003; Rockwell & Dunham, 2006), and in the treatment of substance abuse (Feen-Calligan, 1999; Groterath, 1999; Mahoney, 1999).

Whether in the area of training, assessment, or treatment of substance abuse, art therapy typically is conceived of as an adjunctive approach rather than as a central treatment, and the literature has been characterized by isolated studies describing single techniques (Allen, 1985; Cox & Price, 1990; Luzzatto, 1987). Art therapy has been described as helpful in amplifying feelings of unmanageability (Cox & Price, 1990; Wadeson, 2000), confronting shame (Johnson, 1990; Wilson, 2003), and enhancing spirituality (Chickerneo, 1993; Feen-Calligan, 1995; Miller, 1995). Another goal of art therapy in substance abuse programs has been to clarify the internal and external worlds of persons using substances in order to augment future behavioral choices (Hanes, 2007; Luzzatto, 1987). Finally, art therapy has been used effectively to educate professional health care workers about the types and intensity of difficulties induced by substance use and to change previously negative attitudes towards persons who use substances (Adelman & Castricone, 1986; Biley, 2006).

Art therapists, at times, have bristled against demands to deliver art therapy services in the context of a disease model of substance abuse disorder founded upon the 12-Step treatment approach (Allen, 1985; Horay, 2006; Mahoney, 1999). Attempts at formulating integrated approaches to art therapy and substance abuse disorder were made by Horay (2006), Feen-Calligan (1999), and Matto, Corcoran, and Fassler (2003). Matto and her colleagues (2003) elegantly explained the numerous ways that the goals of art therapy and solution-focused therapy dovetail to produce an effective art therapy treatment for substance abuse disorder. The article is full of meaningful comparisons and practical suggestions but it does not represent an overarching theory of how and why art therapy is uniquely effective; the article supports art therapy as a valuable technique in solution-focused therapy. Matto (2002) published a more comprehensive explanation of art therapy in the service of substance abuse and she did a fine job of explaining the therapeutic benefits of art therapy in short-term inpatient settings. Springham (1999) eloquently described how art therapy can be used in the context of object relations theory to help substance dependent patients negotiate the therapeutic journey between narcissistic frustration and instant gratification. Images were said to convey the narcissistic need often obscured by the "false self" presented in treatment.

Horay (2006) decried the amount of emphasis in the art therapy literature on 12-Step doctrine, especially the use of art therapy for breaking through defenses and increasing patients' feelings of unmanageability as pronounced in the first of the 12 Steps. The author stated that a wider range of focus was needed when employing art therapy in substance abuse treatment programs, emphasizing the lack of attention to patients' feelings of ambivalence towards recovery. Horay described how art therapy could be implemented in a stages-of-change therapeutic model that would address ambivalence at each phase along the road to recovery. Again, art therapy was examined and explained as a technique to be used in the context of a larger psychological theory; it was not promoted as a wide-ranging treatment in its own right.

Feen-Calligan (1999) attempted to formulate a "grounded" theory of substance abuse treatment and to discover an underlying principle descriptive of the approach. Her research was "grounded" in the interview process; she interviewed treatment providers and patients to find that enlightenment was central to their understanding of art therapy applied to substance abuse treatment. Enlightenment was defined as understanding important aspects of recovery and their application in individual's lives (Feen-Calligan, 1999). Feen-Calligan concluded her study by stating, "Finding the most effective treatment for each individual is a challenge. Art therapy deserves consideration for its potential to contribute to the treatment, the relative happiness of each individual living life without drugs and alcohol" (p. 158). Art therapy can be a powerful treatment for substance abuse disorders, but this theoretical article lacked well-articulated practical suggestions as to how it might be applied.

Although Feen-Calligan (1999), Matto and colleagues (2003), and Horay (2006) attempted to place art therapy treatment in a broader context within chemical dependency treatment, the effect is less than satisfying. Comprehensive and individualized treatment protocols are recommended, but the basis for most substance abuse treatment programs remains a 12-Step model with a disease focus (Breslin, Reed & Malone, 2003; Matto, 2002). The unique contributions of art therapy are not recognized, and common questions in the field of substance abuse treatment linger. Such questions include: why doesn't treatment work? Or, why doesn't treatment work the first time? And, why doesn't the same treatment work for everyone? (Breslin et al., 2003; Moore, 1983). Therapists treating substance abuse disorder stress the importance of thorough assessment and individualized treatment plans (Breslin et al., 2003; Feen-Calligan, 1999; Matto, 2002). However, what seems more prevalent is that time and monetary constraints force patients to join ongoing treatment groups sometimes by choice and other times by necessity (Cox & Price, 1990; Johnson, 1990; Luzzatto, 1987). This sort of one-size-fits-all treatment approach characteristic of many inpatient treatment programs may contribute to the high rates of relapse and revolving door treatment.

Art therapy conceived of within the context of the Expressive Therapies Continuum (ETC) can provide assessment and treatment information that highlights unique patient strengths and individual needs that must be therapeutically addressed, even in the context of a uniform treatment program (Hinz, in press). This chapter proposes that the Expressive Therapies

Continuum provides a theoretical and practical manner of approaching the assessment and treatment of substance abuse disorders. It offers a framework for the assessment of chemical dependency, as well as a structure for formulating individual treatment goals that can exist within any substance abuse treatment program. The ETC offers a way to conceive of art therapy as an integral part of comprehensive treatment for substance abuse disorder rather than as an isolated technique.

Introduction to the Expressive Therapies Continuum

As originally conceived, the Expressive Therapies Continuum describes persons' interactions with art media or other experiential activities in order to process information and form images (Kagin & Lusebrink, 1978; Lusebrink, 1990). The ETC organizes media interactions into a developmental hierarchy of information processing and image formation strategies from simple kinesthetic experiences at one end, to complex symbol mastery at the other. The ETC consists of four levels of increasingly complex processing. The first three levels are bipolar as shown in Figure 4.1. The two components of these first three bipolar levels have an interdependent relationship: as activity with the component on one side of the level increases, activity with the other component decreases. The therapeutic use of these associations will be demonstrated later in this chapter. The fourth level, the Creative level, can occur with the use of any single component of the ETC or can represent the integration of functioning at all levels. Patients generally demonstrate a preference for one type of information processing; this preference could be related to the origin of the substance abuse disorder or it could be a consequence of it. Understanding these preferences can help art therapists devise individualized and effective treatment plans.

Each component of the Expressive Therapies Continuum has a distinct healing role as well as a unique emergent function (Kagin & Lusebrink, 1978; Lusebrink, 1990, 1991). The emergent function of each ETC component is the activity that arises out of work with a certain component process. Often art making experiences evoke more complex processing of information and/or images, and frequently movement to a higher level of the ETC. The fact that one type of functioning possibly evokes a higher-level process can complicate the prescription of "pure" expressive experiences. However, projecting the progress of emergent components, along with knowledge of their healing properties, helps guide art therapists to provide the most effective therapeutic interventions. Healing functions are those processes considered therapeutic about working at a particular level of the ETC. Lusebrink (1990) discussed the healing functions of each component and they are presented in Table 4.1 along with their relationships to substance abuse treatment goals.

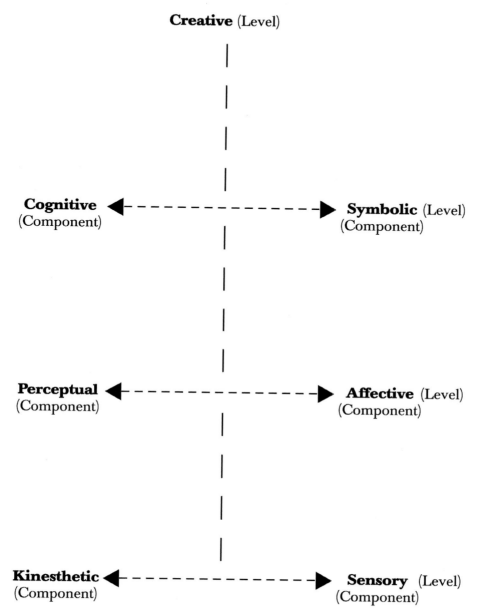

Creative (Level)

Cognitive ← - - - - - - - - - - - - - - → **Symbolic** (Level)
(Component)   (Component)

Perceptual ← - - - - - - - - - - - - - → **Affective** (Level)
(Component)   (Component)

Kinesthetic ← - - - - - - - - - - - - → **Sensory** (Level)
(Component)   (Component)

Figure 4.1. The Expressive Therapies Continuum: A Developmental Hierarchy of Information Processing and Image Formation. All rights reserved. Reprinted with permission of the American Art Therapy Association, Inc. (AATA). Originally published in *Art Therapy: Journal of the American Art Therapy Association 25*(1), 38–40.

Healing Functions of the Expressive Therapies Continuum

Kinesthetic/Sensory Level. Referring back to the developmental hierarchy of the Expressive Therapies Continuum as expressed in Figure 4.1, the first level of the ETC is the Kinesthetic/Sensory Level and it represents the simplest form of information processing. Information processing begins as it does in infancy with input taken in and processed through movement and the senses. Kinesthetic feedback from motor action, as well as internal and external sensation, provides information through sensorimotor feedback loops (Piaget, 1954). The healing function of the Kinesthetic component is rhythmic motion and energy release. Individuals can use art experiences to release the build-up of tension often experienced as a prelude to substance use. Head (1975) mentioned that years of substance use could have physical and psychological anesthetizing effects which kinesthetic movement can counteract. In addition, the author mentioned the sensory stimulation provided by art experiences as another way that patients often "awaken" using art. Clay work and scribble drawings emphasize the energy release of the Kinesthetic component. Kinesthetic/Sensory activity can be used to evoke Perceptual/Affective processes, as these are the emergent functions of the first level of the ETC.

The healing function of the Sensory component of the Expressive Therapies Continuum is awareness of internal and external sensations. Sensory awareness promoted by art experiences may help individuals become more tolerant of internal and external sensations and less dependent on substances to manage or provide sensation. Kaplan (as cited in Moore, 1983) provided her adolescent chemical dependency group with a sensory experience by asking group members to adorn partners' faces with a special paint made from cold cream, cornstarch, and food coloring. Other sensory experiences include relating aromas and odors to pleasant and unpleasant using experiences, experiencing the tactile qualities of art materials, and mixing paint colors. What can emerge from work with the Sensory component is awareness of the emotional input from the next highest level of the ETC.

Perceptual/Affective Level. Moving up the developmental hierarchy, information processing/image formation occurs on the Perceptual/Affective Level. The healing function of the Perceptual component of the Expressive Therapies Continuum is a focus on formal visual elements and organization. Highlighting formal visual elements such as line, shape, and color through perceptually-oriented art experiences can emphasize organization. Through the process of isomorphism, work with the Perceptual component can augment internal organization. As a result, individuals may feel fewer urges to use substances to manage what previously felt like chaotic inner experiences. In addition, the use of Perceptual processes can help patients visualize their

TABLE 4.1. HEALING AND EMERGENT FUNCTIONS OF
ETC COMPONENTS RELATED TO SUBSTANCE USE.

Expressive Therapies Component	Healing Function	Healing Function as related to Substance Abuse Treatment	Therapeutic Use of the ETC Component
Kinesthetic	Energy release; Rhythm	Stress reduction; Bodily awareness	Clay work; Scribble drawings
Sensory	Awareness of internal and external sensations	May help individual become less dependent upon substance for providing or managing sensation	Face paint, Aroma associations; Mixing paint colors
Perceptual	Focus on form and organization	Promotes awareness of internal organization; helps patients visualize problems in concrete terms in order to heighten awareness and bring about needed change	Self in the world drawing (Luzzatto, 1987); Changing point of view drawing (Lusebrink, 1990)
Affective	Awareness of appropriate affect	Learning to identify discriminate, express, and soothe emotions without substances	Pro and con collage (Horay, 2006); 4 primary emotions
Cognitive	Generalization of concrete experiences	Thinking through consequences of actions (especially substance use) without experiencing them	Incident drawings (Cox & Price, 1990); Future incident drawings; Cartooning, Life books
Symbolic	Formation and mastery of personal symbols	Learning about and integrating previously disowned or unknown parts of self	Self-portraits (Hanes, 2007); Self-symbols Mandala drawings; Mask-making
Creative	Creative expression related to self-actualization	Reduction of shame; access to higher self; interdependence on others; increased self-actualization	Any single or integrative art experience

situation in concrete terms in order to heighten awareness and bring about needed change. Luzzatto (1987) used a Perceptual experience to help patients visualize themselves and the world. According to Luzzatto, if patients were encouraged to visualize negative views of themselves and the world in concrete forms, they were less likely to project this negativity onto the therapist and therapeutic process. The Changing Point of View drawing (Lusebrink, 1990) is a Perceptual activity that has patients create an image, and in response make an extreme close-up view of one aspect of the first image, and a bird's-eye view of the original image. These two different perspectives rendered through two different perceptual experiences help patients recognize that their view of a situation colors its meaning and significance.

The healing function of the Affective component of the Expressive Therapies Continuum is increased awareness of appropriate affect. Art therapy most often has been identified as a safe therapeutic method of helping chemically dependent individuals express affect (Chickerneo, 1993; Horay, 2006; Moore, 1983; Virshup, 1985). Before they can express affect; however, patients in recovery from chemical dependency also may need education in identifying, discriminating, and soothing emotions. Identifying and discriminating emotions can be accomplished by having patients depict four different primary emotions (sad, mad, glad, and afraid) as distinctly as possible from one another (Hinz, 2006). Further, Horay (2006) demonstrated how pro and con collages could be used to access, identify, and express the many diverse and often ambivalent feelings brought up throughout substance abuse recovery. Art, instead of substance use, can be a way to express and soothe previously troublesome emotions. The emergent function of the Perceptual/Affective level can be the ability to engage in complex cause and effect thinking, especially concerning emotions or the ability to create and master symbols.

Cognitive/Symbolic Level. Cognitive/Symbolic functioning is represented at the third level of the Expressive Therapies Continuum. Information processed on the Cognitive/Symbolic level is sophisticated and sometimes mysterious; it requires intuitive recognition, planning, and complex cognitive action. Cox and Price (1990) used incident drawings to help patients examine the consequences of their past actions. Cognitively-oriented art therapy tasks such as cartooning, future life books, or future incident drawings can teach cause and effect thinking and help patients to think through the consequence of potential future actions. Future life books require that patients write their life stories from past through an unknown future, writing, and illustrating the possible consequences of various life choices, including substance use. Patients can benefit from thinking through the complex chain of events that begins with a trigger emotion or situation and often ends in using. Research demonstrates that emotional triggers can be anticipated and prepared for to reduce the likelihood of relapse (Ekman, 2003).

The healing component of the Symbolic component of the Expressive Therapies Continuum is learning about and integrating previously disowned or unknown parts of the self. Often feelings of shame surrounding childhood issues and past behavior prompts substance abuse as patients attempt to reject personality characteristics, past experiences, or current needs (Johnson, 1990; Wilson, 2003). Hanes (2007) discussed the spontaneous and planned use of self-portraits as a method for helping patients accept disowned parts of themselves. Other forms of Symbolic expression include self-symbols, mandala drawings, and mask making. These art experiences can enhance the acceptance and integration of shadow qualities or other disowned aspects of the self that previously motivated substance use.

Creative Level. The Creative level can exist at any or all of the levels of the Expressive Therapies Continuum. For example, painting to music can be a soothing, sensory experience used to help an individual achieve serenity. Thus, patients can create a relaxed state from the simple experience of painting to music. The creative moment can be explained by saying that the media experience helped bring about an inner sense of calm. Alternatively, a Creative experience might combine elements from all levels of the ETC. Thus, painting to music might begin as a Sensory experience as described above and change into a more integrative experience. As the paintbrush moves paint over the paper, lines appear which allow forms to be perceived. The Sensory experience becomes a Perceptual experience when these forms become part of the creative tapestry. A Symbolic experience can be achieved if randomly created forms take on meaning, thus producing personal symbols. In this instance, all levels of the ETC are represented in one creative experience. Creativity in substance abuse treatment is conceived of as a path for individuals to reconnect with their higher selves and other people, and as an antidote to shame (Johnson, 1990). According to Wilson (2003), creative experiences not only allow patients to heal the crippling effects of shame, but also set the stage for self-actualization.

Assessment Within the Expressive Therapies Continuum Framework

The starting point in providing effective art therapy is a comprehensive assessment of patient needs as well as patient strengths. Based upon such an assessment, individualized treatment goals can be formulated which best address unique patient concerns. One premise of the Expressive Therapies Continuum is that problems in living are caused by overuse or underuse of component functions. One goal of successful art therapy treatment is for patients to be able to take in and process information using all levels and with all component of the ETC (Lusebrink, 1990). By using the ETC as a framework for assessment, art therapists can establish patients' preferred method of information processing—Kinesthetic, Sensory, Perceptual,

Affective, Cognitive or Symbolic—as well as determine any overuse or under-use of component functions. With these predilections and aversions as a starting point, it is possible to devise effective individualized treatments that help patients (1) reduce dependence on overused functions, (2) increase the use of underutilized or blocked components, and (3) begin using all channels to receive and process information (Hinz, in press). Finally, patients can be aided to express themselves creatively such that integrated functioning occurs to replace with increasing frequency, the need to use substances for self-expression.

Similar to the assessment procedures described by Matto (2002), assessment of individuals in the context of the Expressive Therapies Continuum examines patients' preferences for and interactions with art media, their statements and behaviors during the art-making process, and the finished art product itself. These aspects of the first art therapy session(s) will give suggestions as to how patients prefer to receive and process information, as well as where there might be overuse or underuse of component functions that might be related to substance use or other difficulties. Observation of the creative process, listening to self-talk, and style elements from the finished art product can help pinpoint to preferences for symbol use, elaborate or impoverished cognitive processes, splurges of or avoidance of affect, perceptual focus, sensory stimulation, and or an orientation toward action (Hinz, in press). Figure 4.2 demonstrates that media preferences also can indicate the level of the ETC where patients currently are most comfortable processing information. Fluid media are likely to call up affective experiences whereas resistive media will evoke cognitive processes. Thus, directing media choices and use can be one method of helping patients meet treatment goals (Cox & Price, 1990; Feen-Calligan, 1995; Lusebrink, 1990). Resistive media can augment cognitive functioning and fluid media can be implemented when increased affective functioning is a desired therapeutic outcome. For example, in order to make their incident drawings more emotionally compelling, Cox and Price (1990) used paint to stimulate affect. The authors reported that the unmanageability of paint highlighted chemically dependent patients' awareness of their lack of ability to manage their lives while using.

The Expressive Therapies Continuum as a Framework for Substance Abuse Treatment

The theoretical structure of the Expressive Therapies Continuum supports the use of art therapy in a variety of complex and comprehensive ways, not merely as a technique to facilitate the expression of emotion. Therapeutic goals related to the ETC may consist of the release of tension, self-soothing, and relaxation on the Kinesthetic/Sensory level. On the Perceptual/Affective

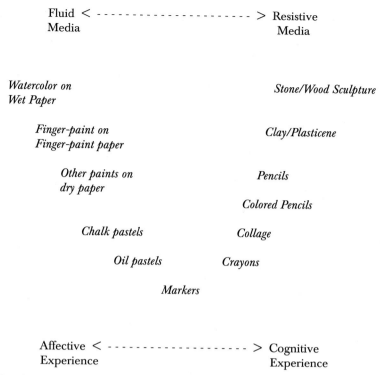

Figure 4.2. Media Properties and Affective or Cognitive Experience. Reproduced by permission of Jessica Kingsley, Publishers from: Hinz (2006) *Drawing From Within: Using Art to Treat Eating Disorders.*

level, goals might include clarification of relations between parts of a problem, expression and containment of emotions, reintegration of affect as a guide to behavior, and perceiving order out of the chaos of emotions often flooding the substance-abusing individual. Cognitive/Symbolic goals could be conceptualized as increasing planning and problem-solving abilities, supporting greater decision making skills, promoting cause and effect thinking, consolidating personal meaning through symbol mastery, and deepening personal meaning via understanding universal themes. The Creative level allows for shame reduction and the expression of spirituality. Creative use of art media sets the stage for self-actualization experiences.

Because they can change and direct media use, art therapists can vary therapeutic experiences provided in treatment centers in ways that traditional verbal therapists cannot. Art therapists have the ability to provide different experiences or materials to their patients in order to individualize treatment protocols. Customizing media provided to patients can be one way to individualize art therapy treatment even within a structured art therapy program. As was stated above, Cox and Price (1990) used tempera paints in their incident drawings with chemically dependent adolescents in order to provoke feelings of unmanageability. It is not hard to imagine that there would be patients for whom paintings such as these would be overly affectively evocative. Consequently, patients who would benefit from gaining cognitive control over emotions could use colored pencils instead of paint in the same incident drawing experience.

Patients naturally will wonder why some are being offered one type of media and others another. The prescription of media use can be thoughtfully explained to actively enlist patients as partners in formulating and implementing treatment goals. Accordingly, patients will understand that media have the ability to evoke different responses, and that the considered use of art media will be one part of individualized treatment planning. Media for use in group art therapy can be laid out along a continuum from most resistive and likely to promote cognitive responding (e.g., pencil), to most fluid and likely to promote affective processing (e.g., paint). This type of media presentation can aid in the assessment of patients assigned to inpatient art therapy groups without prior information. A new patient's choice of media from this continuum can give one piece of assessment information to aid in ascertaining preferred level of ETC, overused and underused ETC components, and to devise effective art interventions.

Table 4.2 contains information about the overuse and underuse of Expressive Therapies Continuum component functions and implications for substance use disorder. For example, a preference for the Cognitive component of the Expressive Therapies Continuum often is noted among chemically dependent patients. Intricate verbal rationalizations and intellectualization are used to support the denial that maintains substance abuse (Wadeson, 2000). Stylistically, drawings made by chemically dependent patients typically avoid color, present just the right details of the disorder, but avoid the affect associated with it (Wadeson, 2000). Patients such as this use cognitive activity as a means of denying the practical and emotional consequences of substance use. The same materials and methods can be used in a different fashion, perhaps with incident drawings such as those described by Cox and Price (1990) to help patients directly confront the consequences of their substance use. Color could be added gradually to the art therapy process to help overly cognitively involved patients begin to access the affect that has been censored and suppressed.

Alternatively, patients in treatment for chemical dependency might overuse motor behavior to ward off emotions that threaten to overwhelm (Lusebrink, 1990). The constant motion of leg swinging or toe-tapping can be an indication for art therapy work with the Kinesthetic component of the Expressive Therapies Continuum. Wadeson (2000) described an art therapist

TABLE 4.2. OVERUSE AND UNDERUSE OF ETC COMPONENT FUNCTIONS
AND IMPLICATIONS FOR SUBSTANCE USE DISORDER.

ETC Component	Overuse of Component Function	Underuse of Component Function	ETC Directed Intervention	Rationale
Kinesthetic	Hyperactivity; use of activity to ward off emotions (e.g., leg swinging, toe tapping)	Lack of awareness of body; Feeling "uncomfortable in one's skin"	Kinesthetic activities release tension; Affective awareness	Substance use is no longer needed to calm or release tension emerge
Sensory	Highly Sensitive Person uses alcohol to avoid overly stimulating sensations	Sensory Integration Problems	Sensory experiences help actively manage sensory stimulation	Substance use not needed to increase or decrease "sensory diet"
Perceptual	Compulsive behavior; stereotypical images help maintain denial or contain emotion	Disorganization, Overly emotional	Patients "see" their situations differently or impose form & organization	Freedom from compulsivity can occur without substance use
Affective	Overwhelmed by emotions; Inability to think or learn from them	Alexithymia; No words for or awareness of emotions	Affect can be contained or encouraged	Appropriate affective expression reduces need for substances
Cognitive	Intellectualization; Rationalization supports denial of substance use	Decreased cause and effect thinking and other more sophisticated thought processes	Cognitive processes show cause and effect; confront denial of consequences	Increased ability to think through consequences; decreased substance use
Symbolic	Esoteric Thinking overly elaborative symbolic or metaphorical thought; mental confusion	Concrete thought processes; cognitive distortions	Cognitive distortions and esoteric thinking clarified through image	Clear thinking reduces need for substance use

who used clay to stimulate action and emotion in his chemically dependent patients. The goal of Kinesthetic activity such as vigorous clay work or other rhythmic action is the release of tension. What might emerge from such work is the perception of form and increased awareness of inner organization or the experience of emotion. With gentle guidance, emotion can be identified and expressed through art, rather than avoided through further repetitive motion. Again, in the interest of creating the most individualized treatment possible, one patient can be encouraged to use plasticene or clay without all persons in the group having to use it.

The first pictures drawn by patients in substance abuse treatment often include images of substance use and drug paraphernalia (Dickman, Dunn & Wolf, 1996; Wadeson, 1980). These images sometimes are drawn repetitively in a compulsive fashion and thus demonstrate overuse of functioning on the Perceptual component of the Expressive Therapies Continuum. The images of bottles, drugs, and drug paraphernalia are stereotypical images made with the intent to glorify substance use or at least maintain a defensive stance about it. Art therapy can help addicted individuals move away from stereotypical images to fuller emotional expression. The art therapist can encourage patients stuck on the Perceptual component to examine their images carefully and talk about what is actually *seen* rather than what was *intended* when the drawing was conceived. In addition, any slight variation in the formal elements of the image can be used as a point of departure for movement to the next level of the ETC (Hinz, 2006). What can emerge from this manner of looking at an image is the ability to see situations differently (Luzzatto, 1987) and freedom from compulsivity without the use of alcohol or other substances.

Chemically dependent patients who are overly affectively involved demonstrate a preference for paint and other fluid media. They might use the art experiences to overindulge in emotional expression without trying to learn from the experience or move forward. The final art products might not contain any visible form or identifiable symbols; these patients might not be able to comment on anything except the emotion, conjuring no relation of the emotion to causes or consequences of substance use. Movement away from purely affective responding towards the Perceptual component, or movement to the Cognitive/Symbolic level of functioning would help overly emotional patients gain the internal and external structure necessary for therapeutic change. Changing to a more structured media and focusing on form and organization can help move affectively involved patients to the Perceptual component or Cognitive/Symbolic level. With containment of emotion by media and form, the appropriate expression of emotion can begin to replace the use of substances as a means or "excuse" to express affect.

Diverse Art Tasks, Universal Themes

Art therapy groups are unique in that members can work separately on individual issues or projects. There is no verbal group therapy equivalent of each member choosing or being assigned a different task which they come together at the end of the session to discuss. In an art therapy group, when patients' under and overused components are known, media choices, and task instructions can be tailored so that individual patients receive the creative experiences that will be uniquely therapeutic. For example, affectively overwhelmed patients would profit from a perceptual focus on the formal elements of visual expression, which would lead them to an awareness of their own inner organization. Alternatively, careful introduction to the language of emotional expression would help alexithymic patients move beyond rigid organization and dependence on substances to facilitate affective expression.

When group members have had various creative experiences, therapists can artfully guide them to comment on shared symbols, themes, and emotions rather than discuss each art product individually. Thus, the healing component of universality is not forced through the imposition of the same task on each group member, but felt through common emotional themes experienced during the recovery process. An examination of the Expressive Therapies Continuum clarifies some of the reasons that similar treatments do not influence all chemically dependent patients in the same fashion: different preferences and aversions for information processing and image formation will mean that one art experience may overly inhibit or overly stimulate different patients. Devising individualized art therapy treatment plans based on knowledge gained from assessment within the ETC can address some of these concerns. Thus, even in the context of a structured group, various media can be assigned to different therapeutic effects. In a less structured environment, unique individualized therapeutic experiences can be provided.

Conclusion

Because it is a comprehensive theory explaining the relevance of art therapy across all avenues of information processing and image formation, applying the Expressive Therapies Continuum to chemical dependency treatment perhaps requires more work for the art therapist. Nevertheless, this theory reaches well beyond the application of a single art therapy technique to provide individualized and optimally effective art interventions. The increased work stems from greater attention paid to assessment and using assessment information to tailor individual media choices and task instructions. ETC assessment evaluates media preferences, verbal comments, and art-making behavior during the artistic process, as well as stylistic elements of the final art product. Assignment of tasks can be personalized, even within the context of group art therapy, with patients being enlisted as partners in the formulation of therapeutic goals. Task instructions and materials are individually conceived for each patient in order to bring about integrated functioning with all levels and components of the Expressive Therapies Continuum. Experiencing integrated creative functioning provides a foundation for patients to eschew the use of substances and approach self-actualization.

Appendix–Terms

Alexithymia–A condition in which a person has no words for emotions or does not experience emotions.

Component Function–One part of the bipolar levels of the Expressive Therapies Continuum. Components represent methods of information processing information and image formation: kinesthetic, sensory, perceptual, affective, cognitive, and symbolic. Their overuse or underuse can cause difficulties with living.

Emergent Function–The activity that arises out of work with a certain component function. Often art-making experiences evoke more complex processing of information and/or images, and frequently movement to a higher level of the Expressive Therapies Continuum.

Expressive Therapies Continuum–A theoretical and practical framework for describing persons' interactions with art media or other experiential activities in order to process information and form images.

Fluid Media–Media that flows quickly and easily onto the working surface; facilitates the expression of affect in art therapy.

Formal Elements of Visual Expression–Elements of a visual image such as line, shape, color, size, spatial relations, implied energy, and space used that define the expression of an image.

Healing Function–The process considered distinctively therapeutic about working with a particular component of the Expressive Therapies Continuum.

Media Preference–A natural or learned affinity for working with particular art materials.

Stereotypical Images–In chemical dependency treatment, images of bottles, drugs, or drug paraphernalia that do not act as symbols to transmit information, but rather act as defenses against conveying personal information.

Structured Media–Media with inherent organization such as pencil, collage, mosaic, or wood; facilitates cognitive expression in art therapy.

Stylistic Elements–Features of the finished art images such as line quality and color use that point to clients' preferred component of the Expressive Therapies Continuum.

References

Adelman, E., & Castricone, L. (1986). An expressive arts model for substance abuse group training and treatment. *The Arts in Psychotherapy, 13,* 53–59.

Allen, P. B. (1985). Integrating art therapy into an alcoholism treatment program. *American Journal of Art Therapy, 24,* 10–12.

Biley, F. C. (2006). The arts, literature and the attraction paradigm: Changing attitudes towards substance misuse service users. *Journal of Substance Use, 11*(1), 11–21.

Breslin, K. T., Reed, M. R., & Malone, S. B. (2003). A holistic approach to substance abuse treatment. *Journal of Psychoactive Drugs, 35*(2), 247–251.

Chickerneo, N. B. (1993). *Portraits of spirituality in recovery: The use of art in recovery from co-dependency and/or chemical dependency.* Springfield, IL: Charles C Thomas.

Cox, K. L., & Price, K. (1990). Breaking through: Incident drawings with adolescent substance abusers. *The Arts in Psychotherapy, 17*(4), 333–337.

Dickman, S. B., Dunn, J. E., & Wolf, A. W. (1996). The use of art therapy as a predictor of relapse in chemical dependency treatment. *Art Therapy, 13*(4), 232–237.

Ekman, P. (2003). *Emotions revealed.* New York: Henry Holt.

Feen-Calligan, H. (1995). The use of art therapy in treatment programs to promote spiritual recovery from addiction. *Art Therapy, 12*(1), 46–50.

Feen-Calligan, H. (1999). Enlightenment in chemical dependency treatment programs: A grounded theory. In C. A. Malchiodi (Ed.), *Medical art therapy with adults* (pp. 137–161). London: Jessica Kingsley Press.

Forrest, G. (1975). The problems of dependency and the value of art therapy as a means of treating alcoholism. *Art Psychotherapy, 2*(1), 15–43.

Francis, D., Kaiser, D., & Deaver, S. P. (2003). Representations of attachment security in the bird's nest drawings of patients with substance abuse disorders. *Art Therapy, 20*(3), 125–137.

Friedman, A. S., & Glickman, N. W. (1986). Residential program characteristics for completion of treatment by adolescent drug abusers. *Journal of Nervous and Mental Disease, 175*(7), 419–424.

Groterath, A. (1999). Conceptions of addiction and implications for treatment approaches. In D. Waller & J. Mahoney (Eds.), *Treatment of addictions: Current issues for arts therapies* (pp. 14–22). London: Routledge.

Hanes, M. J. (2007). "Face-to-face" with addiction: The spontaneous production of self-portraits in art therapy. *Art Therapy, 24*(1), 33–36.

Head, V. B. (1975). Experiences with art therapy in short-term groups of day clinic addicted patients. *Ontario Psychologist, 7*(4) 42–49.

Hinz, L. D. (in press). *Expressive therapies continuum: A framework for using art in therapy.* New York: Routledge.

Hinz, L. D. (2006). *Drawing from within: Using art to treat eating disorders.* London: Jessica Kingsley Publishers.

Horay, B. J. (2006). Moving towards gray: Art therapy and ambivalence in substance abuse treatment. *Art Therapy, 23*(1), 14–22.

Johnson, L. (1990). Creative therapies in the treatment of addictions: The art of transforming shame. *The Arts in Psychotherapy, 17*(4), 299–308.

Kagin, S. L., & Lusebrink, V. B. (1978). The expressive therapies continuum. *Art Psychotherapy,*

5(4), 171–180.

Lusebrink, V. B. (1990). *Imagery and visual expression in therapy.* New York: Plenum Press.

Lusebrink, V. B. (1991). A systems-oriented approach to the expressive therapies: The expressive therapies continuum. *The Arts in Psychotherapy, 18*(5), 395–403.

Luzzatto, P. (1987). The internal world of drug-abusers: Projective pictures of self-object relationships. *British Journal of Projective Psychology, 32*(2), 22–33.

Mahoney, J. (1999). Art therapy and art activities in alcohol services: A research project. D. Waller & J. Mahoney (Eds.), *Treatment of addictions: Current issues for arts therapies* (pp. 117–140). London: Routledge.

Matto, H. (2002). Integrating art therapy methodology in brief inpatient substance abuse treatment for adults. *Journal of Social Work Practice in the Addictions, 2*(2), 69–83.

Matto, H., Corcoran, J., & Fassler, A. (2003). Integrating solution-focused and art therapies for substance abuse treatment: Guidelines for practice. *The Arts in Psychotherapy, 30*(5), 265–272.

Miller, M. A. (1995). Spirituality, art therapy, and the chemically dependent person. In R. Kus, (Ed.), *Spirituality and chemical dependency* (pp. 135–144). New York: Haworth Press.

Moore, R. W. (1983). Art therapy with substance abusers: A review of the literature. *The Arts in Psychotherapy, 10*(4), 251–260.

Piaget, J. (1954). *The construction of reality in the child.* New York: Basic Books.

Rockwell, P., & Dunham, M. (2006). The utility of the formal elements art therapy scale in assessment of substance use disorder. *Art Therapy, 23*(3), 104–111.

Springham, N. (1999). All things very lovely: Art therapy in a drug and alcohol treatment programme. In D. Waller & J. Mahoney (Eds.), *Treatment of addictions: Current issues for arts therapies* (pp. 141–166). London: Routledge.

Virshup, E. (1985). Group art therapy in a methadone clinic lobby. *Journal of Substance Abuse Treatment, 2*(3), 153–158.

Wadeson, H. (1980). *Art psychotherapy.* New York: John Wiley & Sons.

Wadeson, H. (2000). *Art therapy practice.* New York: John Wiley & Sons.

Wilson, M. (2003). Art therapy in addictions treatment: Creativity and shame reduction. In C. A. Malchiodi (Ed.), *Handbook of art therapy* (pp. 281–293). New York: Guilford Press.

Biography

Lisa D. Hinz, Ph.D., ATR is a clinical psychologist and registered art therapist. She is an adjunct faculty member in the Saint Mary-of-the-Woods College art therapy master's degree program. Dr. Hinz is a consultant to the St. Helena Hospital Center for Health in St. Helena, California where she teaches classes and provides art therapy and psychological services for residents in addiction recovery and lifestyle management programs.

Chapter 5

MULTIFAMILY GROUP ART THERAPY FOR ADOLESCENT SUBSTANCE ABUSE: TIME FOR CREATIVE REPAIR AND RELIEF IN FAMILY RELATIONSHIPS AND ADOLESCENT SELF CARE

SHELLEY A. PERKOULIDIS

S ome 200 million people, or 5 percent of the global population age 15–64, have used illicit drugs at least once in the last 12 months (United Nations, 2006). It is irrefutable that drug and alcohol addiction and abuse costs governments and communities across the world greatly, across families, relationships, productivity, mental health, education, justice system, well-being, and lives each and every day, with adolescents being positioned at a particularly high risk. They are in a position to be helped to break free from this cycle of potential addiction and loss in their futures in a timely manner, with benefits to current and future relationships and maximizing of individual potential.

Family, individual, and group therapy are each utilized extensively in the non-pharmacological treatment of adolescent substance abuse and addiction, and each have been shown in the literature to achieve results within the population (Todd & Selekman, 1991). However, increasing numbers of adolescent substance-related difficulties are presenting at schools, mental health clinics, youth shelters, hospitals, and support services. It is therefore timely and important that we begin to look thoroughly and creatively at what can be done, not only for adolescents, but for their families, during these difficult times to maximize safety and successful outcomes, and utilize learning through research to enhance results for families seeking help in community settings (Robbins, Bachrach & Szapocznik, 2002).

Who is the Adolescent and Family Struggling Most with Substance Misuse and Addiction?

Writing this paper in Australia, I looked to gain a local understanding of an adolescent in Australia at this point in time. In doing so, and learning about what we could offer young people struggling with substance misuse and addiction, I began to think about the adolescents across the world and how my learning and ideas may benefit those within and also outside of the country I work in. As I was exploring a potential way to describe the Australian adolescent or the Australian family attempting to deal with substance misuse and addiction, I realized I could be describing any family in Australia, and indeed around the world. I found no simple way to demographically describe the Australian adolescent or the Australian family that is dealing with substance abuse and addiction. The issue is affecting all types of families and all types of adolescents due to increasing availability, affordability, socialization of drug and alcohol use across community, and celebrity, amongst many other issues (Brunette, Mueser & Drake, 2004).

What Have We Offered Adolescents and Families Dealing with Adolescent Substance Abuse?

In understanding the diverse nature of the population, it became clear that adolescents and their families could benefit from accessible services and flexible programs with a mix of helpful information and individualized work on goals and concrete outcomes. Previous literature also highlights that adolescents and families can potentially benefit from motivational support and drug education; from physical and emotional safety from self/others and dangerous substances; from developmentally appropriate interventions; and from interventions that strongly involve supports and families (Brunette, Mueser & Drake, 2004; Carr, 2000). Liaison and regular communication between services and support people to the benefit of consumers is also important. Intervention programs that reduce and alleviate developmentally appropriate defenses of adolescents, allowing individual processing to occur and the opportunity to work on both what is being thought and felt, but also on what is being done and can be seen within families (e.g., relationship patterns, communication styles, support) are also potentially beneficial in addressing symptoms along with pattern of underlying issues and maladaptive meeting of needs (Carr, 2000; Landgarten, 1987).

With the population demographics being diverse and also clinically dissimilar at times in presentation, currently services are reflecting upon this in real time and attempting to meet demand by offering multiple treatment options or mixing options without empirical consideration, in the hope that less is not more with this population. Consequently, options have often included mixes of individual therapy, family therapy, short and long-term detoxification, rehabilitation, group therapy, peer support, recreational therapies, alternative therapies, harm reduction versus abstinence models, or substance use education, and motivational interviewing techniques (Brunette, Mueser & Drake, 2004; Micucci, 1998; Robbins, Liddle, Turner, Dakof, Alexander, & Kogan, 2006; Weiss, Jeaffee, deMenil, & Cogley, 2004).

Within this complexity inside treatment options, it becomes apparent that knowing what to do or where to go could be overwhelming into itself for families and adolescents, let alone being able to attempt to engage with a service and work through a treatment plan. We as clinicians need to be mindful of this therapeutic minefield we are potentially setting for adolescents and their families if we are to help them access services, use the interventions available well, and prevent further harm from substances. So how do we know what is the most appropriate way of assisting adolescents and their families? We need to step back and closely look at what we already know about what works in this problem area and then examine what the contemporary population knows about their experience and their needs at this point in time.

The Current Therapy Outcomes Landscape
for Adolescents and Their Families

Literature differs in its conclusions regarding the benefits of different therapy modalities (Hogue, Dauber, Stambaugh, Cecero, & Liddle, 2006). Researchers and clinicians have been looking at differentiation factors between interventions in an effort to understand further if and how multiple interventions can produce outcomes for this population; however, are finding continued difficulties in highlighting aspects that continually predict good outcomes (Brunette, Mueser & Drake, 2004; Liddle, Dakof, Turner, Alexander, 2006; Hogue, Liddle, Rowe, Dakof, & Lepann, 1998). Recent research has shown that family therapy is potentially more beneficial in reducing drug-using behaviors over shorter periods of intervention time than CBT or group therapy; however, combinations of family therapy and individual therapy for the adolescent also produce comparable outcomes over long follow-up time (Waldron, Slesnick, Brody, Turner, & Peterson, 2001). Research has also found group and family therapy to be beneficial in treatment for adolescent substance abuse and family therapy to be superior at creating multiple therapeutic alliances across families, more so than individual therapy, and these alliances being beneficial in relation to desired outcomes (Hogue, Dauber, Stambaugh, Cecero & Liddle, 2006; Robbins, Liddle, Turner, Dakof, Alexander & Kogan, 2006).

Whilst evidence bases for practice are telling us that family therapy brings about changes in communication, reduction in adolescent drug use, increases in proactive and pro-social behaviors and also predicts long-term change when therapeutic alliances are strong (Hogue, Dauber, Stambaugh, Cecero & Liddle, 2006; Robbins, Liddle, Turner, Dakof, Alexander & Kogan, 2006), making a move from individual therapy to family therapy in community clinics is a dramatic move for service providers. Adolescent substance abuse has long been treated with a sufferer-focused individualized or peer-based group model, not a systemic one, and one could argue that the two therapeutic orientations and philosophies potentially are not compatible (Bamberg, Findley, & Toumbourou, 2006; Toumbourou, Blyth, Bamberg, Bowes & Douvos, 1997).

Therefore, it is imperative that we carefully consider the potential implications for adolescents, families, and service providers when considering these changes, particularly when we are also aware that families dealing with substance abuse can also be significantly fragile and victims of shame, stigma, and potentially blamed by others for the substance use issues within their family system (Corrigan, Miller & Watson, 2006). This shame and stigma could make it difficult for families to access services, particularly those frequently made more accessible and attractive to adolescents, not adults and subsequently impact upon the forming of the therapeutic alliance and treatment retention. Addressing potential shame, blame, and stigma could be of benefit if addressed within treatment planning (Corrigan, Miller & Watson, 2006; Hogue, Dauber, Stambaugh, Cecero & Liddle, 2006).

However, despite these potential limitations, there is literature showing that more people enter into family therapy than other therapies in this population at this time, also engage better and for longer periods, and achieve sound reductions in problematic behaviors than other therapies, making it non-discountable in treatment planning and best practice (Hogue, Dauber, Stambaugh, Cecero, Liddle, 2006; Robbins, Liddle, Turner, Dakof, Alexander, & Kogan, 2006; Slesnick & Prestopnik, 2005). Therefore, if clinicians can carefully consider how to make family therapy accessible, non-threatening, and practical to different members of families, community agencies could potentially bring family therapy successfully into their current peer group models and individual therapy models, making the most of current research to their client's benefit and potentially improving the longevity of change (Corrigan, Miller & Watson, 2006; Hogue, Dauber, Stambaugh, Cecero & Liddle, 2006). These changes are being indicated by research, but we must be mindful of client need as well. Whilst I may be convinced from my research and practice of the benefits of systemic intervention in this problem area, as a clinician I value the learning that can be gained from research of others. Being a practitioner teaches me that we need to value the client's perceptions and needs too, in the here and now, to ensure therapeutic ideas are going to be compatible with what our client is looking for and what our client is going to feel that will be helpful for them.

What do the Consumers Say?

Most adolescents report using substances because it is fun (Blume, 1993; Cox & Price, 1990). Longer-term use often leads from fun to escaping from issues and pressures and it is within this change that substance use often becomes problematic, addictive, and more risky (Corrigan, Miller & Watson, 2006). Understanding reasons for use is important in maximizing potential for change and in assessment of presentation, need, and subsequent treatment planning (Hogue, Dauber, Stambaugh, Cecero, & Liddle, 2006; Robbins, Liddle, Turner, Dakof, Alexander, & Kogan, 2006). Adolescents also report liking programs that are informative, creative, individualized, helpful, and practical, and build confidence (Brunette, Mueser, & Drake, 2004; Cox & Price, 1990).

Practitioners report enjoying client-driven and empowering work with adolescents and with families and comment that this appears to assist in reducing dropout rates for adolescents and families (Corrigan, Miller & Watson, 2006; Klorer, 1992; Robbins, Liddle, Turner, Dakof, Alexander, & Kogan, 2006; Riley, 2001; Rubin, 2001). But some services and treatment plans often exclude families; aligning and building alliance with only young people and this has been shown to be non-beneficial to long-term goals, treatment retention, outcomes, and developmental needs/phase resolution for adolescents (Diamond & Liddle, 1999). Families report liking to be aware of what is happening for their adolescent, and being involved and informed of what they can do to help out, particularly as many family members can feel helpless, hopeless, and cut-off from others (Robbins, Bachrach, & Szapocznik, 2002).

Where do We Go from Here?

At this point in the review of the literature, it becomes apparent that the history of substance abuse treatment within peer group models and sufferer-focused interventions should not be discounted in its historical importance and significant outcomes for clients of services around the world to date. What is also equally apparent, however, is that these outcomes, and new outcomes in the way of indicators of longer treatment retention and wider reaching change, are being clearly shown to be evident from family therapy with adolescents and significant others in this field. Whilst these two models of intervention have been proposed by some within the literature to be mismatched, it seemed to me that a potential and non-confronting link was also in existence in the literature and this appeared to be extremely relevant to treatment both historically and in more recent times, but lacking in evidence base and systematic review. This link was the utilization of art therapy.

Art Therapy in Family Treatment for Adolescent Substance Abuse: Time for Creative Relationship Building

What makes art therapy different from more traditional approaches is that it can provide more flexibility within the therapeutic relationship. Although the goals may be quite similar, an individual art experience becomes less threatening than a more traditional psychotherapy session. Much of the 'art' of art therapy can also be viewed as the sensitivity with which the therapist guides the person towards self-revelation through the interpretation of fantasy productions. (Wolf, 1975, p. 266)

As explained by Wolf (1975), over 30 years ago, the real "art" of art therapy can be found within the successful utilization of flexibility and insight through creative and fantasy projections and ideals. These are qualities in therapy which are much needed in treatment for families presenting with adolescent substance abuse, as illustrated by literature pointing to the importance of the flexible and changing therapeutic relationships between the therapist and members of the family during therapy and relaxed approaches to goals and symptoms (Hogue, Dauber, Stambaugh, Cecero, & Liddle, 2006; Robbins, Liddle, Turner, Dakof, Alexander, & Kogan, 2006), potentially making art therapy a valid addition to family therapy in this field.

Historically, art therapy has long been utilized in the field of treatment for substance abuse, and found to be helpful in processing incidents of substance use; enhancing motivation; drawing attention to maladaptive behavior patterns; expressing trauma and processing traumatic events; and easing through developmentally appropriate defenses and communication styles not overly adaptive to change or introspection (Atlas, Smith & Sessoms, 1992; Cox & Price, 1990; Landgarten, 1987; Riley, 2001; Rubin, 2001). Art in combination with outdoor activity and song writing are also being shown in the literature to be interesting to the population and assisting in engagement and enhancing outcomes and processing of previous trauma and future planning (Atlas, Smith & Sessoms, 1992; Blume, 1993; Flynn & Stirtzinger, 2001; Klorer, 1992).

At this point in time, art therapy is frequently a part of treatment for adolescent substance abuse; however, it is utilized predominately only with adolescents in individual therapy, and in group therapy with adolescents and their peers (Cox & Price, 1990; Landgarten, 1987; Riley, 2001; Rubin, 2001). Family art therapy does not appear within the literature as a dominant approach to family therapy with this population, but potentially offers a highly adaptive resolution to difficulties in the field which are being shown in the literature to hinder outcomes for this work. At the time of writing, the family art therapy literature was pointing to benefits in the areas of enhancing communication and collaborative goal building, limiting opportunity for aggressive communication within therapy sessions, and allowing families to increase understanding of overt and covert communications and actions, moving subtly through family changes and stages relevant to growth, and longevity of the family system (Landgarten, 1987; Riley, 2001; Rubin, 2001). The apparent opportunity for family members to learn to tolerate the company of each other within a different environment and activity also allows for opportunity for consideration, collaboration, and change (Rubin, 2001).

These benefits, if coupled with those found in parent groups and individual and group adolescent therapy, could also potentially be further enhanced. If clinicians could also develop therapy which would mix these benefits in a way that could also attempt to address factors such as shame, isolation, and hopelessness, which have been shown to impede therapy within this population (Corrigan, Miller & Watson, 2006; Klorer, 1992; Robbins, Liddle, Turner, Dakof, Alexander & Kogan, 2006), outcomes could again be enhanced or therapy made available to a greater number of families in a time and cost-effective manner.

Overall, review of the literature highlights that this population can find therapy a difficult activity and process to engage and remain in. This difficulty coupled with sound results across some therapy modalities, illustrates a need to make therapy as accessible as practical. There is great potential in the linking the positive outcomes of group therapy and family therapy within this population, and in beginning to maximize and also empirically clarify the potential benefits of art therapy within the population. It is the author's opinion that further clinical research is needed in the area of art therapy with families dealing with adolescent substance abuse, and also that in light of the experiential findings in existence currently; there is validity in exploring the potential of linking art, group, and family therapy in this field with multifamily group art therapy.

Multifamily Group Art Therapy for Adolescent Substance Abuse

Researcher and practitioners first began exploring the use of multi-family group therapy in mental health settings in the 1960s and 1970s with some successful outcomes for clients and their families (e.g., Laqueur, 1976; Laqueur, LaBurt & Morong, 1964). In the last decade, there has again been research and practice interest in this form of therapy, and this modality of treatment has been again producing reported benefits for clients and interest from researchers across various areas of mental health (e.g., Asen, 2002; Asen & Schuff, 2006; Lemmens, Eisler, Migerode, Heireman & Demytenaere, 2007) and most recently, in New Zealand in a substance misuse treatment setting (Schafer, 2008). It appears that short-term multifamily group programs may be a way to allow families to access therapy in a way that is not as isolating or anxiety-provoking as individual family therapy can be. This type of intervention also potentially captures the benefits previously shown of parent support groups and education groups, of family therapy and of peer-based adolescent group therapy too (Joanning, Thomas, Quinn, & Mullen, 1992; Todd & Selekman, 1991; Weiss, Jaffee & deMenil, Cogley, 2004).

The potential for linking families with other families, reducing shame effects, and also accessing peer links for adolescents in an environment that potentially is lessening negative impacts of cultural acceptance of substance use than that within peer-only groups is all evident within such a model as multifamily group therapy. To then add the medium of art therapy could also create opportunity for enrichment in family system understanding and change and opportunity to clarify and learn more previous research outcomes highlighting the benefits of art therapy for individuals and families in this population. The playfulness of art-making is also likely to be an adolescent friendly way of communicating, but deep exploration of metaphor, change, developmental need, and systemic factors can be addressed readily if families are supported by appropriately trained professionals, equipped with understanding of the group process and expectations, and available and willing (Landgerten, 1987; Makin, 2000; Riley, 2001; Rubin, 2001). The potential themes and considerations for a multifamily art therapy intervention could include the following:

- *Non-directive art therapy:* Exploring themes, events, and processes within families and across families with tangible art making representing their struggles with substance misuse.
- *Family roles and developmental change:* Art-making such as sculpturing and collage of family roles and household structure, used to capture family dynamics and roles and facilitate changes within families necessary in progressing successfully through adolescence.
- *Peer awareness and social skill building:* Art-making exploring parental and older sibling collective wisdom and new ideas from adolescents in relation to building supportive peer relationships, fostering safe independence from family, and ways to maintain helpful family communication and support between adolescents and their parents.
- *Use of family and adolescent appropriate art media within groups:* The use of

uncomplicated and limited (not too many choices of) media has been shown to be helpful with families and adolescents, as has the use of technology informed therapy (computer art, digital collage, email art, and communication).

- *Substance education and harm reduction education:* Use of art-making to explore impacts of substances on body systems via completion of body outlines and health matters (strengths and difficulties) identified via drawing on tangible body drawings with education and re-mapping of health bodies or goals for changes in health.
- *Support for positive behavioral interventions and debriefing in a multifamily context:* Use of art-making and role-playing in exploration of behavioral interventions and safety plans, with collective debriefing and shared ideas regarding the often ongoing battle to maintain safety and change maladaptive behavioral patterns in family interactions.

Conclusions and Considerations

Services and individual practitioners are continuing to explore effective treatment options in relation to client need in the area of substance misuse. Government is also continuing to build on knowledge of drug use and problematic behaviors and establish programs for preventative education and family communication. Group therapy and family therapy could be explored further in the substance use treatment literature, particularly the area of multifamily group art therapy. Art therapy, the benefits of which can be extended via individual, group or family therapy settings, offers unique opportunity for adolescents and their families to learn about themselves and their relationships, to improve communication through alternative means, break down defensive barriers and improve listening to others needs via tangible expression of want and need. It is hoped that through this medium of art-making, new opportunities can be gained outside the therapy room for adolescent and family understanding, resilience, and healthy development and well-being and with this, increased clinical research will be produced which will allow more practitioners to then extend the benefits of art therapy to their clients as a clear, empirically proven and undeniable part of the their models of best practice.

References

Asen, E. (2002). Multiple family therapy: An overview. *Journal of Family Therapy, 24,* 3–16.

Asen, E., & Schuff, H. (2006). Psychosis and multiple family group therapy. *Journal of Family Therapy, 28,* 58–72.

Atlas. J. A, Smith, P., & Sessoms, L. (1992). Art and poetry in brief therapy of hospitalized adolescents. *The Arts in Psychotherapy, 19,* 279–283.

Bamberg, J., Findley, S., & Toumbourou, J. (2006). The BEST Plus approach to assisting families recover from youth substance problems. *Youth Studies Australia, 25*(2), 25–32.

Blume, T. W. (1993). Social role negotiation skills for substance abusing adolescents: A group model. *Journal of Substance Abuse Treatment, 11*(3), 197–204.

Brunette, M. F., Mueser, K. T., & Drake, R. E. (2004). A review of research on residential programs for people with severe mental illness and co-occuring substance use disorders. *Drug & Alcohol Review, 23*, 471–481.

Carr, A. (2000). *Family therapy: Concepts, process and practice.* London: Wiley.

Corrigan, P. W., Miller, F. E., & Watson, A. S. (2006). Blame, shame, and contamination: The impact of mental illness and drug dependence on family members. *Journal of Family Psychology, 20*(2), 239–246.

Cox, K. L., & Price, K. (1990). Breaking through: Incident drawings with adolescent substance abusers. *The Arts in Psychotherapy, 17*, 333–337.

Diamond, G. S., & Liddle, H. A. (1999). Transforming negative parent-adolescent interactions: From Impasse to dialogue. *Family Process, 38*(1), 1999.

Flynn, C., & Stirtzinger, R. (2001). Understanding a regressed adolescent boy through story writing and Winnicott's intermediate area. *The Arts in Psychotherapy, 28*, 299–309

Hogue, A., Dauber, S., Stambaugh, L. F., Cecero, J. J., & Liddle, H. A. (2006). Early therapeutic alliance and treatment outcome in individual and family therapy for adolescent behaviour problems. *Journal of Consulting & Clinical Psychology, 74*(1), 121–129.

Hogue, A., Liddle, H. A., Rowe, C., Turner, R. M., Dakof, G. A., & LePann, K. (1998). Treatment adherence and differentiation in individual versus family therapy for adolescent substance abuse. *Journal of Counselling Psychology, 45*(1), 104–114.

Joanning, H., Thomas, F., Quinn, W., & Mullen, R. (1992). Treating adolescent drug abuse: A comparision of family systems therapy, group therapy, and family drug education. *Journal of Marital and Family Therapy, 18*(4), 345–356.

Klorer, G. P. (1992). Leaping beyond traditional boundaries: Art therapy and a wilderness stress challenge program for adolescents. *The Arts in Psychotherapy, 19*, 285–287.

Landgarten, H. B. (1987). *Family art psychotherapy: A clinical guide and casebook.* Brunner/Mazel: New York.

Laqueur, H. P. (1976). Multiple family therapy. In P. Guerin (Ed.). *Family therapy: Theory and practice* (pp. 405–416). New York: Gardner Press.

Laqueur, H. P., LaBurt, H. A., & Morong, E. (1964). Multiple family therapy: Further developments. *International Journal of Social Psychiatry, 10*, 69–80.

Lemmens, G., Eisler, I., Migerode, L., Heireman, M., & Demytenaere, K. (2007). Family discussion group therapy for major depression: A brief systemic multifamily group intervention for hoptalized patients and their family members. *Journal of Family Therapy, 29*, 49–68.

Makin, S. R. (2000). *Therapeutic art directives and resources: Activities and initiatives for individuals and groups.* London: Jessica Kingsley.

Micucci, J. A. (1998). *The adolescent in family therapy: Breaking the cycle of conflict and control.* New York: The Guilford Press.

Riley, S. (2001). *Group process made visible: Group art therapy.* London: Brunner-Routledge.

Robbins, M. S., Bachrach, K., & Szapocznik, J. (2002). Bridging the research-practice gap in adolescent substance abuse treatment: The case of brief strategic family therapy. *Journal of Substance Abuse Treatment, 23*, 123–132.

Robbins, M. S., Liddle, H. A., Turner, C., Dakof, G. A., Alexander, J. F., & Kogan, S. M. (2006). Adolescent and parent therapeutic alliances as predictors of dropout in multidimensional family therapy. *Journal of Family Psychology, 20*(1), 108–116.

Rubin, J. R. (2001). *Approaches to art therapy: Theory and technique* (2nd ed). London: Brunner-

Routledge.

Schafer, G. (2008). Multiple family group therapy in a drug and alcohol rehabilitation centre. *Australian and New Zealand Journal of Family Therapy, 29*(1), 17–24.

Slesnick, N., & Prestopnik, J. L. (2005). Ecologically based family therapy outcome with substance abusing runaway adolescents. *Journal of Adolescence, 28,* 277–298.

Toumbourou, J. W., Blyth, A., Bamberg, J., Bowes, G., & Douvos, T. (1997). Behaviour exchange systems training: The 'BEST' approach for parents stressed by adolescent drug problems. *Australian and New Zealand Journal of Family Therapy, 18*(2), 92–98.

Todd, T. C., & Selekman, M. D. (1991). *Family therapy approaches with adolescent substance abusers.* London: Allyn & Bacon.

United Nations. (2006). *World drug report 2006.* United Nations Publications: New York/Geneva.

Waldron, H. B., Slesnick, N., Brody, J. L., Turner, C. W., & Peterson, T. R. (2001). Treatment outcomes for adolescent substance abuse at 4 and 7-month assessments. *Journal of Consulting and Clinical Psychology, 69*(5), 802–813.

Weiss, R. D., Jeaffee, W. B., de Menil, V. P., & Cogley, C. B. (2004). Group therapy for substance use disorders: What do we know? *Harvard Review of Psychiatry, 12*(6), 339–350.

Wolf, R. (1975). Art psychotherapy with acting out adolescents: An innovative approach to special education. *Art Psychotherapy, 2,* 255–266.

Biography

Shelley A. Perkoulidis is an Art Therapist and a Registered Psychologist in Australia. She holds a B.Sc (Psych); P.Grad Dip (Psych); MA (Couns Psych) and MMH (Art Therapy) and is a Member of the Australian Psychological Society (MAPS). Shelley specializes in parent-infant, child, adolescent and family therapy, with particular interest in the use of art therapy and play therapy within evidence-informed practice. She is currently employed within Queensland Government Child and Youth Mental Health Services on the Sunshine Coast in Queensland, Australia and is a private practitioner in Noosa, Queensland, Australia, providing child, adolescent, individual and family therapy and also supervision and training for professionals. Shelley can be contacted via email: shelley.perkoulidis@gmail.com

Chapter 6

COMIC ADDICT: A QUALITATIVE STUDY OF THE BENEFITS OF ADDRESSING AMBIVALENCE THROUGH COMIC/CARTOON DRAWING WITH CLIENTS IN IN-PATIENT TREATMENT FOR CHEMICAL DEPENDENCY

Katherine M. Fernandez

This chapter describes a heuristic process of comic drawing that was used to express and address ambivalence in adult clients within an inpatient treatment facility that have experienced varying severities of chemical dependency. Using case examples, I will present the potential benefits of comic drawing seen in male and female art therapy groups, as well as differentiate forms of comic expression between genders. I will suggest possible and further uses of the comic drawing method and future research questions. Comic drawing and ambivalence have been understudied in the fields of art therapy and addiction. I will explore the role of humor in the comic drawing process and suggest that comic drawing be used as a vehicle for laughter and joy in the group-sharing session and in family therapy. I will illustrate how the comic creation process can enable self-exploration and self-transformation, increase self-empowerment, and motivate change. I will deconstruct and elaborate on the framework of 12-Step group dynamics and propose that the comic art therapy group be appropriately adapted to address ambivalence. Using examples from the groups, I will discuss the comic art process as a means to distance and regulate the self and self-identity, while the art product acts as a medium for communication and interaction within the group (Vickers, 2004).

For more than half a century, the response to clinical treatment of addiction in the United States has reflected the 12-Step model of Alcoholics

Anonymous (A.A.). The majority of art therapy academic works adopt a fixed adherence to the 12-Step model, a focus on using art-making to confront client denial and an implied sense of absolute transformation once the client admits powerlessness (Horay, 2006). The first step in the twelve steps of Alcoholics Anonymous (2001) is "We admit we are powerless over alcohol and drugs and that our lives have become unmanageable." Denial is seen as a major "roadblock" to recovery and as a precipitous factor in relapse occurrence (Hanes, 2007). Entry into and maintenance of a 12-Step program or residential treatment program revolves strictly around rejection of and breaking through denial. Confrontational art therapies have been used as a way to "break down the client's resistance to substance abuse treatment by storming the ramparts of defense" (Allen, 1985). Cox and Price (1990) suggest that "combining art expression with work centered around issues of unmanageability, being out of control, and powerlessness can foster the admission of alcoholism/drug treatment." Self-portraiture may represent the individual's need to face up to something that is hard to accept (Dalley, Rifkind & Terry, 1993). Hanes (2007) agreed that a spontaneous frontal self-portrait reflects the individual's effort to come face-to-face with his or her addictive nature.

According to the A.A. model, denial is the ultimate self-deception that underlies all of the alcoholic's problems. But "denial" in chemical dependency treatment has become interconnected with the term "honesty." Honesty to self and others has been the preferred and promoted mechanism for removing denial and the key to beginning to eliminate one's problems. The first step to accepting powerlessness is to identify as an alcoholic and to introduce oneself to the group. Kurtz (1982) posits that acceptance of powerlessness through the admission and identification as "an alcoholic" and the ability to identify oneself by one's limitations is the acceptance of personal fundamental finitude. William Barrett (1958) philosophically explains *finitude* as the presence of the *not* in the very being of any individual human, the limitations of what we *cannot be* or *cannot do*. For the client who has experienced chemical dependence, this is the realization that continuing to use substances will likely end his/her life—the acute acceptance of being an alcoholic/addict that *cannot* drink/use, of *not being* recovered if one *can* drink/use. However, finitude is not the sum of human limitations but rather, the core of human *being*, where positive and negative existences interpenetrate. Barrett postulates that human strength coincides with human pathos, human vision with human blindness, human happiness with human suffering, and human truth with human untruth (Barrett, 1958; Kurtz, 1983).

While the philosophical concept of *finitude* underscores the interpenetration of positive and negative elements of human existence, the standard therapeutic modalities of recovery treatment can fail to adequately acknowledge that interpenetration. Many have agreed that the client's ambivalent attitude toward giving up their substance of choice makes it difficult to work with them (Waller & Mahoney, 1999). In fact, therapeutic treatment policies have been constructed to refuse service to "active addicts." The problem with equating confrontation of denial with an acceptance of addiction that results in the clarity, serenity, and sanctity of recovery–a road out of delusion–is that this ideology in itself *is* the ultimate delusion. With the goal of absolute transformation as the potential treatment outcome, it becomes the therapist's responsibility to "do something (Waller & Mahony, 1999), inspire insight, transformation, alleviate symptoms, and offer solutions." Improving target symptoms can be a result of effective treatment, but therapy that has positive consequences for a wide range of life problems beyond the target problems is relapse prevention. As one recovering alcoholic with ten years of sobriety so eloquently stated, "giving up the bottle was the first release of suffering, but life is a series of unending releases–the first release, rehab, was the easiest."

Confronting denial of addiction (negative) does not, in practice, always generate sobriety (positive) in the recovering addict. Acceptance and honesty are not mutually inclusive. It is possible and quite common that one might honestly accept their addiction and continue to use despite that awareness or even because of it. Does acceptance/realization always mean the ability to change one's behavior? Ambivalence, defined as feeling uncertain or having fluctuating feelings caused by inability to make a choice or by a simultaneous desire to say or do two opposite or conflicting things, lies at the root of personal fundamental finitude. Lipkus et al. (2005) suggests that ambivalence may serve as a strong cue that a person is reconsidering the decision to use alcohol or drugs. The opposing positive and negative beliefs and feelings are experienced as conflict management strategies (Weber, Baron & Loomes, 2003). The difficult issues of shame, guilt, and loss when examined tend to reinforce ambivalence to change. Ignoring or minimizing ambivalence precludes admission of limitations and powerlessness. Denying ambivalence forestalls the acceptance of guilt, shame, and loss that underlies addiction, denial of addiction, and the difficulty of recovery.

According to Prochaska and Norcross (2001), only a small percentage of clients that enter treatment remain sober. The Trans Theoretical Model (TTM), developed by Prochaska and DiClemente (1984), suggests that 80 percent of clients in treatment settings are either in precontemplation or contemplation stages of change (Horay, 2006). It has been shown that clients in precontemplation stages will manifest higher rates of drop-out (Callaghan et al., 2005). The Trans Theoretical Model suggests that ambivalence naturally occurs as people progress from inaction or precontemplation to the engagement of any change-related behaviors. Getting stuck in ambivalence or approach-avoidance conflicts are difficult to resolve on one's own. Clinical styles that acknowledge and induce feelings of ambivalence may be useful in developing motivation to change (Callaghan et al., 2005; Lipkus et al., 2005). Motivational Interviewing (MI), *a client-centered, directive method for enhancing intrinsic motivation to change by exploring and resolving ambivalence,* developed by Miller and Rollnick (2002) is one of the most contemporary approaches to enhancing clients' motivation to change. Miller and Rollnick state that motivation is in many ways an interpersonal process influenced by interaction with other people. The principles of MI, expressing empathy, developing discrepancy, and rolling with resistance (Miller & Rollnick, 2002) have been effective in the addiction treatment domain. Developing discrepancy most accurately describes the process of dealing with ambivalence. Discrepancy is what underlies the perceived importance of change. The difference between two perceptions and the degree of discrepancy determines the importance for change. The proposed method of comic drawing emphasizes that induction and examination of ambivalence is a useful construct from which to explore the desire to stop drug use and difficult emotions that continue even after gainful sobriety. This form of art therapy is based on the stages of change and motivational interviewing models of addiction treatment, which have had significant impact on social functioning, suggesting that the comic drawing process has positive consequences for a wide range of life problems beyond target problems.

The Use of Comic Drawing in Group Therapy

Since the establishment of the 12-Step group movement in the 1930s, addiction specialists have embraced it as an effective treatment modality (Flores, 2004). Group addiction therapy is synonymous with the 12-Step method of recovery. Art therapists have also embraced this movement in theory and practice. There is a paucity of professional art therapy literature in the United States that approaches drug and alcohol treatment without reliance on the AA model. Wadeson (2000) offered a selection of current views within the field in her book *Art Therapy Practice.* Foss (as cited in Wadeson, 2000) emphasized the "here and now" art-making process through clay sculpture with the goal of emotional release, sense of accomplishment, and the opportunity to work successfully through frustration. Wolff's master's thesis describes the use of "addiction monsters" to confront denial of substance abuse (as cited in Wadeson, 2000). Importantly, she acknowledged that the images created symbolized the continuous attraction the client has for drugs rather than the unambiguous images of personal transformation. Albert-Puleo (as cited in Wadeson, 2000) advocated for the encouragement of client resistance to strengthen it. He argues that the root of substance abuse is a learned narcissistic withdrawal defending against anger and unpleasant feelings. The process of addressing ambivalence through comic drawing is appropriate for group art therapy. It offers the client the opportunity to independently create and control the art object, the self-image, as well as regulate the release and presentation of the self-image to the group.

However, the dynamics of the group play a critical role in the expression of ambivalent thought and emotion. It is important to note that even within American addiction treatment programs or therapies that offer other primary modalities of treatment, the 12-Step model and dynamics may manifest in the group therapy because of its prominent cultural presence. Also, the art object can become infused with the influences of involvement in A.A. It is crucial that we understand the dynamics of the A.A. group, its implication and possible adaptations for a successful art therapy group that addresses ambivalence.

I propose that an understanding of Kurtz's (1983) dependence-independence explanation of the leaderless organization of A.A. fellowship is a paradox that reflects Barrett's (1958) concept of personal fundamental finitude and can be accentuated to promote ambivalent expression. Additionally, the corrective language of A.A. can be examined and acknowledged within the group in an effort to promote ambivalent language in the comic-making process. Finally, the intrinsic Higher Power dilemma of A.A. can be used to explain the use of a comic character to explore ambivalent identity and motivation. These adaptations can help to combat the barriers to expressing ambivalence within the art therapy group.

Dependence/Independence Paradox. Alcoholics Anonymous has been one of the most effective self-help groups for addiction and has expanded to include many specialized addiction groups (i.e., gambling, overeating, sex, spending, narcotics). The reciprocity of dependence and independence is the central focus of the A.A. group. Human dependence and human independence are mutually related, not only between people but within people (Kurtz, 1983). The group enables and fulfills each member. The group also antagonizes and exacerbates the social inadequacies of the addict. The interpenetration of dependence and independence is the irony of *all* human existence (Kurtz, 1983). For example, the periodic need for dependence reoccurs intertwined with the need for independence, breathing, eating, and sleeping. Dependence is a way of asserting independence; one can be truly dependant only when exercising real dependence (Kurtz, 1982). Independence is a way of reinforcing dependence; one can only be truly independent when acknowledging dependence. This is exemplified by the leaderless structure of A.A. groups.* A.A. groups that are built around the concept of "fellow-

---

*The leaderless group was replicated in the comic art sessions. The facilitator is a recovering alcoholic and created the comic drawing as a tool for her own recovery. A therapist with personal experience with addiction may be able to use their experience to simulate a leaderless group.

ship"–The Society of Alcoholics Anonymous–reflects the need for the understanding of we (interdependence and dependence) and the alcoholic's need to think of one's self as a part of society. Winship (1999) suggests that addiction is a social problem in which the interpersonal field of relationships underpins the cause of addiction. Individuals must learn to rely on the group as a whole: ninety meetings in ninety days is often the prescription to the new member given by the group. It is the responsibility of the alcoholic to carry the message to other alcoholics. Freud (1922) wrote about groups with leaders and without leaders. In place of the leader is an "idea" or "abstraction."

Ambivalent Expression. In A.A., the substitute leader is the 12 steps and traditions. Inclusion in the group is the purported primary message: "The only requirement for drinking is an *honest desire* to stop drinking" (Alcoholics Anonymous, 2001). It is important to note that an honest desire is marked by ambivalent expression and vocabulary rather than direct action. The corrective language and confrontation of A.A. vernacular (i.e., keep it simple) is conducive for combating denial but not for supporting ambivalence, promoting discrepancy, or developing motivation to change. A.A.'s treatment involves the systematic manipulation of an individual's life to provide a new vision of that life and of the world. The purpose of the vision is to provide new coherence, meaning, and implications for behavior. The alcoholic must discover a new past to confirm what must ultimately be a self-diagnosis. Confrontation, critique, and question of ambivalent thinking and expression within the group that encourages and addresses ambivalence must be reserved.

> *We had to find a power by which we could live, and it had to be a Power greater than ourselves.* (Alcoholics Anonymous, 2001)

This statement grows out of the promotion of spiritual reconstruction and group confession, the product of The Oxford Movement developed by Frank Buchman, a Lutheran minister (Weegmann, 2004). The religiosity of the Oxford groups presented obstacles to attracting and retaining alcoholics. There are well-researched ideas on the spiritual dimension of A.A., among them the spiritual/existential ideas of Carl Jung, for whom alcoholism was a "spiritual disease." The ideology of A.A. as influenced by Dr. William Silkworth, includes medical categorization of alcoholism, describing the illness as a disease of the mind and an allergy of the body (Weegmann, 2004). However, substance abuse is prevalently co-morbid, making it difficult to comprehend that a heterogeneous group is afflicted with one disease.

The Higher Power Dilemma. The secular terminology of A.A. came to include "Higher Power or Power greater than ourselves." The first steps of sobriety do not require classic belief in a traditional "God" but does require that the alcoholic accept his powerlessness, what Kurtz (1979) terms his "not God-ness." The A.A. group is clearly such a "Higher Power." The alcoholic/addict is expected to surrender his narcissistic belief of control over people, places, and things to the Powerful Whole of the group. But what would be the result if this rather than surrendering absolute control, this control were transferred to the creation of realistic self-image? Historically, it has been the concept of divinity, the notion of the deity that includes the idea of absolute control. If narcissism is at the root of obsessive-compulsive substance abuse it seems necessary to invoke the avatar as a method for identity control, reformation, and eventual transformation. The comic character can be used in this way.

The word avatar is Sanskrit for the passing down or over to describe the descent of a deity to the earth. The avatar in cartoon form, is the embodiment of a collection of attitudes, beliefs, principles, and views of life. When personified, the "attitude, principle, view" has a higher power of controlling the self-image and a higher power for passing down or letting go. This process has the ability to empower change. The encoding of symbols to form a character mirrors the internal self-concept (Hatfield, 2005). This collection makes visual the prerequisites self-contemplation and self-consciousness. It is important to remember that such a simplified portrait, a caricature, does not constitute a literal representation. It is crucial for the therapist to recognize that the chemically dependent individual can have various levels of insight and readiness to alter world views or sense of self (George, 1990; Stevens-Smith & Smith, 1998). Whether discrepancies are explored and developed has to do with incongruities among aspects of the person's own experiences and values (Miller & Rollnick, 2002). "Self-portraiture gives us access to an intimate situation in which we see the artist at close quarters from a privileged position in the place of the artist himself and through his own eyes" (Kinneir, 1980, p.15). Therapist flexibility, toleration of uncertainty, silence to generate anxiety-free thoughtfulness, and an ability to refrain from arguing and providing solutions (Miller & Rollnick, 1991), are powerful tools to assist in addressing ambivalence through comic drawing.

Comic Drawing: The Process

Constructing a comic strip is like looking at yourself in water
but then leaving your reflection behind.
Barnaby Richards, comic artist (as cited in Bell & Sinclair, 2005, p. 6)

If ambivalence is the result of identifying with opposing positive and negative beliefs and feelings trapped in cyclical indecision, autobiographical comic drawing is a release of self-expression through exploration and transformation of self-identity with the power to motivate change. Creating the cartoon self in his/her surrounding cartoon environment forces a raw autobiographical image to weave the internal self-image and external self-expression into the coarse facts of the outer-world. Indeed, the process of becoming a parody of oneself requires having knowledge of how one looks or has looked to others. For the alcoholic/addict this means grappling with how the chemically dependant self "looks" and the impact that impression has made on his/her environment. Further, the alcoholic/addict in early recovery must transform that "look" and "impact" to represent, in pictorial form, how he/she experienced him/herself when using their substance and how they experience themselves in the moment. It is important to note that the cartoon character is an avatar, an embodiment or personification as a principle, attitude, or view of life/addiction and not a representation of the artist as a full person.

In the following paragraphs, I elucidate the ways in which this comic drawing processes brings about insight and facilitates motivation to change. It is with ambivalence that I retell the experiences and "re-draw" the drawings for the reader. Because the cartoon self-representation and self-recognition involves simplification, the highly simplified images invite "viewer involvement and interpretation," (McCloud, 1993, p. 34) what E.H. Gombrich (1972, p. 17) terms the "beholder's share." Gombrich states, "We tend to project life and expression onto the arrested image and supplement from our own experience what is not actually present" (p.17). I have attempted to describe only factual and firsthand information.

The character development drawing session was designed to assist clients in the creation of a cartoon or exaggerated representation of their drinking/using self. It was specifically stated that the character does not need to look like a person. The character may take any conceivable form (e.g., an animal, a shape, a word). The only requirement is that the character should feel like *your character*. Once completed, participants are asked to give their character a name.

The objectification of the self through the creation of the exaggerated self-representation informs an autobiography that warrants control over self-image. Often the self-image becomes a stereotypical self-depiction. For example, one client depicted her character as a "sly fox" trapped on a circular path in a crowded forest of pines. Another client depicted her character as a dull brown mountain range in the middle of a happy pink haze. Others created more literal representations—self-portraits: a man wearing name brand clothes; his North Carolina hat engulfed in red and orange flames; a woman with a black tear falling from her eye and baring her black heart as a disconnected audience watches her perform; an emaciated alien creature with sunken, sullen eyes. Common means of representing the self as an addict/alcoholic were sunken, red, or bloodshot eyes, afflictions to the head (i.e., flames, fumes, swirling forces), disturbed balance (i.e., falling, stumbling), disappointed and disconnected others, ruinous environments or surroundings, animalistic nature (i.e., wild animals, intemperate actions).

After the character development session, clients reported feeling depressed, sad, "It wasn't much fun and caused shame." One client stated that the process was "creepy." Another noted that the process brought up "good memories at first, then horrible memories." Historically, the caricature in comic art is a form of alienation or estrangement, through which the cartoonist, autobiographer regards himself as other, as a distinct character to be seen or heard (Hatfield, 2005). Again, the expression of internal self- image requires being able to see one's self through one's own eyes. As Forrest (1975) stated, "Most alcoholics . . . cannot find the means to be aware of their feelings or of themselves as a complete entity because of the alienation and separation they feel, both from the world and their bodies." However, the process of becoming a parody of one's self facilitates a more detached (stereotypic) view, leaving the client open to experiencing difficult emotions rather than engaging defense mechanisms. The client is not being confronted with their problem but rather exploring and experiencing the ways in which they see themselves, a prerequisite for transformation. The client is able to achieve at once a sense of self-intimacy and critical distance.

In another session participants are asked to create a character for recovery, to have their comic characters interact with recovery, or to transform their original character into a recovered character. Vibrant spaces and object (i.e., flowers, fields, rainbows), smiling, clear-eyed faces, and supportive others were common depictions. For example, one client depicted his recovered client as a large bright flower, another client drew his character running through a field toward a rainbow, and another character was transformed into a wide-eyed girl carrying balloons. A client stated that this session, "made me realize how dumb my 'using' days were, and how bright my future can be."

The cartoon stereotype provides insight into the culture of addiction, as well as the oversimplification and set conceptions of addiction of recovery. These stereotypic selves act as hoped-for selves, the addict in active addiction or the addict in recovery. I propose that the stereotypic portrait/self-image reflects the impetus of ambivalence. At one end of the spectrum there is the depiction of the shameful, isolated, desperate addict, at the other the hope, happiness, and glory of recovery. Moving towards the gray (Horay, 2006) of ambivalence is the goal of the next art therapy session.

Participants are asked to create a scene or comic strip using their character from session one. The drawing is to tell a story about good and bad memories of using. Fantasies of using or invented memories are acceptable references for drawing in this session. Instructions are given to create a second character for the participant's substance of choice and to have the self-referential comic character interact with the substance-using character.

For example, one client remembered having fun playing cards while drinking and drugging with his friends and girlfriend. He described the party and mapped out the apartment in his drawing. During this episode, he remembered grabbing a bottle in anger and blacking out. His character holds a bottle of Old English in one hand and dollar bills fly out of the other hand. His head is surrounded in red and orange flames. His character's mouth is open. A bubble contains the words, "Fuck you guys you are all just using me." He explained to the group that when he "came to" everyone was afraid that the police were coming. The friends that surround his character are

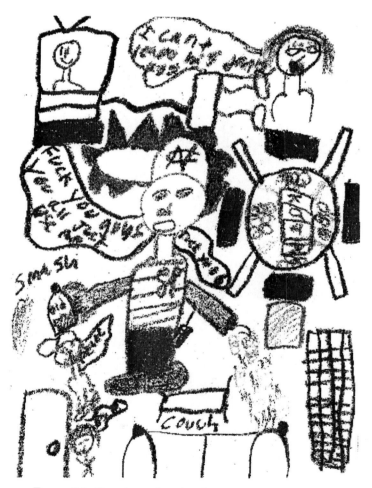

Figure 6.1. Drawing using the character from session 1.

headed for the door, exclaiming, "peace," and "bye," except for one. He told the group that his best friend hid his money during his blackout. He stated that, "she hid my money so no one would steal it, but she took five dollars for cigarettes, but that's okay, I didn't mind." He shared with the group, "I realized that I can be really nice or an asshole when I am drunk or when I am sober." For this participant, the self-referential character from session one became the character for his substance of choice. The drawing session allowed this participant to express ambivalence; the fun of alcohol use versus its cost, being taken advantage of versus being cared for, being the same person whether intoxicated or sober. In exposing his ambivalent feelings, the group offered support for his desire and motivation to change. He later admitted, "I have more control over my anger when I am sober."

Rather than alienating, the self-caricature set in an external (autobiographical) environment, enables the artist to recognize and externalizes his or her subjectivity (Hatfield, 2005), to discover self-understanding and self-transformation. Through the creation of a self-referential image/character, a narrative and visual story can emerge that is both fictional and biographical. In fact, McNiff (1992) states that all self-portraiture is paired with portraiture of the imagination, what one can and cannot be, both autobiographical and fictional. This guided session allows the client to create what McNiff (1992) calls *imaginal realism,* a direct presentation of the life of imagination by the person who is experiencing it. Through the creation of a *vicarious entity,* that can now express, describe, and develop language for fantasies and/or memories of using and dissatisfaction with sobriety and drug use, safely choose actions and consequences, and clearly investigate their feelings about change. The client can use this technique to maintain sobriety, even once outside the inpatient treatment program.

Speiglman (1977) argues that the narrative has the power to individualize the stereotype. Committing the exaggerated characterization of the artist's internal self-concept, what the artist knows of themselves, can reveal internal attitudes, allowing him/her the opportunity for expression, while the objectified character reflects how authentically the artist presents and describes what he/she knows of him/herself. The character that is given language has the power to conflate both expression and description. All art creation is a process of choice, exploration, and selection. Comic art or comics include these processes and the process of discarding successive stereotypic "selves" (Hatfield, 2005): A tool for developing discrepancy.

The Use of Humor

Cartoons can be funny, but of course not all cartoons are funny. There is nothing funny about the trauma, loss, and shame that many addicts experience. The phrase "there is nothing funny about the truth" comes to mind. The truth is often painful, confrontational. Mark Twain (1897) explained,

> *Truth is stranger than fiction, but it is because Fiction is obliged to stick to possibilities; Truth isn't (p. 156).*

The trauma of addiction makes it difficult to establish and maintain coherence—the ways in which the mind integrates the identity and the experience through narrative processes (Siegle, 1999). The fictional element of the comic drawing process can help to develop coherence. The scrutiny of truth through fiction enables selection and control of overwhelming negative emotion. The integration of humor enables reconciliation between the incongruity of reality and fantasy, the reception of personal limitation—what one can and cannot be. Uekermann, Channon, Winkel, Schlebusch, and Daum (2006) explain the requirement of false belief necessary for the expression and understanding of humor. Humor requires theory of mind: The ability to reason about mental states to predict and understand other people's behavior on the basis of their mental states. Uekermann and colleagues (2006) suggest that theory of mind is assessed by false belief tasks which require that the individual has a false belief. Therefore, if one can create a false memory, as was suggested in the false memories or fantasies comic strip activity, and integrate that memory into identity expression there is potential for the resolution of incongruity, the release of shame, loss, guilt, remorse, through joy, mirth, and humor.

The comic drawing art therapy groups revealed the potential for the use of humor in art therapy as a mechanism for releasing negative emotion. A female client, in her mid-twenties participated in two of the three comic drawing sessions. During her first session (addict comic character creation) she was very timid, did not share freely with the group, had difficulty making eye contact with others. She looked very down and she had a hard time drawing but tried. She did not share her drawing with the group, but stated "It is difficult to think about the past." She wrote in the survey that she had felt slow and like she didn't belong. Her counselor later reported that she was struggling with her learning disability and past abuse. After the first session, she seemed very depressed. In the following session, she made a beautiful picture. She did not include characters but as she was drawing squealed a few times in delight over the materials. She seemed to be able to be freer and more child-like. During the process, she looked up at me and said, "I am tensed." I repeated what she said. She shrugged her shoulders and said, "yeah, I am tensed," she chuckled and said, "I am not used to it that's all." She shared her picture with the group, a fuzzy pink background, with brown jagged mountains that represented her hardships, and a big flower blooming out of the corner representing her growth. She said it was hard to think about her past, that it was really hard for her to draw, that she felt like she couldn't draw last time, but she really liked how this picture turned out. She wanted to use more sheets of paper next time. "It was hard to pick just one topic."

As with all the clients at this in-patient center, there are many potential confounding variables that may be influencing this young woman's transformation. They are offered outside A.A. group involvement opportunities, many clients received proper diagnosis and medication for co-morbid disorder, and the length of her stay and prolonged involvement in group and individual therapy cannot be ignored. I do not presume to attribute transformation solely to the comic drawing process. However, in the creative moment, this client who had previously been so devoid of emotional expression simultaneously experienced and expressed tension/pain and laughter. Humor, joy, and mirth can be experienced at the same moment as discomfort, pain, and loss. Learning to "hold" both emotions, incongruous emotions, without taking compulsive action, is a crucial part to maintaining sobriety and preventing relapse.

The induction of positive emotions helps to reduce psychological distress and arousal caused by negative emotions (Fredrickson, 1998). Humor provides important psychological benefits by inducing a positive emotional state that can be shared by a group of individuals. Humor is a form of play that enables fun and derives emotional pleasure from incongruities. The benefits of humor include positive, emotional association, uses of humor for social communication, more creative problem solving, more efficient organization, and memory, higher levels of pro-social behavior and influence, tension relief, and coping (Isen, 2003, Martin, 2007). Sociologist Michael Mulkay (1988) suggested that humor be viewed as a mode of interpersonal communication. Because humor involves playing with incongruities and contradictory ideas and coveys multiple meanings at once, humor is a useful tool in communication in situations where more serious and direct modes run the risk of being too confrontational.

Spontaneous laughter was also observed as a mode of social interaction during drawing sessions. Often, clients would turn to each other and point out exaggerated features of their characters and share moments of spontaneous laughter. Although many of the comics and their content were not funny, the comic format seemed to be associated with the idea of the Sunday "funnies." The awkward use of drawing tools (pens, pencils, markers, and pastels) in creating a comic character can naturally produce laughter. It is much like an out-of-body experience, like watching an exercise tape and trying to mimic what you see someone else doing, imagining that personification of yourself, but not being able to physically contort or control your body to replicate the exact movement or form, while at the same time having a visual image of how ridiculous you look in comparison. The act of independently creating and controlling the creation of the self-image and the incongruity of needing to depend on the eyes of others to validate the self-image, whether stereotypical or authentic, inspires an understanding of limitation that can find expression in spontaneous shared laughter.

Humor played a powerful role in the sharing of the art object with the group, but also with family members. One woman drew her character as an emaciated alien whose arms were the full length of her body. After completing the drawing, she stated feeling that the process was "creepy." After some time, she shared her drawing with another client who had not taken part in the comic drawing session. In sharing her drawing, she made fun of the parody of herself, sharing laughter with her co-resident. In the following session, she said that she had given her drawing to her boyfriend, who said that "at first he was disturbed by it, then we laughed about it. There was lightness in how difficult it was."

Thus, humor used in self-deprecating ways can be positive if it provides insight. Christopher Lasch (1978), author of *The Culture of Narcissism*, writes that pathological narcissism is not akin to traditional narcissism—hedonism and self-centered sense of self—but rather very weak sense of self. He criticizes the "confessional mode" of presenting personal experience without reflection, stating that "undigested forms" of experience solicit "salacious curiosity" rather than search for deep understanding. Humor without insight, exploration of the humorous, is far from honest, it "waives the right to be taken seriously," and can attract undeserved attention and sympathy. The social play of humor can be used to communicate a variety of messages, some congenial and pro-social, while others more aggressive and coercive. While the appropriate use of humor can offer psychological benefits and a tool for the release of negative emotions, the inappropriate use of humor can have deleterious effects on the recovery process. The main distinction between useful humor (growth) and ineffective humor (defense) in addiction is the ability to look within the self and engage cognitive thought and humor to resolve incongruities that prevent growth.

Humor and laughter are not always benevolent. Some traditional theories suggest that aggression is an essential element of all humor and laughter. Humor can be used in aggressive and hostile ways: Teasing, joking, ridicule, or sarcasm can exclude individuals from a group, reinforce power and status differences, and suppress behavior that does not conform to the group.

An example of coercive and dismissive humor is seen in the comic drawing by a young man who joined the comic drawing group in its second session. His counselor reported that he had been having trouble with appropriate social interaction with his co-residents. He drew a comic scene of his character interacting with recovery. His character, a stick figure, with a large head stands in a large field that is dotted with flowers and trees. One black mark indicates a squinting eye, while the other eye is covered with hair. A word bubble escapes from his wide smile stating "We're clean." He is speaking to the character beside him. The character beside him is his depiction of the co-resident sitting beside him in the group. The co-resident's head is slightly smaller than his own, has larger back eyes and speckles on top of his head indicate shorn hair. The co-resident's smile is not as large and a word bubble states, "Hell yea." This expression seemed sarcastic. The sharing of this drawing made the whole group burst into laughter. The laughter seemed to be pointed at the client.

This is the only drawing from both sessions that incorporates the client in relation to another client. The self-identity in relation to the present group expressed through comic drawing is an interesting avenue to explore, which could potentially reveal the group identity and expose the group dynamics that are productive and counterproductive for the individual. However, this young man's comic drawing attempts to incorporate another client's recovered identity to support his undiscovered recovery. When he explains his picture to the group, he states, "This is me and my buddy enjoying nature." The dismissal of recovery and the attempt to persuade the viewer and the other character in the picture that "we are clean" does not represent the humor that is created from resolution of fantasy and truth, but the harmful humor that is found in adherence to and operation out of fantasy.

The use of humor in therapy is severely understudied. More research is needed to examine the various forms humor can take (i.e., nervous humor, aggressive humor, self-deprecating humor, authentic humor) and the use of humor in resolving or inhibiting resolution of negative emotion in chemically dependant clients in early recover. The role of humor in socialization, the ways in which humor can benefit or interrupt productive group work and specifically how the benefits of humor can be experienced through art therapy needs further study. In addition, the therapist's use of humor and ability to facilitate laughter and joyful expression at appropriate times during addiction therapy needs further study. The study of humor's role in the comic drawing process was secondary to the understanding of ambivalence and motivation to change through the comic process. However, during the course of the session it became apparent that humor played a crucial role in the release of negative emotions, the interaction of individuals within the group, and the ability to share one's experience with others. The type of humor expressed also seemed to be congruent with the client's position in the stages of change. The above observations are only the beginning of a necessary exploration of the use of humor in art therapy within the addiction treatment setting.

Gendered Expression in Comic Drawing

There is a vast amount of research and theorizing on addiction in men. Only within the past decade has an emerging literature on female addiction sharpened the awareness of gender specificity in the ways that males and females use drugs. There is an even greater paucity of research on gender specificity in creative therapy expression. This study was conducted with gender segregated groups ranging in age, severity of addiction, and comorbidity. During the three session process, themes surfaced in each group that may shed some light on the differences of gender expression as it applies to comic drawing.

It is a common cultural belief that men are less communicative and less emotionally expressive than women. Barbee (1996) explored the use of art therapy with males experiencing major depression. He examined depression through the lens of "sex role expectation." Adherence to traditional masculine role expectations can result in a negative psychological state known as gender-role conflict (O'Neil, 1981). Research looking at gender-role conflict has confirmed that men who subscribe to more traditional gender roles exhibit more restrictive emotionality, view their problems as signs of weakness, and thus are less likely to acknowledge their experiences of trauma, mental distress, or helplessness. Osherson and Krugman (1990) stated that the denial of weakness and the attenuation of powerful emotions in order to control expressivity leads to emotional pain and distress in men, but also what is felt as a dangerous reluctance to express and expose the pain to others. The strain resulting from this disinclination can ultimately find expression in anger, violence, substance abuse, and other characteristics of a male depressive syndrome (Barbee, 1996; Cochran & Rabinowitz, 2000; Trombetta, 2007). One common symptom of depression for men is alyxtheimia, which is the inability to identify or express an emotion or experience, the inability to verbally communicate affect (Krystal, 1988). Trombetta (2007) posits that while alyxtithymia primarily refers to lack of words, it may also apply to the use of words to defensively deny, disguise, or reattribute the affects being experienced. This lack of words and the defensive vocabulary help to distinguish the ambivalent vocabulary.

For example, one client used a sea otter to depict his character. The sea otter was meant to represent the playfulness and fun that he experienced when he was drinking. He illustrated a blackout incident. The sea otter lies on the ground with birds circling his head. He has fallen off his bike, and tread marks cover his body, fins, and face. He drew alcohol as a band conductor. A word bubble hangs over the conductor's head stating RIGHT THIS WAY! This may be a case in which humor and comic drawing may be a more useful tool for the therapist than for the client, in assessing his desire

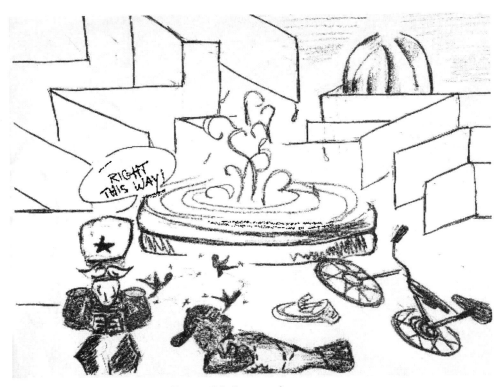

Figure 6.2. Image of sea otter.

or lack of desire to discontinue substance use. This client did not seem to be in the precontemplation stages of change, there were very few ambivalent expressions. He did not see his drinking as a problem. He said about his drawing, "I didn't feel threatened during this blackout session. I was out for only a short time. I did have chain marks on my face (laughter). It was a long time ago, I disassociate myself from this. It feels more like a story." The therapist's ability to recognize the use of humor that informs the client's defensive vocabulary can guide a motivational interview about the client's thoughts on moderation rather than abstinence in an effort to induce honest ambivalence. It is important to note that progression through the stages of change is not unidirectional and not a rapid process.

For men, the incorporation of additional characters in the comic drawing seems to allow for self-expression through vicarious expression. Trombetta (2007) noticed that male clients resistant to self-disclosure often used comics, tattoos, and graffiti style imagery in their artwork. This was evident in the comic process. Males had an easier time creating comic strips and successive characters. Interestingly, their drawings also typically included more language than their female cohort. Females tended to use labels rather than the thought or word bubbles associated with comic drawing. Their drawings more commonly contained comic scenes with their self-image as the main character. Males met the task of constructing a comic with little resistance, while females often stated being confused and having difficulty with the task although their art objects ultimately addressed the suggested assignment. While this difference could be attributed to greater male exposure to comics and comic books as boys, it is also likely that the vicarious nature of the process provides men with a safe and acceptable forum for self-expression.

One client depicts his overdose experience in the form of a comic strip. In the first frame of his comic strip, he is wearing a hat of horns, he tells the group that "he is the devil in this comic strip." He is flanked by bottles of pills labeled soma and xanax. The pill bottles are open and additional pills fly toward the character. In addition to the labels, the words XANAX! And SOMA! surround his head.

In the second frame, he lies on a bed, his once empty eyes have been transformed into small x's. His arm rests along side his lifeless body. There is an underdrawing of a hand that has been filled in. The arm becomes a small handless oval surrounded by the blackness of his upper body. The

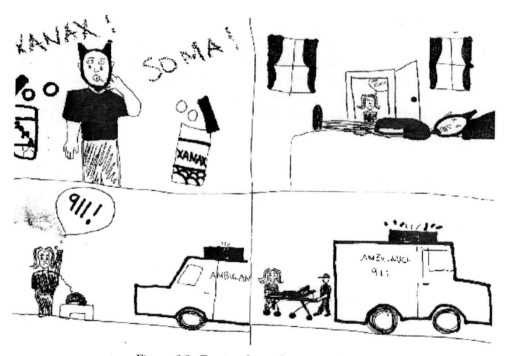

Figure 6.3. Comic of overdose experience.

hand is but a phantom. In the background, his girlfriend stands bound by the doorway. She is frowning and a thought bubble contains the words, "oh know." It is presumptuous to assume that this is anything more than a misspelling. However, the "beholder's share" makes interpretations irresistible. This man has not only expressed helplessness, but has also acknowledged that his girlfriend "knows," that his girlfriend no-s his helplessness. In the third frame the self-referential character is absent. We are shown the girlfriend with black tears falling from both eyes, she holds a phone and another thought bubble is filled with thick black numerals, "911!" His helplessness has become an emergency. The ambulance arrives and the character is loaded on a stretcher as his girlfriend, helplessly stands by. In group, the participant shared his feelings directly, "this session made me feel like shit, feel bad. I hurt my family and the people I care about." The opportunity to present and narrate his fictional autobiographic in a safe, ambivalence supporting environment allowed this male client to regulate and express his guilt and shame with direct vocabulary and awareness of his impact on others (his loved ones, as well as the group).

As mentioned previously, research on gender specificity in creative therapy expression is lacking. What is known is that it is likely that among women, depression, borderline personality, eating disorders, and post-traumatic stress disorder related to sexual abuse precede substance abuse (Staussner, 1997). Given the differences in gender role socialization for women and men, it is not surprising that women's drawings also tended to focus on relationships to their families.

For example, one female client incorporated family members into all three of her comic drawings. In the first drawing, she portrayed her addict self as a fox, which she labeled "Forlorn Fox" but called "Sly Fox." The fox is standing beside a circular path that encloses a forest of pines. Her husband, in human form, is walking on the path behind her, frowning and lines drawn around his head indicate that he is drunk. Her drunken self-image is of a wild animal, while her husband's image is human. A black cloud hangs over the forest. In the background, her children, also human forms, smile and hold hands in the yard surrounded by trees and a big house. The sun shines over this background scene.

When asked if she had experienced any difficult emotions or memories during this drawing session, she stated that she had and that maybe the process helped indirectly through thinking about her character's surroundings and mental state. In the second comic drawing session, she re-drew the forest. The fox is now exploring the pines and is far from the beaten path that encircles them. The fox holds a container of alcohol facing away from her children who are now inside the circle among the pines and their expressions are of disappointment and sadness. Her husband is outside of the circle at the

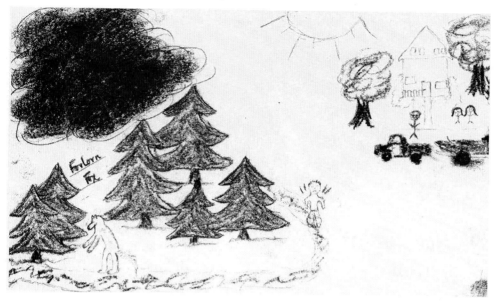

Figure 6.4. Forlorn fox.

far right border of the paper, it seems as though he is walking off the page. He is smiling and carrying a beer can. The client expressed feeling loneliness and abandonment to the group. She stated that this drawing brought about a realization, "I was alone then and I am alone now."

In the third drawing session, the client transformed herself into human

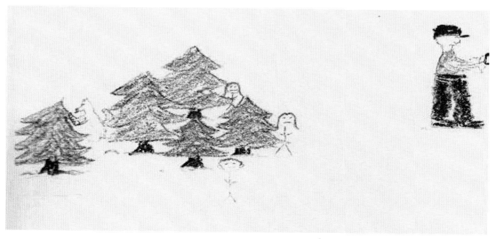

Figure 6.5. Expression of loneliness and abandonment.

form. Her drawing is a map of the inside of her house. Her children sit on a couch facing a fireplace and she approaches with hot chocolate for everyone. Her husband is not in the drawing. During this session, she stated that she did not experience any difficult feelings or memories. She had taken time to look at all three of her drawings and stated, "I recognized things in the pictures that I hadn't intentionally tried to depict but weren't necessarily untrue based on my perspective." While the client did not incorporate words in the comic drawings, she was able to recognize difficult emotions through visual representation of herself, her environment, her mental state, and her loved ones, and verbalize to the group her interpretation of those emotions. Ultimately, she created her story of transformation.

As illustrated above, women can also experience gender role strain due to the process of social gendering. Anderson, Stevens, and Pfost (2001) suggest that for alcoholic women, the discrepancy between traditional feminine sex-role identity and their participation in a traditionally male-dominated activity such as excessive drinking creates a discrepancy between their perceived femininity when intoxicated versus when sober. While intoxicated, the

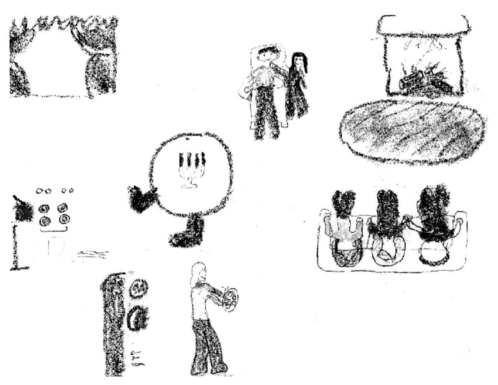

Figure 6.6. Map of client's house.

female client's self-image was of a wild animal. This may also be related to why studies of alcoholics point to the likelihood of depression as secondary to alcoholism in men and primary in women (Helzer & Pryzbeck, 1988). The wild animal was always depicted near her human husband. When the fox was the subject of her drawings, the client reported feelings of loneliness and abandonment. When sober, the fox transformed into a woman with long hair and curves and reported feelings of contentment and peace. She drew herself in the act of maternal caregiving within her home. Her husband was absent from this scene. Her femininity could be revealed only in his absence.

The sex-role identity discrepancy may be associated with the common theme of body-image in women's drawings. Full views, rather than portraits were used in the women's artwork. The female client, who depicted herself as an emaciated alien, with a crack pipe weighing on her shoulder in her first two drawings, was transformed into a healthy girl holding balloons that represented the lightness of recovery.

Conclusion and Future Uses

I shed my shortcomings and existed in an imaginary world as I wished
I could have done in reality. This served as a therapeutic outlet because
I put into words and pictures the things I longed to say or do.
Mulholland (2004, p. 42)

The proposed three session comic drawing process can be a safe avenue for addressing ambivalence and an alternative to confrontational therapies. Creation of self-image, regulation of self-expression, and the integration of appropriate humor within an ambivalence supporting group has the power to motivate change. Learning to cope with ambivalent emotion through independent expression, dependence on social interaction, and the use of humor as a mechanism for understanding simultaneous emotion enables the client to feel empowered, to release negative emotions, and possibly prevent relapse. Further, the comic-making process can be used to enhance family sessions, engage less verbal patients, stimulate communication about ambivalence in detoxification settings, and can naturally be adapted for use with chemically dependant adolescent clients.

The use of other art forms to address ambivalence through the use of an avatar should be explored. Two-dimensional mediums such as autobiographical photography could provide an even clearer "through other's eyes" self-image experience for the client in early recovery. Three-dimensional, virtual mediums should also be explored. The virtual avatar that is so popular in electronic culture could be used for those who feel inadequate in their creative abilities. The phenomena of the avatar in virtual reality has the potential to inform further research on self-expression and identity and the use of vicarious characters in fictional settings, as well as the implications of a fictional character or self-parody and social interaction.

Comic drawing and ambivalence have been understudied in the fields of art therapy and addiction. While this chapter opens the discussion and exploration of the comic drawing process in treatment with individuals who have chemical dependency, much more research is needed to expand on the use of comics to induce ambivalent expression and motivate change. A more prolonged series of comic drawing sessions would provide more data and insight into the creative and verbal expressions of ambivalence. An in-depth analysis of group therapy and the adaptability of current addiction group therapies to address ambivalence are needed, as is research on the leaderless group and the replication of such an art therapy group dynamic.

Appendix–Terms

Alyxtheimia: the inability to identify or express an emotion or experience, the inability to verbally communicate affect (Krystal, 1988).

Ambivalence: feeling uncertain or having fluctuating feelings caused by inability to make a choice or by a simultaneous desire to say or do two opposite or conflicting things (*The American Heritage Dictionary of the English Language,* 2000).

Avatar: the passing down or over to describe the descent of a deity to the earth (*The American Heritage Dictionary of the English Language,* 2000). The avatar in cartoon form, is the embodiment of a collection of attitudes, beliefs, principles, and views of life. When personified, the "attitude, principle, view" has a higher power of controlling the self-image and a higher power for passing down or letting go.

Discrepancy: the difference between two perceptions (Miller & Rollnick, 2002).

Imaginal Realism: a direct presentation of the life of imagination by the person who is experiencing it (McNiff, 1992).

Personal fundamental finitude: the presence of the not in the very being of any individual human, the limitations of what we *cannot be* or *cannot do* (Barrett, 1975).

Theory of Mind: the ability to reason about mental states to predict and understand other people's behavior on the basis of their mental states (Uekermann et al., 2006).

Vicarious Entity: a character/form created by the client to express, describe, and develop language for fantasies and/or memories.

References

Alcoholics Anonymous World Services, Inc. (2001). *Alcoholics anonymous: The story of how many thousands of men and women have recovered from alcoholism.* New York: Alcoholics Anonymous World Services, Inc.

The American Heritage Dictionary of the English Language. (2000). Boston: Houghton Mifflin Company

Allen, P. B. (1985). Integrating art therapy into an alcoholism treatment program. *American Journal of Art Therapy, 24,* 10–12.

Anderson, R. M., Stevens, M. J., & Pfost, K. S. (2001). Sex role strain in alcoholic women. *Substance Use & Misuse, 36,* 653–662.

Barbee, M. (1996). Men's roles and their experience of depression. *Art Therapy: Journal of the American Art Therapy Association, 13,* 31–36.

Barrett, W. (1958). *Irrational man: A study in existential philosophy.* Garden City, NY: Doubleday.

Bell R. & Sinclair, M. (2005). *Pictures and words: New comic art and narrative illustration.* New Haven, CT: Yale University Press.

Cochran, S., & Rabinowitz, F. (2000). *Men and depression: Clinical and empirical perspectives.* San Diego, CA: Academic Press.

Cox, K. & Price, K. (1990). Breaking through: Incident drawings with adolescent substance abusers. *The Arts in Psychotherapy, 17,* 333–337.

Callaghan , R. C., Hathaway, A., Cunningham, J. A., Vettese, L. C., Wyatt, S., & Taylor, L. (2005). Does stage-of-change predict dropout in culturally diverse sample of adolescents admitted to inpatient substance abuse treatment? A test of the transtheoretical model. *Addictive Behaviors, 30,* 1834–1847.

Dalely, T., Rifkind, G., & Terry, K. (1993). *Three voices of art therapy: Image, client, therapist.* London: Routledge.

Flores, P. (2004). Addiction as an attachment disorder: Implications for group psychotherapy. In B. Reading & M. Weegmann (Eds.), *Group psychotherapy & addiction* (pp. 1–18). Philadephia, PA: Whurr Publishers.

Forrest, G. (1975). The problems of dependency and the value of art therapy as a means to treating alcoholism. *Arts Psychotherapy, 2,* 15–43.

Fredrickson, B. L. & Levenson, R. W. (1998). Positive emotions speed recovery from the cardiovascular sequelae of negative emotions. *Cognition and Emotion, 12,* 191–220.

Freud, S. (1922). *Group psychology and the analysis of the ego.* (J. Strachey, Trans.). New York and London: W.W. Norton & Company.

George, R. (1990). *Counseling the chemically dependant: Theory and practice.* Boston: Allyn and Bacon.

Gombrich, E. H. (1972) The Mask and the face: The perception of physiognomic likeness in life and in art. In E. H. Gombrich, J. E. Hochberg, & M. Black (Eds.), *Art perception, and reality* (pp. 1–46). Baltimore: John Hopkins University Press.

Hanes, M.J. (2007). "Face to face" with addiction: The spontaneous production of self-portraits in art therapy. *Journal of the American Art Therapy Association, 24,* 33–36.

Hatfield, C. (2005). *Alternative comics: An emerging literature.* Jackson, MS: University Press of Mississippi.

Helzer, J. F., & Pryzbeck, T. R. (1988). The co-occurance of alcoholism and other psychiatric disorders in the general population and its impact on treatment. *Journal of Studies of Abnormal Psychology, 86,* 609–614.

Horay, B. J. (2006). Moving towards gray: Art therapy and ambivalence in substance abuse treatment. *Journal of the American Art Therapy Association, 23,* 14–22.

Isen, A. M. (2003). Positive affect as a source of human strength. In L. G. Aspinwall & U. M. Staudinger (Eds.), *A psychology of human strengths: Fundamental questions and future directions for a positive psychology (pp. 179–195). Washington D.C.: American Psychological Association.*

Kinneir, J. (1980). *The artist by himself: Self-portrait drawings from youth to old age.* New York: St. Martin's Press.

Krystal, H. (1988). *Integration and self-healing: Affect-trauma-alexithymia.* Hillsdale, NJ: Analytic Press.

Kurtz, E. (1979). *Not-God: A history of Alcoholics Anonymous.* Center City, MN: Hazelden.

Kurtz, E. (1982). Why A.A. works: The intellectual significance of alcoholics anonymous. *Journal of Studies on Alcohol, 43,* 38–80.

Kurtz, E. (1983). Why A.A. works: The intellectual significance of alcoholics anonymous, part two. *Journal of Studies on Alcohol, 43,* 57–70.

Lasch, C. (1978). *The culture of narcissism: American life in an age of diminishing expectations.* New York: Norton.

Lipkus, I., Pollak, K., McBride, C., Schwartz-Bloom, R., Lyna, P., & Bloom, P. (2005). Assessing attitudinal ambivalence towards smoking and association with desire to quit among teen smokers. *Psychology and Health, 20,* 373–387.

Martin, R. A. (2007). *The psychology of humor: An integrative approach.* California: Elsevier Academic Press.

McCloud, S. (1993). *Understanding comics.* Northhampton, MA: Tundra Publishing.

McNiff, S. (1992). Imaginal Realism. In *Art as medicine* (pp. 66–73). Boston, MA: Shambhala.

Miller, W. R., & Rollnick, S. (2002). *Motivational interviewing: Preparing people for change* (2nd ed.). New York: The Guilford Press.

Miller, W. R., & Rollnick, S. (1991). *Motivational interviewing: Preparing people to change addictive behavior.* New York: Guilford Press.

Mulkay, M. (1988). *On humor: Its nature and its place in modern society.* New York: Basil Blackwell.

Mulholland, M. J. (2004). Comics as art therapy. *Art Therapy: Journal of the American Art Therapy Association, 21,* 42–43.

O'Neil, J.M. (1981). Patterns of gender role conflict and strain: Sexism and fear of femininity in men's lives. *Personnel and Guidance Journal, 60,* 203–210.

Osherson, S., & Krugman, S. (1990). Men, shame, and psychotherapy. *Psychotherapy, 27,* 327–339.

Prochaska, J. O., & DiClemente, C. C. (1984). *The transtheoretical approach: Crossing boundaries of therapy.* Malabar, FL: Krieger Publishing Co.

Prochaska, J. O., & Norcross, J. C. (2001). Stages of change. *Psychotherapy, 38,* 443–448.

Richards, B. (2005). Foreward. In R. Bell & M. Sinclair (Eds.), *Pictures and words: New comic art and narrative illustration* (p. 6). Connecticut: Yale University Press.

Schaverien, J. (1990). The scapegoat and the talisman: Transference in art therapy. In T. Dalley, C. Case, J. Schaverien, F. Weir, D. Halliday, P. Hall, & D. Waller (Eds.), *Images of art therapy: New developments in theory and practice* (2nd ed.) (pp. 74–108). London: Routledge.

Siegle, D. (1999). *The developing mind toward a neurobiology of interpersonal experience.* New York: The Guilford Press.

Staussner, S. (1997). Gender and substance abuse. In S. Staussner & E. Zelvin (Eds.), *Gender and addictions* (pp. 5–27). Northvale, NJ: Jason Aronson Inc.

Stevens-Smith, P., & Smith, R. (1998). *Substance abuse counseling: Theory and practice.* Columbus, OH: Merrill.

Speigelman, A. (1977). *Breakdown: From Maus to now: An anthology of strips by Art Spiegelman.* New York: Belier Press.

Trombetta, R. (2007). Art therapy, men, and the expressivity gap. *Art Therapy: Journal of the American Art Therapy Association, 23,* 29–32.

Twain, M. (1897). *Following the equator: A journey around the world.* Hartford, CT: American Publishing Company.

Uekermann, J., Channon, S., Winkel, K., Schlebusch, P., & Daum, I. (2006). Theory of mind, humor processing and executive functioning in alcoholism. *Addiction, 102,* 232–240.

Vickers, L. (2004). One-off art therapy in in-patient detoxification. In B. Reading & M. Weegmann (Eds.), *Group psychotherapy & addiction* (pp. 117–132). Philadelphia, PA: Whurr Publishers.

Wadeson, H. (2000). *Art therapy practice: Innovative approaches with diverse populations.* New York: John Wiley & Sons.

Waller, D., & Mahony, J. (Eds.) (1999). *Treatment of addiction: Current issues for art therapies.* New York: Routeldge.

Weber, E.U., Baron, J., Loomes, G. (2001). *Conflict and tradeoffs in decision-making.* Cambridge, UK: Cambridge University Press.

Weegmann, M. (2004). Alcoholics Anonymous: group therapy without the group therapist. In B. Reading & M. Weegmann (Eds.), *Group psychotherapy & addiction* (pp. 27–41). Philadelphia, PA: Whurr Publishers.

Winship, G. (1999). Addiction as an attachment disorder: Implications for group psychotherapy. In D. Waller & J. Mahony (Eds.), *Treatment of addiction: Current issues for art therapies* (pp. 46–59). London: Routledge.

Biography

Katherin Fernandez has developed and facilitated creative and educational programming for a diverse population of at-risk, low-income, urban children and adolescents and their families through community centers, the public school system, alternative schooling sites, and correctional centers in Madison, Wisconsin. Katherin has worked with adolescents and adults that have experienced chemical dependency, both through a non-profit organization offering creative programming and employment support and through internship at an inpatient treatment center. Her educational achievements include a Bachelor's of Fine Arts Degree from The School of the Art Institute of Chicago. She completed post-baccalaureate work with a Clinical Counseling concentration at Edgewood College in Madison, WI. She is currently a graduate student in the Counseling Psychology at the University of Wisconsin–Madison. Katherin began making comics as a part of her own recovery from alcoholism. Her artwork has been shown in art galleries in Wisconsin and Illinois. Katherin can be contacted at fernheit@msn.com.

The author wishes to dedicate this chapter to Siriano
for his contribution, his sense of humor, and courage.

Chapter 7

ALL BOTTLED UP: PLAY THERAPY WITH CHILDREN EXPOSED TO ADDICTION

BRIAN L. BETHEL

Childhood is supposed to be a time of laughter, a time for learning, and a time of innocence. However, for the millions of children who live with a parent addicted to drugs or alcohol, they become robbed of these basic rights. For these children, childhood becomes a time of chaos, a time of confusion, and often a time of danger. Tragically, the impact that parental addiction may have on a child's life can precipitate years of struggles. This chapter will offer an overview regarding the impact of parental addiction on the lives of children. Additionally, a rationale for the use of play therapy for working with children exposed to addiction in the family will be provided. Case examples will illustrate the implementation of play therapy techniques in addressing the treatment goals when working with children affected by family addiction.

The disease of addiction has unfortunately become a common occurrence in the American society. Grant (2000) reported that an estimated 9, 700, 000 children under the age of 17 are living with an alcoholic. This translates to one in every four children being exposed to alcohol abuse or dependency within his or her family unit. While these figures appear overwhelming, Edwards (2003) suggested that these figures are probably conservative given the stigma and secrecy that accompanies alcoholism.

Families touched by addiction often develop boundary issues and accept role assignments that greatly reinforce the instability within the family system (Werner et al., 1999). Although substance abuse affects the entire family, it has only been in recent years that these efforts have been expanded to include the children of substance abusing parents (Lambie & Sias, 2005). Historically, the addict within family systems has been viewed as the identified patient and has received most of the attention. As recently as 2000, Thompson and Rudolph (2000) asserted that society has offered little attention to family members in addictive homes as the treatment of the addict typically takes precedent.

As Werner and colleagues (1999) reported substance abuse is not unlike other chronic illness. However, families of addicts may not recognize the impact the addict may play on the entire family system. All family systems strive to achieve a sense of homeostasis. Nichols and Schwartz (2003) affirmed that all members within a family system will compensate to attain this sense of balance. Regrettably, children living in alcoholic homes regularly use unhealthy measures to obtain this homeostasis. It would not be uncommon for family members to minimize denial or rationalize an addict's behavior. Tragically, these attempts to justify an addict's behavior only serve to fuel the disease of addiction (Kinney, 2003). Therefore, it is important for professionals to challenge families in gaining a better awareness of their personal contributions to the family disease of addiction.

Children who are raised in addictive homes confront a number of obstacles. Specifically, the disease of addiction will only serve to distort any traditional values of healthy families (Hawkins, 1997). As early as 1981, the rules for families of addicts were being examined. Black (1981) highlighted the three most common rules that family members adapt when living with an addict. Family members frequently prescribe to the following: "Don't talk, Don't trust, and Don't feel." Each of these rules only serves to perpetuate the progression of the disease of addiction.

George (1990) discussed the numerous consequences for children who accept these rigid beliefs. As a result of the "don't trust" rule, children become fearful of discussing their thoughts and live each day of their lives in a constant state of secrecy. As long as secrets exist, the addict is permitted to continue their substance addiction. Similarly, children are taught by the addict not to trust outsiders. Consequently, the "don't trust" rule is designed to restrict communication to anyone outside of the family unit. George (1990) reported that the "don't feel" rule as the most detrimental for children of addicts. Children who choose to live by this rule are forced to deny their emotions and as a result may experience a lack of coping skills.

More recent writings have expanded on the rigidity associated with rules in alcoholic homes. Ruben (2001) discussed the inflexible beliefs that often infect the alcoholic family. Children of alcoholics are not permitted to discuss problems that exist within the family unit. This secrecy correlates with the understanding that all feelings within the addictive family should be suppressed. Consequently, children living in an addictive environment become isolated. Unfortunately, children of addicts frequently adopt the rule of limiting their communication. The addict works hard to reinforce the closed family system and thus limits the possibility of intervention from outsiders (Edwards, 2003). These unspoken rules are designed to maintain the secrecy that helps to enable the cycle of addiction.

Research has suggested that nothing in the addict family is done in moderation (Kinney, 2003). The addict commonly attempts to blame others within the family unit when something bad happens. Tragically, children growing up in this environment adopt the philosophy that regardless of what they do, it is never good enough. Likewise, individuals living in these chaotic environments are forced to accept the belief that their personal needs are irrelevant. Despite the need to live up to these unrealistic expectations, children of alcoholics do not allow themselves the possibility of fun or relaxation. Children of addicts accept the need of constantly trying to prove their self-worth. Lastly, children in addictive homes adhere to the rule of avoiding conflict at all costs (Ruben, 2001).

Similarly, the literature has documented various personality characteristics that children of addicts may adopt as a means of survival. Lambie and Sias (2005) reported that children of alcoholics may develop inflexible roles in an effort to negotiate the harmful feelings within the family unit. These roles were first introduced by Wegscheider-Cruse (1981) and have been discussed in the literature for the last three decades. Lambie and Sias (2005) identified the roles of the addict family as the chief enabler, the family hero, the family scapegoat, the lost child, and the family mascot. Each of these roles is designed to assist the family in achieving a sense of balance. Although family members may utilize these roles as a shield to guard against the emotional costs of living in addictive homes, it is important to note that these roles have not been validated by any empirical data (van Wormer & Davis, 2003). Consequently, these roles are generalizations and should only be used to obtain a basic framework of family functioning.

The chief enabler has been described as the individual who protects the addict from the potential consequences of addiction. Typically, the chief enabler is the partner of the addict and will offer a number of rationalizations to deny the severity of the addiction (Lambie & Sias, 2005). Although the chief enabler may appear responsible and in control, the enabler's ongoing attempts to regulate the addict's behavior only serves to precipitate chaos within the family system (Werner, Joffe & Graham, 1999).

The role of the family hero is designed to bring pride to the family. This individual attempts to take the focus from the addict via his or her successes. The hero, who is typically the firstborn, will often excel at school and work (Lambie & Sias, 2005). The family hero is very achievement-oriented and may be viewed as a "people pleaser." Despite the success of the family hero, their attempts to bring pride to the family system never stop the addict from using. Consequently, the family hero habitually views himself or herself as a failure (Werner, Joffe & Graham, 1999).

Unlike the family hero, the family scapegoat attempts to take the focus from the addict by acting out. This individual is viewed by the family system as the troublemaker. As long as the focus can remain on the family scapegoat, the addict's behavior will go undetected (Lambie & Sias, 2005). The family scapegoat is more often brought to the attention of mental health professionals due to his or her high risk for destructive behaviors. Although labels of being defiant and resistant may be used to describe the scapegoat, it should be noted that this individual is commonly experiencing a great deal of pain. The child's inappropriate behavioral issues could be viewed as an external expression of their anger and emotional trauma (Werner, Joffe & Graham, 1999).

The lost child adapts to the addict within the family by isolating himself or herself. These children are usually overlooked as they are not discipline problems. In contrast to the scapegoat, the lost child is predictably the last child seen by mental health professionals. Unfortunately, the lack of attention for these children put them at high risk for self-injurious behaviors (Lambie & Sias, 2005).

Humor and comic relief are used by the family mascot as a means of taking the focus from the addict. The family mascot is often the youngest child within the family unit and strives to get his or her needs met through humor (Werner, Joffe & Graham, 1999). Moreover, the family mascot offers humor to the chaotic family in an effort to alleviate the pain of others (Sciarra, 2004; van Wormer & Davis, 2003).

Children living in addictive homes also experience more direct effects of the disease of addiction. These children frequently become victims of abuse and neglect (Thompson & Rudolph, 2000). Studies have documented the link between parental addiction and child abuse and neglect and validated the belief that physical and sexual abuse are more common for children living in addictive homes (Bijur et al., 1992). More specific estimates reveal that children living with a parent addicted to drugs and/or alcohol are three times more likely to be abused and four times more likely to be neglected than are children of non-substance abusing parents (Reid, Macchetto & Foster, 1999). Additional studies have shown that substance abuse is a factor for at least half of the families in the child welfare system (Werner et al., 1999).

Likewise, children raised in addictive homes encounter a number of psychological challenges. Kinney (2003) suggested children living in addictive homes tend to blame themselves for the chaos that exists in the addictive family. As a result, these children may develop feelings of guilt, low self-esteem, and feel that they were unable to "fix" their family (Arman, 2000). Several mental health diagnoses have been link to a child's exposure to addiction. Specifically, children of addicts commonly experience post-traumatic stress disorder, sleep disturbances, nightmares, anxiety, and depression. Regressive behaviors such as crying, bed-wetting, and developmental deficits are also documented for children exposed to parental addiction (Kinney, 2003).

Similarly, Lambie and Sias (2005) highlighted several issues that children of addicts may present in their academic environments. Children of addicts are more likely to be identified with learning disabilities, exhibit lower academic achievement scores, and be truant compared with their peers. These children also are identified more frequently as delinquent and have a higher drop-out rate than children of non-substance abusing parents (Arman, 2000). The literature has also widely supported the cyclical effect of addiction. Numerous studies have found a genetic predisposition to the mutigenerational disease of addiction (Black, 1981; Brook et al., 2003; Kinney, 2003; Lambie & Sias, 2003). It is estimated that children of addicts are four times more likely to develop an addiction problem (Brook et al., 2003).

Given the diverse impact that family addiction can have on children, treatment efforts can be challenging for mental health professionals. Group counseling, individual counseling, and family counseling have all been cited as effective intervention for children from addictive homes (Thompson & Rudolph, 2000). However, Ficaro (1999) offered specific treatment goals for children of addicts and opined that these goals are paramount over the specific intervention format. Specifically, professionals working with children impacted by family addiction should work toward establishing trust, demonstrating an understanding of how children are affected by parental addiction, providing children with the opportunity to express their feelings, providing educational resources, and assisting children with developing alternative coping skills (Ficaro, 1999).

Based upon the philosophy the addiction is a family disease, research has also promoted the inclusion of the family in the child's course of treatment. Kumpfer and colleagues (2003) encourage the implementation of family counseling as part of the treatment for children of addicts. The authors suggest behavioral parent training, in-home family support, brief family therapy, and family education as appropriate models of intervention.

Given the complexity of challenges that children of addictive home experience, professionals should move cautiously through the counseling process. As a result, counseling professionals should explore the use of a variety of treatment options (Ficaro, 1999). Therefore, individuals working with children from addictive homes should explore additional modalities for treatment.

Rationale for Play Therapy

Unlike traditional therapeutic models, play therapy does not require children to cognitively re-visit past traumatic events. Therefore, clinicians can use play therapy as an avenue for children to regain a sense of mastery and control over their environment without necessarily reliving the trauma that they have experienced (Kauson, Cangelosi & Schaefer, 1997). This is particularly helpful when working with children traumatized by addiction in the family. As Smith and Landreth (2003) stated, children can be allowed to use play as a means of communicating and gaining control over their traumatic past.

Play therapy offers a unique approach for working with children and adolescents by offering individuals a non-threatening environment in which they can work to regain some sense of stability. With the specialization of play therapists and play therapy techniques, these theories have been popularly implemented over the last fifty years (Kauson et al., 1997). Similarly, Landreth, Homeyer, Glover, and Sweeney (1996) concluded that play therapy is an effective tool for counseling children with a variety of issues. Gil (1994) also stated that most child therapists agree that play therapy is the most effective medium for treating children.

The history of play therapy dates back to as early as 1920 (Gil, 1991). However, Virginia Axline is perhaps the most commonly recognized for the application of child-centered therapy techniques via play in her work with children (Axline, 1947). Child-centered therapy or non-directive therapy grew out of the work of Carl Rogers. This model emphasized the philosophies of unconditional positive regard and being present with the child as foundations of this theory (Rogers, 1980).

Landreth expanded on Axline's work and identified the term child-centered play therapy using these same standards. Similar to the work of Rogers, child-centered play therapy focuses on the relationship between the clinician and the child (Landreth, 1991). The use of child-centered play therapy when working with children exposed to addiction has also been documented in the play therapy literature (Johnson et al., 1999).

Conversely, directive play therapy techniques are typically best implemented to address specific therapeutic goals. Literature has suggested the implementation of directive play therapy techniques to assist children with a variety of issues. Moe (1993) offered the use of directive play therapy techniques for individuals impacted by addiction within the home. The use of directive play therapy techniques may prove beneficial in assisting children in developing safety plans.

Filial play therapy is an additional intervention when working with children and families. B.G. Guerney, (1964) first developed filial play therapy as a means of involving parents in the treatment of children with emotional and behavioral difficulties. Yet, this practice has been applied in treating a variety of issues. The use of filial play therapy when working with children of alcoholics has also been documented in the literature (Johnson et al., 1999).

Case Illustrations

The first case example will show how the use of sandtray work can assist clinicians in normalized feelings associated with a child's reactions to parental addiction. Moreover, the case provided will offer readers an example of how sandtray techniques could be implemented in treatment of families with addiction issues. The use of sandtray provides a non-threatening approach for children to discuss the experiences.

Josh was eight years old when he first came to the attention of the community mental health center. The identified child was referred to counseling by his officials at his school and the local juvenile court system. According to court documents, Josh had been ordered to counseling after he threatened to beat up a teacher at his school. School records indicated that Josh was failing and had numerous school infractions.

Likewise, Josh's mother stated that he was a "discipline problem" at home. By contrast, Josh's mother stated throughout the initial session that Josh's older sister was an excellent student and very responsible. The child presented himself with resistance throughout the initial session and was argumentative with his mother.

The child was seen individually during the second session and was asked to complete a sandtray. Josh was given the directive of creating his work in the sand via the use of minatures. Josh was very selective in determining the minatures to include in his sandtray. Upon completion of the sandtray, the child offered a detailed explanation of his world. This was the first report of any additional issues in the home. Figure 7.1 is a photograph of Josh's sandtray.

The following was the information Josh provided about his sandtray. The child pointed to the various animal minatures included in the container and reported "my house is like a zoo." He went on to elaborate that "my mom never knows when my dad is coming home and my dad always yells." Josh used a child figure surrounded by police officers to represent himself. The police were recently contacted by the school after the child threatened to become physically violent at school. Josh went on to explain that his father drank often and surrounded his father's minature with bottles. Josh used a female minature with two children to symbolize his mother and a superhero figure to represent his sister. The child said "my sister does everything right and I just get yelled at." Ironically, all the figures that represented Josh's family were turned away from Josh.

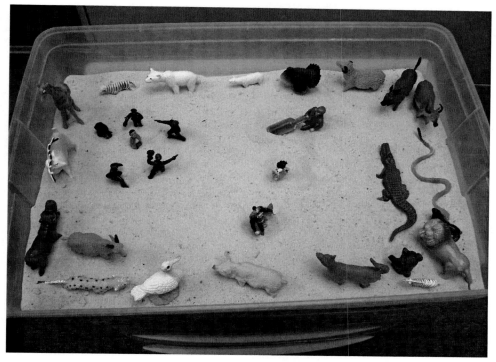

Figure 7.1. The zoo.

Although Josh presented himself in counseling with some initial resistance, the sandtray provided him the opportunity to discuss family issues in a non-threatening environment. Josh was more enthusiastic to talk about the minatures versus talking about himself. This initial sandtray served to be very diagnostic regarding the roles of the family. Directive questions were provided to assist Josh in identification of specific coping mechanism. For example, what can the child do to avoid having the police called? What do you think the child would like to say to the other people in the sandtray? Josh's mother and sister were eventually included in the counseling process. Photographs of Josh's sandtray provided an avenue for discussing the roles in additive family. Fortunately, this prompted Josh's mother and sister to seek individualized treatment. A family sandtray (Gil, 1994) was completed with Josh, his mother and his sister. This was part of the family's preparation to confront their father regarding his alcoholism. Figure 7.2 is a photograph of the family's sandtray. As shown in the photograph, the "zoo" is now contained and the family members stand united.

The second case example will offer specific techniques in assessing a

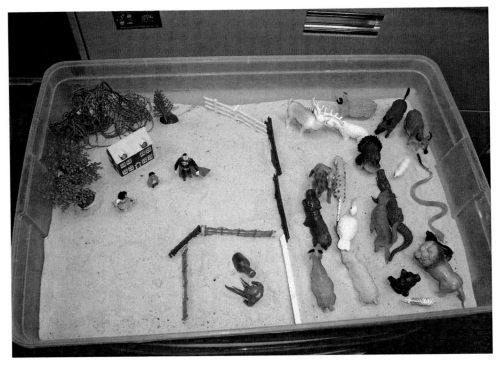

Figure 7.2. Family united.

child's view of his relationships with family members. The use of a self-por-trait (Costas & Landreth, 1999) will be demonstrated. As indicated in the case example, this technique can provide a variety of benefits for working with children confronting issues related to parental addiction. The second case example involves a child who also experiences a parent addicted to alcohol.

Logan was eight years old when he was referred to counseling by the local child welfare agency. Logan and his siblings had been placed in foster care due to physical abuse allegations and neglect by his alcoholic mother. Unlike his siblings, Logan was very quiet and often isolated himself. This behavior was a concern for child welfare officials. Logan also contributed minimally to counseling sessions and was very defiant in addressing his feelings. Therefore, the course of Logan's treatment remained non-directive. It was during the child's third session that he was asked to draw a self-portrait. Figure 7.3 is a photograph of the child's self-portrait.

Although Logan had continually been minimal in his communication, the self-portrait provided him with the opportunity to address his feelings of anger, depression, loneliness, and fear. At the completion of Logan's draw-ing, he openly talked about drawing a "storm with lots of wind in front of his

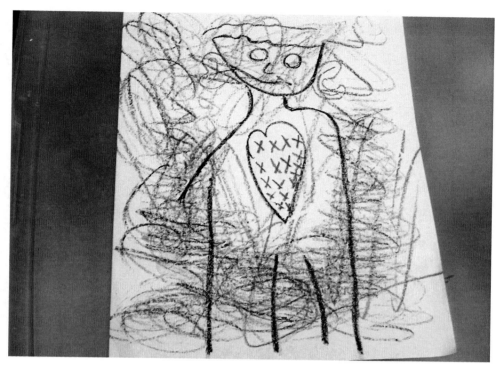

Figure 7.3. The storm.

body." Logan provided more detail in saying "The storm makes me confused 'cause it has lots of feelings in it." It appeared much easier for Logan to talk about the picture versus talking directly about himself.

The child's self-portrait became an integral piece of counseling. Throughout the child's counseling experience, he would reference "the storm" of his self-portrait when he struggled with coping with his mother's alcoholism. Logan's foster mother also participated in the child's counseling session. Through the use of filial therapy, Logan's foster care provider was taught the importance of recognizing Logan's emotions through his play. This technique encouraged the child to utilize his foster mother as a source of support.

A second self-portrait was completed midway through treatment. Although the second self-portrait continues to exhibit signs of emotional trauma, the storm is absent. This was significant for Logan's counselor and foster mother as a sign of progress. Logan continued to openly discuss his feelings with his foster family and siblings. Figure 7.4 is a photograph of Logan's second self-portrait.

In summary, counseling children can be extremely challenging. As Gil

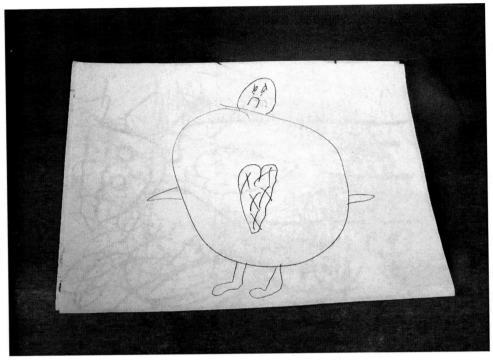

Figure 7.4. Sadness.

(1991) stated, the work with children can be both very rewarding and yet challenging. Children who are exposed to family addiction often share their traumatic experiences and this can present countertransferences issues for clinicians. Therefore, clinicians should be strongly advised to establish appropriate boundaries and utilize appropriate self-care practices.

The treatment of children of addicts is a complex and often challenging task. It is important that clinicians explore all available options when counseling this challenging population. Play therapy provides one modality for the treatment of children who have endured the experience of living in an addictive environment. Play therapy offers a variety of techniques to assist clinicians in the normalization of the traumatic experience as well as addressing specific symptoms that children may present. The use of play therapy provides children with unique opportunities for addressing traumatic issues.

In conclusion, play therapy can have a key role in assisting children from addictive families in developing alternative coping mechanisms, increasing support systems, and expressing the emotional costs of their experience. In offering children a non-threatening environment, play therapy often serves to allow children the opportunity to gain mastery over their experience without reliving the traumatic past. Professionals who are dedicated to serving children have the opportunity to utilize play therapy in assisting children of addicts who frequently find themselves all bottled up.

Appendix—Terms

Play Therapy: the systematic use of a theoretical model to establish an interpersonal process wherein trained play therapists use the therapeutic powers of play to help client prevent or resolve psychosocial difficulties and achieve optimal growth and development.

Substance Addiction: is a dependence on a substance, such as drugs and/or alcohol.

Child-Centered Play Therapy: is the method of play therapy developed by Virginia Axline, an associate of Carl Rogers. CCPT follows the principles of Client-Centered Therapy of creating a non-judgmental, emotionally supportive therapeutic atmosphere, but with clear boundaries that provide the child with psychological safety to permit the learning of emotional and behavioral self-regulation.

Directive Play Therapy: Specific play therapy techniques implemented to address a specific therapeutic goal.

Filial Play Therapy: The filial approach emphasizes a structured training program for parents in which they learn how to employ child-centered play sessions in the home.

References

Arman, H. F. (2000). A small group model for working with elementary school children of alcoholics. *Professional School Counseling, 3*(4), 290–294.

Association for Play Therapy. (2008). About Play Therapy. Play Therapy Defined. Retrieved June 01, 2008 from www.a4pt.org.

Axline, V. (1947). *Play Therapy: The inner dynamics of childhood.* Cambridge, MA: Houghton Mifflin Company.

Bijur, P. E., Kurzon, M., Overpeck, M.D., & Scheidt, P. C. (1992). Parental alcohol use, problem drinking, and children's injuries. *JAMA 267,* 3166–3171.

Black, C. (1981). Innocent bystanders at risk: The children of alcoholics. *Alcoholism,* Jan-Feb.

Brook, D. W., Brook, J. S., Rubenstone, E., Zhang, C., Singer, M., & Duke, M.R. (2003). Alcohol use in adolescents whose fathers abuse drugs. *Journal of Addictive Disease, 2*(1), 11–43.

Costas, M., & Landreth, G. (1999) Filial therapy with nonoffending parents of children who have been sexually abused. *International Journal of Play Therapy, 8,* 43–66.

Edwards, J. T. (2003). *Working with families: Guidelines and techniques* (6th ed). Durham, NC: Foundation Place Publishing.

Ficaro, R. C. (1999). The many losses of children in substance-disordered families individual and group interventions. In N. B. Webb (Ed.) *Play therapy with children in crisis individual, group, and family treatment* (pp. 294–317). New York, NY: Guilford Press.

George, R. (1990). *Counseling the chemically dependent: Theory and practice.* Boston: Allyn and Bacon.

Gil, E. (1991). *The healing power of play.* New York, NY: Guilford Press.

Gil, E. (1994). *Play in family therapy.* New York: The Guilford Press.

Grant, G. F. (2000). Estimates of US children exposed to alcohol abuse and dependence in the family. *American Journal of Public Health, 90*(1), 112–116.

Guerney, B. G. (1964). Filial therapy: Description and rationale. *Journal of Consulting Psychology, 20,* 304–310.

Hawkins, C. A. (1997). Disruption of family rituals as a mediator of the relationship between parental drinking and adult adjustment in offspring. *Addictive Behavior, 22*(2), 219–231.

Johnson L., Bruhn, R., Winek, J., Krepps, J., & Wiley, K. (1999). The Use of Child-Centered Play Therapy and Filial Therapy with Head Start Families: A Brief Report. *Journal of Marital and Family Therapy 25*(2), 169–176.

Kauson, H.G., Cangelosi, D., & Schaefer, C. E. (1997). *The playing cure.* Northvale, NJ: Jason Aronson, Inc.

Kinney, J. (2003). *Loosening the grip: A handbook of alcohol information.* New York: McGraw-Hill.

Kumpfer, K. L., Alvarado, R. & Whiteside, H. O. (2003). Family-based interventions for substance use and misuse prevention. *Substance Use & Misuse, 38*(11–13), 1759–1787.

Lambie, G. W., & Sias S. M. (2005). Children of alcoholics: Implications for professional school counseling. *Professional School Counseling 8*(3), 266–273.

Landreth, G. L. (1991). *Play therapy: The art of the relationship.* Muncie, IN: Accelerated Development, Inc.

Landreth, G.L., Homeyer, L., Glover, G., & Sweeney, D. (1996). *Play therapy interventions with children's problems.* Northvale, NJ:Jason Aronson.

Moe, J. (1993). *Discovery finding the buried treasure.* Dallas TX: Imagine Works.

Nichols, M. R., & Schwartz, R. C. (2003). *Family therapy: Concepts and methods* (6th ed.). Boston: Pearson Allyn and Bacon.

Reid, J., Macchetto, P., & Foster, S. (1999). *No safe haven: Children of substance-abusing parents.* New York: Columbia University Center on Addiction and Substance Abuse.

Rogers, C. L. (1980). *On becoming a person.* Boston, MA: Houghton Mifflin.

Ruben D. H. (2001). *Treating adult children of alcoholics: A behavioral approach.* San Diego, CA: Academic Press.

Sciarra, D. T. (2004). *School counseling: Foundations and contemporary issues.* Pacific Grove, CA: Brooks/Cole Thompson Learning.

Smith, N., & Landredth, G. (2003). Intensive Filial Play Therapy with child witnesses of domestic violence. *International Journal of Play Therapy, 12*(1), 67–88.

Thompson, C. L., & Rudolph, L. B. (2000). *Counseling children* (5th. ed). Belmont, CA: Brooks/Cole.

van Wormer, K., & Davis, D. R. (2003). *Addiction treatment: A strengths perspective.* Pacific Grove, CA: Brooks/Cole Thomson Learning.

Wegscheider-Cruse, S. (1981). *Another chance: Hope and help for the alcoholic family.* Palo Alto, CA: Science and Behavior Books.

Werner, M.J., Joffe, A., Graham, A.V. (1999). Screening, early identification, and office-based intervention with children and youth living in substance-abusing families. *Pediatrics, 103,* 1099–1112.

Biography

Brian L. Bethel is the Outpatient Services Director for a community mental health center in south central Ohio. In additional to his supervisory role, Mr. Bethel specializes in the therapeutic treatment of children, adolescents, and families. He is a Licensed Professional Counselor with Supervisory Endorsement (PCC-S) and a Licensed Chemical Dependency Counselor (LCDC) with the state of Ohio as well as a Registered Play Therapist-Supervisor. Mr. Bethel earned a masters degrees in clinical counseling and rehabilitation counseling from Ohio University and is currently completing doctorial studies in Counselor Education and Supervision.

Chapter 8

CHEMICAL DEPENDENCE, PLAY THERAPY, AND FILIAL THERAPY: REPAIRING THE PARENT-CHILD RELATIONSHIP

STEPHEN DEMANCHICK

Introduction

"Well, next time something goes south with your kids don't look at me, man. Ain't my problem. I didn't do it. I wish I did!" says the drug dealer standing at the corner of a mini-mart parking lot (Office of National Drug Control Policy 2008, Drug dealer public service announcement). The drug dealer in this commercial is complaining about the fact that the teens who used to buy their drugs from him are now getting high for free simply by raiding their parents medicine cabinets. What are parents to do, you ask? The Office of National Drug Control Policy (2008a) suggests that parents and families need to protect their prescriptions, discard old prescriptions, set limits and boundaries for children, and act as good role models; however, this problem continues to grow. The 2006 National Survey on Drug Use and Health (NSDUH) indicates that about seven million people aged 12 or older responded that they used doctor prescribed psychotherapeutic medications for non-medicinal purposes in the past month (Substance Abuse and Mental Health Services Administration, 2007). In 2005, 4.7 people responded similarly to the recreational use of these drugs. It was reported in the results from the same survey that 55.7 percent of those who used pain relievers in a non-medical fashion obtained those drugs from family members or friends (Substance Abuse and Mental Health Services Administration, 2007).

The message here is that drug use and abuse is pervasive and growing with its own life and trends. Prescription drugs that may be easy to obtain from physicians, friends, or family members pose a great risk and threat of addiction to adults and children. Years ago, inhalants such as spray paint, lacquer, and paint thinner garnered attention on investigative television shows as the current drug of choice for many young people. In 2006, nearly 800,000 people aged 12 and over reported that they used inhalants for the first time at some point during that year (Substance Abuse and Mental Health Services Administration, 2007). In addition, use of the commonly thought of drugs such as alcohol, cocaine, marijuana, and heroin does not seem to be going away. Further findings from the 2006 National Survey on Drug Use and Health indicate that four million individuals aged 12 and over received some form of help to deal with a problem related to the use of alcohol or drugs (Substance Abuse and Mental Health Services Administration, 2007). According to the survey, the most popular sites for receiving help included the self-help group, the outpatient rehabilitation center, and the outpatient mental health center. Among the most frequent substances for which help was given were alcohol, marijuana, cocaine, pain relievers, and stimulants.

While the concern over adolescent substance use is a salient issue, it is imperative that we continue to consider the impact of parental substance abuse and its effect on the family system. Interviews with 70 opiate addicts in a methadone treatment program describe the effects of parental drug use on children (Kohler, Brown, Haertzen & Michaelson, 1994). For example, several addicts reported that their children experienced disruptive events in several areas (living circumstances, physical and sexual abuse, disability of parents and other adults in the home, or prolonged separation from the parent) prior to the child turning 19 years of age. Kohler and colleagues found that 14 percent of parents had a child placed in foster care, adoptive care, or a group home. Seven percent of parents had a child in a juvenile detention facility. Sixty percent had a child receive overnight hospitalization for a medical condition and 1 percent reported that the stay was for psychiatric care. Beyond disruptions in living situations, 46 percent of parents reported that they had struck a child with excessive force. Twenty-four percent of parents reported that they received mental health treatment since the birth of their child (Kohler, Brown, Haertzen & Michaelson, 1994).

The difficulties faced by children and parents when one or both of the adults in the family system are using drugs can be immense. Johnson and Leff (1999) contend that children with substance-abusing parents are at risk of developing problem behaviors because of the various factors that they are exposed to. While parents who use substances put themselves in jeopardy both emotionally and physically, Johnson and Leff argue that for children, "the single most potent risk factor is their parent's substance-abusing behavior; this single risk factor can place children of substance abusers at biologic, psychological, and environmental risk" (p.1086). For example, children of alcoholics face a greater risk of developing alcohol-related problems later in life (Belcher & Shinitzky, 1998; Erickson, 2007; Molina, 2006).

Moreover, the presence of substance use within the family system threatens to prevent and/or erode the bond between parent and child. In a review of research, Suchman, Mayes, Conti, Slade, and Rounsaville (2004) highlight that mothers who are dependent on drugs exhibit decreases in sensitivity and responsiveness, lack knowledge of child development, respond harshly or critically, exhibit low levels of tolerance, and often are at more risk for losing their children to foster care. The parent-child bond, as stated by the National Institute of Drug Abuse (NIDA) is the "bedrock of the relationship between parent and child" and further NIDA recommends that family-based prevention programs must focus on developing parent-child relationships and increasing the level of bonding within the parent-child unit (National Institute of Drug Abuse 2004, n.p.).

It is clear that substance use and abuse within a family is highly damaging, growth-defeating, and has deleterious effects. When one or more parents are using, children can suffer psychological and biological damage that can last throughout the course of development. More pertinent to this chapter, the relationship between parents and children can be strained or damaged and left untreated, may go on to suffer permanent damage. Therefore the purpose of this chapter is to apply the tenets of child-centered play therapy (CCPT) and filial therapy (FT) as a way to repair the bond between parent and child as well as offer suggestions on how to use CCPT to help children of substance-abusing parents to become more emotionally healthy. It should be noted that the model presented in this chapter is not intended to be used with parents who are currently using, rather these models are put forth as a way to help parents in recovery or non-using parents help build their relationship with their child. As noted earlier in this chapter, parents who are in the midst of substance use often do not have the capability to be fully sensitive, empathic, accepting, and non-judgmental in relationship with their child and the models presented are deeply and fervently built around these relational skills.

Child-Centered Play Therapy

Rogers' (1951, 1959) theoretical postulates of personality development and client-centered therapy provide a basis for the theory and practice of child-centered play therapy (Guerney, 2001; Landreth, 2002). In both his 1951 book entitled Client-Centered Therapy and his 1959 chapter in Koch's *Psychology: A Study of Science, Vol. 3,* Rogers clearly articulated a position on personality development that is fundamental to understanding child-centered play therapy.

Landreth (2002) cites Rogers (1951) frequently in order to present the conception of personality development in child-centered play therapy. Landreth highlights the person, phenomenal field, and the self as three core constructs that provide a basis to personality development within a child-centered play therapy context. The person is simply all that the child is, including her thoughts, feelings, behaviors, and physiology. The phenomenal field "includes all that is experienced by the organism, whether or not these experiences are consciously perceived" (Rogers, 1951, p. 483). The self according to Rogers (1959), develops from a discriminate part of one's experience that becomes forefront in awareness. Self-concept is the image of that awareness of self that is continuously changing in contrast to social relationships and environmental factors.

Rogers stated that individuals live within a "changing world of experience (phenomenal field) in which the individual is at the center" (1951, p.483). As an organized whole or total system of the person, the individual reacts to his perceptions of experience. Rogers argued against the notion of an absolute reality; rather he espoused the notion that for any individual reality is constituted by what is perceived.

Therefore, a fundamental concept underlying Rogers' theory is critical; individuals are continually striving towards self-actualization and enhanced experiencing. Landreth (2002) stated that, "The resulting behavior is basically the goal-directed, emotionally influenced attempt of the child to satisfy her needs as experienced. Therefore, the best vantage point for understanding the child's behavior is from the child's internal frame of reference" (p. 64).

Since the fundamental drive of the individual is toward a greater state of actualization, the behaviors displayed by the individual usually fit within one's concept of self. Behaviors that do not match the self-concept are not adopted. Personal difficulty or maladjustment occurs when one's experiences differ from one's self-concept. As Rogers (1951) stated, "Any experience which is inconsistent with the organization or structure of self may be perceived as a threat, and the more of these perceptions there are, the more rigidly the self-structure is organized to maintain itself" (p. 515). For example, a young boy who displays a highly sensitive and often volatile relational style perceives that other children often make too many mistakes and are going to get in trouble. His self-concept dictates that he is a "good" boy who is justified in correcting others actions. Socially, he finds it hard to make friends and his mother suggests that he relax and just have fun doing what the other boys are doing. However, the experience of "doing what the other boys do" and the behaviors associated with that contradict his self-concept so they are dismissed. Environmental tensions increase because the boy finds it hard to make friends and often gets picked on by other boys. He often feels depressed and lonely. Tensions increase with his parents because they are overwhelmed by the boy's lack of social cohesion and related difficulty in school. Perhaps anxiety about school is becoming an issue and the boy often remarks, "I hate school because nobody likes me." Evaluative statements from his mother such as, "You tell on other kids too much" and "You should-n't be so worried about what they are doing" result in the boy becoming more anxious and distraught in his relationship with his mother as he shouts back, "I don't tell too much. They are doing bad things and I don't want them to get in trouble." The boy does not accept the feedback from his moth-er because it poses a threat to his self-concept. Acceptance of himself as a tat-tletale is diametrically opposed to his self-concept of being justified in help-ing to keep other kids on the right path.

Rogers (1951) stated that only in the right conditions, in which no threat is present to the self-concept, can the individual begin to review experiences, revise them and integrate new experiences into the self-concept. As Landreth (2002) points out, the new more integrated self-concept becomes increasing-ly open to new experiences and more positive. Further, this helps the indi-vidual relate better to others.

Virginia Axline (1947, 1969), a student of Carl Rogers, postulated a non-directive or child-centered play therapy that builds on Rogers' notion that individuals are constantly striving, seeking need fulfillment, and self-actual-izing (Kirschenbaum, 1979). Axline posited that in an optimal environment such as the playroom, the child can use toys to "play out his feelings" while being exposed to empathy, structured limits, and acceptance, thus allowing the child to work through inner conflict (Axline, 1947, p. 9). This resulting decrease in inner conflict facilitates the child's self-actualization, growth, development, and the release of blocked emotion.

Filial Therapy

Suchman and colleagues (2004) presented several reasons why parent skills training programs fall short of helping parents to develop relationships with their children and in turn foster the psychological development of their children. The authors suggested that these types of programs may over-focus on behavior management techniques and are less interested in helping par-ents to develop their ability to be responsive, available, and in tune with their children. Filial therapy, on the other hand, is the polar opposite to these con-tentions.

Originally developed by Bernard Guerney in 1964, filial therapy, at its core, seeks to strengthen the parent-child relationship, not by employing a steadfast list of behavioral techniques but rather by helping the parent and child to connect on a deeply personal, emotional, and individual level through the implementation of play sessions. Filial therapy is about enhancing familial relationships through play and creating intentionally different ways of being within the parent-child dyad. Since the development of filial therapy, it has been adapted and used by all types of non-professional helpers (Vanfleet, 1994; Vanfleet & Guerney, 2003). Guerney (1964) wrote, "The parent-child relationship is nearly always the most significant one in a child's life. Therefore, if a child were provided the experiences of expression, insight, and adult acceptance in the presence of such power people as parents, every bit of success the parent achieves in carrying out the therapeutic role should be many more times more powerful that that of a therapist doing the same thing" (p. 309). This is an important message to put forth. Parents often represent the most meaningful and deepest relationships in a child's life. Even in stressful times or in less than positive familial relationships, one would find it difficult to argue that the parent-child connection could ever be completely lost.

The theory and practice of filial therapy is grounded in child-centered play therapy. Fundamentally, the parent learns the skills used by the child-centered play therapist to help the child become more emotionally expressive while fostering the relationship between both individuals. The 10 million dollar question still looms large at this point; what does the child-centered play therapist or parent do with a child?

Axline (1947) developed eight basic principles that guide the practice of child-centered play therapy and are equally inherent in the practice of filial therapy: (1) Build rapport with the child, (2) Accept the child unconditionally, (3) Establish a sense of permissiveness, (4) Reflect the child's feelings, (5) Maintain respect for the child, (6) Let the child lead the way, (7) Do not hurry the child, and (8) Establish limits as needed (pp. 73–74). As Landreth (2002) points out, the practice of child-centered play therapy and/or filial therapy can be more closely characterized as a personal style or way of being in relationship to children rather than a cadre of techniques employed with precision and skill at just the right time. Just as Rogers (1957) stressed empathy, genuineness, and unconditional positive regard as the conditions needed for change within therapy, so too did Axline make them a crucial part of her conceptions about play therapy.

In child-centered play therapy, the course of treatment is often 20–25 sessions; however, in filial therapy, parents can learn the method in roughly 10 weeks and continue using the model as long as it is beneficial to both the parent and the child. These particular forms of play therapy are often used with children between ages 3 and 11 because fantasy/expressive play is still perceived as fun and interesting. Play also becomes an important vehicle for self-expression because young children do not typically have the verbal skills to express themselves as would be expected in traditional talk therapy. Some skills that the parent learns and uses include empathic responding, the use of structuring statements, tracking responses, and limit-setting statements (Guerney, 1983; Landreth, 2002; Moustakas, 1973).

Empathic responses are parent responses that address the thoughts and feelings of the child (Guerney, 1983). Some examples of these responses are, "You just hate the toys in this room" or "You feel so frustrated when those blocks won't stand up the way that you want." Tracking statements are responses that capture more of the content of the play rather than the underlying feelings. An example of a tracking statement might be "It looks like you are stacking those blocks." Tracking statements indicate to the child that the parent is paying attention and involved (Landreth, 2002).

Structuring statements are those that inform the child about length of the play session and what the child can do within a session (Guerney, 1983). In my own work, I include an opening statement such as, "In the playroom you can say anything that you want to, do almost anything that you want to do and when we come to something that you cannot do, I will let you know." The use of opening statements allows the child to experience both a sense of structure and freedom.

As is evident from my example of an opening statement, limits are not stated at the outset. Less burden is placed upon the child and expression is facilitated when limits are stated when they arise rather than listed in the beginning of a play session (Axline, 1969; Guerney, 1983). As Guerney notes, limits in child-centered therapy are extremely important to keep individuals safe, help the child to build self-control, and show the child that the parent is not uncaring and lax. Limits on a child's behavior during a session are few and often prevent the child from destroying property or hurting himself or an adult (Axline, 1969; Guerney, 1983; Landreth, 2002).

The process of setting limits can vary. Guerney (1983) advocates for a three-step phase. For example, a child in the playroom decides that he wants to break the arm off of a plastic doll. In Guerney's model, the therapist would state the limit to the child, "In here, you cannot break the toys." If the child continues to try, then the therapist would state the limit again and offer a consequence such as ending the session. If the child tries a third time, then the consequence is imposed. Landreth's (2002) limit-setting process is similar; however, he adds an additional step of targeting an alternative behavior. For example, if a child attempts to paint the wall the therapist might say, "In here you cannot paint the wall. If you would like to paint, you can paint on the canvas in the corner."

Guerney (1983) provides the following guidelines when choosing toys that can be used in a session. She states that the toys that are selected should encourage the expression of difficult, real world feelings such as anger and dependence; toys should be able to be used in various ways; and they should also encourage use by more than one person. Dolls of different sizes, for example, are ideal because they can represent a family constellation, be used to denote power struggles, and can be utilized in many fantasy play situations. In addition, a game with rules is discouraged because although more than one person can use it, it does not usually promote creative, symbolic, and imaginative expression of feelings. Landreth (2002) posits the same guidelines as Guerney and also stresses that toys should be sturdy, promote exploratory play, and be selected carefully for their symbolic quality rather than amassed for the sake of having a numerous amount of toys available. Axline's (1947, 1969) original list of suggested toys is still useful today. Some examples of appropriate playroom toys are a doll house, family dolls, a baby bottle, eating/cooking utensils, clay, paints, water, sand, toy soldiers, little cars, and action figures. Landreth suggests many of the same toys and goes further to categorize toys into three different areas: (a) real-life toys, (b) acting-out aggressive release toys, and (c) toys for creative expression and emotional release.

Filial Therapy Research

Three studies with Asian parents and their children (Jang, 2000; Yuen, Landreth & Baggerly, 2002; Yuen-Fan Chau & Landreth, 1997) attempted to demonstrate the positive effects of child-centered play therapy techniques in the parent-child relationship. Yuen-Fan Chau and Landreth (1997) taught child-centered play therapy techniques to Chinese parents over the course of ten weeks and asked them to conduct play sessions with one of their children at home. Employing a control group design, Yuen-Fan Chau and Landreth randomly assigned 18 parents to the experimental group and 16 parents to the control group. Pre- and post-tests of the Porter Parental Acceptance Scale (PPAS) (Porter, 1954) and the Parenting Stress Index (PSI) (Abidin, 1983) were completed by the parents. The PPAS is a 40-item self-report assessment designed to measure parental acceptance characterized by behaviors displayed and feelings expressed towards one's children. The PSI is a 101-item self-report assessment designed to measure stress levels in parent-child relationships. Research on both measures indicates adequate reliability and validity (Abidin, 1997; Burchinal, Hawkes & Gardner, 1957; Porter, 1954). Study results indicate that the experimental group showed a significant increase in parental acceptance ($F (1,31) = 146.43$, $p < .05$) and a significant decrease in parent-child relational stress ($F (1,31) = 74.6$, $p < .05$) when compared to the control group.

Yuen, Landreth, and Baggerly (2002) also employed a control group design similar to Yuen-Fan Chau and Landreth (1997) in order to demonstrate positive effects of filial therapy with immigrant Chinese parents. The

18 parents in the experimental group and 17 parents in the control group were administered pre- and post-test measures of the PPAS and the PSI. Between pre- and post-test measure, parents were trained in the same way as Yuen-Fan Chau and Landreth's study and asked to conduct child-centered play therapy sessions at home. Study results indicate that the experimental group showed a significant increase in parental acceptance ($F_{(1,35)} = 6.580$, $p < .05$) and a significant decrease in parent-child relational stress ($F_{(1,35)} = 18.56$, $p < .05$) when compared to the control group.

Results from a study conducted by Jang (2000) do not support the findings previously mentioned. Jang did not find significant differences between experimental and control group scores on the PPAS and the PSI after filial training. However, Jang reports that interview data collected during the course of the study provide support that filial training had a positive effect for the Korean parents in her study. In regard to parental stress, the author claims that parents reported increases in feelings of acceptance and unconditional love for their children. Although not statistically significant, Jang states that the direction of change for pre- and post-test measure was positive.

In addition to these three studies, other filial research studies with similar designs show statistically significant differences in parental acceptance and parent-child stress with parents of chronically ill children (Tew, Landreth, Joiner & Solt, 2002), with single parents (Bratton & Landreth, 1995), and with parents whose children are experiencing learning difficulties (Kale & Landreth, 1999). However, a critical examination of these six studies highlights the issues of small sample size and generalizability. These studies employ relatively small numbers ($N < 30$) in each experimental and control group. As Kale and Landreth note, larger and more diverse samples are "desirable and necessary for greater generalization of findings" (p. 51). However, when taken together as a whole, the results in these studies continue to build a strong case for the provision of filial therapy.

The Case of Tim, Anna, Roger, and Katie

Tim met Anna in their senior year of college. Both were bright and energetic with abundant potential for positive growth. After graduating from college, Tim asked Anna to marry him and without hesitation they moved back to Anna's hometown. Shortly after this transition, they were married and Tim went to work as an apprentice engineer and Anna began her career as a high school English teacher. For many years, they were happy and content. They had many friends and participated in various community events and local get-togethers. Five years into their marriage and with stable careers and financial freedom, they decided to have a child. In October of that year, Roger was born.

The first few years of Rogers' life went extremely well for Tim and Anna. They almost seemed like the picture perfect family. Anna had quit her job to stay home with Roger and they even considered having another child. Almost three years to the date of Rogers' birth, Katie was born.

When Katie turned one year old, Roger developed a particularly troubling case of asthma that kept Tim and Anna up for most nights and in an almost constant state of fear. Tim's job required him to travel rather frequently and most times, Anna had full responsibility for the children. Although she longed to get back into teaching, the thought of leaving her children was an impossibility and she found herself having less and less contact with the out-side world. With Tim gone on a consistent basis, Anna felt the impinging pangs of stress and anxiety creeping up on her. When Tim came home, they found themselves arguing about the kids, their relationship, about responsibilities, about money, and about sex. The image of the picture perfect family had become a façade for those who looked on.

Anna had never been a big drinker. Her father had struggled with alcohol dependency for many years and he eventually died at age 65 from a heart attack. While she enjoyed the occasional cocktail, she never felt the urge to drink excessively; however, that began to change.

With the increasing feelings of stress, anxiety, and depression welling up in her about her kids and her marriage, Anna found that a couple glasses of wine at night helped her to relax after the kids were asleep. It was only a cou-ple glasses at night maybe once or twice a week at first. Those two nights turned into four after awhile and gradually increased to seven before too long. After awhile, a couple glasses turned into a half a bottle and then a full bottle before bed. She found herself taking a drink during the day when the kids went down for a nap in order to "take the edge off," as she liked to say.

Anna's drinking became steadily worse during the following year and she would often wake up with a hangover. She seemed to be woken up in the morning by her children's cries rather than by an alarm clock. The kids were often plunked down in front of the TV with breakfast so Anna could nap. Eventually Anna had such a difficult time functioning in the morning that she was barely able to attend to any of her children's needs. Drinking wine turned into drinking whatever was available while trying to hide it from Tim.

One afternoon, Tim returned home to find his kids in the front yard while Anna was passed out on the living room sofa. He suspected that this prob-lem had been going on for some time but was hesitant to ask for a divorce because of the kids. He thought that if he could stay home more he could compensate for Anna's problems.

Anna drank more and more and became increasingly belligerent and argumentative. The once sweet Anna had changed and Tim barely recog-nized her. Her relationships with her young children became strained as they grew and she was hardly available to them in any meaningful way. Roger and Katie both exhibited emotional and behavioral problems as a result of the constant chaos, the lack of structure, Tim's overcompensation for Anna, and Anna's lack of availability. The family was in crisis.

Case Discussion

After a considerable amount of time, Anna eventually sought help for alcoholism at an inpatient treatment facility after being confronted by Tim and other family members in an intervention setting. Anna has been sober for about 8 months now and wants to mend fences with her children, Roger and Katie now 8 and 5 years old respectively. At this point they do not trust her or feel a particular connection to her but both are extremely clingy with Tim. Tim wants to repair his relationship with Anna as well but also feels distrust and anxiety.

Among the many possible options for therapeutic intervention with this family, one might consider individual counseling for each member of the family, couples counseling for Anna and Tim or perhaps one might consider a family therapy approach. Within the context of repairing Anna's relationship with her children, child-centered play therapy and filial therapy may seem like a viable and worthwhile option.

The first step in working with this family would be to assess and understand the emotional and behavioral worlds of Roger and Katie. Given that they are both experiencing emotional and behavioral difficulties at this point in their lives, it would be most effective and ethically sound to begin individual child-centered play therapy with both children. Before we can think about having Anna conduct play sessions at home, it is imperative to allow the children to experience individual play therapy sessions in order to work through some of their issues and achieve some level of stability before having the parent work with the child.

Since the child leads the way in the play session, the process of the child-centered encounter will look different depending on the child. Landreth (2002) notes several objectives for the child during the course of therapy such as, "developing a more positive self-concept, becoming more self-directive, self-accepting, and self-responsible, experiencing more self-control and personal decision-making, being more sensitive to the process of coping, increasing self-trust, and developing internal evaluative ability" (p. 88). While it may seem that the therapist is a passive player on the child's journey, she is not. As both Axline (1969) and Guerney (1983) point out, the therapist engages with the child, participates actively in the child's play, and works to help the child become more emotionally expressive.

For both Roger and Katie, we would employ a mix of toys that foster aggressive play (e.g., bop bag, alligator puppet, plastic sword), nurturing play (e.g., a baby doll, a baby bottle), real-life play (e.g., plastic food, a kitchen set), tactile/construction play (e.g., sand, water, legos), family play/role play (e.g., dress-up clothes, family dolls, a doll house), and art/music play (e.g., paints, markers, a drum, small keyboard). The sessions themselves would be led by the children and each child would have the opportunity to play out difficulties pertinent to them. The child-centered play therapist does not direct the session to fit a preconceived notion of what might be problematic for a child. Even in the case of Roger and Katie, our professional mind might long to have each child play out a family dynamic because we are quite certain that this is where the trouble lies but using this model we make no assumptions that we know more about what hurts than the child does.

For both Roger and Katie, the act of playing and the special relationship with the therapist can allow these children to be expressive in many ways. We may notice a wide array of themes that emerge from the play including power and control, aggression and nurturing, and loss. It is our best hope that child play therapy will affect Roger and Katie on two levels. First, we want the relationship that we form with them to be different from other relationships that they have experienced. Their relationship with Anna has been marked with feelings of disappointment, loss, stress, worry, and uncertainty. The relationship we form with them will be characterized by empathy, acceptance, genuineness, warmth, and caring. We work to place responsibility and decision-making squarely on the shoulders of the child. Further, we would work to set consistent limits throughout the session to convey predictability and safety. This attitude is critical to help the child express the most difficult of emotions. For these children it may be angry feelings toward Anna, feelings of inadequacy or low self-concept, or feelings of sadness and loss. In child-centered play therapy, we want to create a space for experiencing so that the child can show us how they perceive themselves in the moment.

Second, we want the child to be affected by the act of playing. As Schaefer (1993, 2003) noted, play has many therapeutic benefits. Play can allow the child to express difficult emotions symbolically rather than verbally. Further, play can be cathartic and also help the child to achieve mastery over difficult emotions by playing them out over and over again. Through play, children have the opportunity to try out different roles and emotions and experiment with new ways of being. Further, play allows a child the opportunity to solve problems, improve self-control, feel more competent, and have fun. For example, our work with Katie may highlight her need to replay a relationship in which a doll is abandoned in a forest and left without a mother. In this play, the doll is lost, sad, and crying. As the play continues the doll must learn to care for itself even though she is scared and longing for contact with others.

Once each child has had a chance for emotional expression through individual play therapy and the family dynamic seems conducive to parent-child work, we can begin teaching Anna how to play with her child. In Anna's case, we would want to be assured that she is sober, is serious about rebuilding her relationship, and has spent some time in individual therapy working on her own issues. Fundamentally, one must make sure that the child will be emotionally safe and the parent is willing and able to become emotionally and physically available to the child.

Using the 10 session filial therapy model for training parents entitled, *Child-Parent Relationship Therapy* (Bratton, Landreth, Kellam & Blackard, 2006), we can begin teaching Anna a child-centered way of being. Bratton and colleagues (2006) have created an easy to follow and comprehensive treatment protocol for teaching parents filial therapy. It should be noted that therapists interested in this work should receive training in filial therapy prior to attempting it. Additionally, Bratton et al. have designed this protocol to be used with groups of parents but the approach can be adapted to work with individuals and couples as well.

As noted earlier in this chapter, drug dependent parents often lack the ability to be present and available for their children in a growth-promoting fashion. Filial therapy, in turn, will challenge the parent to adapt a new way of being and as Bratton and colleagues state, "In this special relationship there are no reprimands, put-downs, evaluations, requirements, or judgments" (p. 186). The suggestion here is that we will aim to reverse the parental behaviors that often characterize the parent-child relationship when substance abuse is involved. In the *Child-Parent Relationship Therapy* model, parents are asked to conduct 30-minute play sessions once a week. Among the various concepts that they will be exposed to, parents learn how to conduct a play session, reflect a child's thoughts and feelings, pay attention to a child, recognize emotions, set limits in a clear, consistent, and empathic manner, recognize special qualities about their children, let the child lead, and encourage decision-making and responsibility. It is critical that parents feel successful and positive in this work so the trainer works hard not to be critical of the parent but rather the trainer seeks to capitalize on the parent's strengths and desires to improve the relationship with their child.

Conceptually, this model can offer the recovering parent the opportunity to learn or relearn a healthy parenting style based on the child's needs and the child's primary mode of communication. Moreover, this approach can reinvigorate the loss of fun or joy that is often missing in these eroded parent-child relationships. For Anna, life had become about her and her addiction and the joy she once experienced with her children had long since disappeared. The filial therapy puts the relationship first and allows both parent and child to experience each other in a genuine and real way. For addicted parents, their addiction and ingrained patterns of behavior may make this approach tenuous. Currently, there is a dearth of research and practice literature regarding filial therapy with parents in recovery that keeps this work largely in the conceptual realm. This chapter is written with the hope that those who work with families suffering with addiction will be intrigued with the concept of filial therapy so that our collective knowledge about this work will be expanded in the years to come.

Appendix–Terms

Child-centered Play Therapy–Child-centered play therapy is a form of play therapy developed by Virginia Axline. Therapists using this form of therapy let the child lead, respond empathically, set consistent limits, and encourage symbolic and expressive play.

Filial Therapy–A form of child-centered play therapy in which a child's parent assumes a role similar to that of the child-centered play therapist in order to facilitate the play session with their child.

Empathic Responses–Empathic responses are child-centered play therapist responses that address the thoughts and feelings of the child (Guerney, 1983).

Tracking Statements–Tracking statements are child-centered play therapist statements that capture more of the content of the play rather than the underlying feelings.

References

Abidin, R. (1983). *Parenting stress index.* Charlottesville, VA: Pediatric Psychology Press.

Abidin, R. R. (1997). The Parenting Stress Index: A measure of the parent-child system. In C. P. Zalaquett and R. J. Woods (Eds.), *Evaluating stress* (pp. 271–291). Lathan, MD: University Press of America.

Axline, V. M. (1947). *Play therapy.* Boston: Houghton Mifflin Company.

Axline, V. M. (1969). *Play therapy* (Revised ed.). NY: Ballantine Books.

Belcher, H. M. E., & Shinitzky, H. E. (1998) Substance abuse in children: Prediction, protection, and prevention. *Archives of Pediatrics and Adolescent Medicine, 152*(10), 952–960.

Bratton, S. C., Landreth, G. L., Kellam, T., & Blackard, S. R. (2006) *Child parent relationship therapy (CPRT) treatment manual.* NY: Routledge.

Burchinal, L., Hawkes, G., & Gardner, B., (1957). The relationship between parental acceptance and adjustment of children. *Child Development, 28,* 67–77.

Erickson, C. K. (2007). *The science of addiction.* NY: W.W. Norton and Company.

Guerney, B. G., Jr. (1964). Filial therapy: Description and rationale. *Journal of Consulting Psychology, 28*(4), 303–310.

Guerney, L. (1983). Client-centered (nondirective) play therapy. In C. E. Schaefer & K. J. O'Conner (Eds.), *Handbook of play therapy* (pp. 21–64). NY: John Wiley and Sons.

Guerney, L. (2001). Child-centered play therapy. *International Journal of Play Therapy, 10*(2), 13–31.

Jang, M. (2000). Effectiveness of filial therapy for Korean parents. *International Journal of Play Therapy, 9*(2), 39–56.

Johnson, J. L., & Leff, M. (1999). Children of substance abusers: Overview of research findings. *Pediatrics, 103,* 1085–1099.

Kale, A. L., & Landreth, G. L. (1999). Filial therapy with parents of children experiencing learning difficulties. *International Journal of Play Therapy, 8*(2), 35–56.

Kirschenbaum, H. (1979) *On becoming Carl Rogers.* New York: Delacorte Press.

Kohler, A. F., Brown, B. S., Haertzen, C. A., & Michaelson, B. S. (1994). Children of substance abusers: The life experiences of children of opiate addicts in methadone clinics. *American Journal of Drug & Alcohol Abuse, 20*(2), 159–171.

Landreth, G. L. (2002). *Play therapy: The art of the relationship* (2nd ed.). NY: Brunner-Routledge.

Molina, B. S. G. (2006). High risk adolescent and young adult populations: Consumption and consequences. In M. Galanter (Ed.), *Alcohol problems in adolescents and young adults: Epidemiology, neurobiology, prevention, and treatment* (pp. 49–65). NY: Springer.

Moustakas, C. E. (1973). *Children in play therapy.* NY: Jason Aronson, Inc.

National Institute on Drug Abuse. (2004). *NIDA info facts: Lessons from prevention research.* Retrieved on April 18, 2006 from http://www.nida.nih.gov/infofacts/Infofaxindex.html

Office of National Drug Control Policy. (2008). *Drug dealer.* Retrieved April 26, 2008 from http://www.theantidrug.com

Office of National Drug Control Policy. (2008a). *What you can do? Tips for preventing RX abuse.* Retrieved April 26, 2008 from http://www.theantidrug.com/drug_info/prescription_what_can_you_do.asp

Porter, B. (1954). Measurement of parental acceptance of children. *Journal of Home Economics, 46,* 176–182.

Rogers, C. R. (1951). *Client-centered therapy: Its current practice, implications, and theory.* Boston: Houghton Mifflin.

Rogers, C. R. (1957). The necessary and sufficient conditions of therapeutic personality change. *Journal of Consulting Psychology, 21*(2), 95–103.

Rogers, C. R. (1959). A theory of therapy, personality and interpersonal relationships as developed in the client-centered framework. In Koch, S. (Ed.). *Psychology: A study of a science. Vol. III. Formulations of the person and the social context* (pp. 184–256). New York: McGraw Hill.

Schaefer, C. E. (1993). What is play and why is it therapeutic? In C. E. Schaefer (Ed.), *Therapeutic powers of play* (pp. 1–16). Northvale, NJ: Jason Aronson, Inc.

Schaefer, C. E. (Ed.). (2003). *Foundations of play therapy.* Hoboken, NJ: John Wiley and Sons.

Substance Abuse and Mental Health Services Administration. (2007). *Results from the 2006 National Survey on Drug Use and Health: National Findings* (Office of Applied Studies, NSDUH Series H-32, DHHS Publication No. SMA 07-4293). Rockville, MD. Retrieved April 15, 2008 from http://www.oas.samhsa.gov/nsduh/2k6nsduh/2k6results.pdf

Suchman, N., Mayes, L., Conti, J., Slade, A., & Rounsaville, B. (2004). Rethinking parenting interventions for drug-dependent mothers: From behavior management to fostering emotional bonds. *Journal of Substance Abuse, 27,* 179–185.

Tew, K., Landreth, G., Joiner, K. D., & Solt, K. D. (2002). Filial therapy with parents of chronically ill children. *International Journal of Play Therapy, 11*(1), 79–100.

Vanfleet, R. (1994). *Filial therapy: Strengthening parent-child relationships through play.* Sarasota, FL: Professional Resource Press.

Vanfleet, R., & Guerney, L. (2003). *Casebook of filial therapy.* Boiling Springs, PA: Play Therapy Press.

Yuen, T., Landreth, G., & Baggerly, J. (2002). Filial therapy with immigrant Chinese families. *International Journal of Play Therapy, 11*(2), 63–90.

Yuen-Fan Chau, I., & Landreth, G. L. (1997). Filial therapy with Chinese parents: Effects on parental empathic interactions, parental acceptance of child, and parental stress. *International Journal of Play Therapy, 6*(2), 75–92.

Biography

Stephen P. Demanchick, Ph.D., LMHC is an Assistant Professor for the Creative Arts Department at Nazareth College. He earned his Ph.D. in Counselor Education from the University of Rochester in October 2007. Stephen is also a NIRE certified child-centered play therapist.

Chapter 9

SONGS, MUSIC AND SOBRIETY: AN OVERVIEW OF MUSIC THERAPY IN SUBSTANCE ABUSE

ANNIE HEIDERSCHEIT

The Incidence and Impact of Chemical Dependency

Chemical dependency is perhaps the most common disease encountered by modern medicine. In 1991, the United States Surgeon General announced that according to the Department of Health and Human Services and the Substance Abuse and Mental Health Services Administration, "An estimated 18 million adult Americans have medical, social, and personal problems directly related to the use of alcohol, as do several million adolescents for whom alcohol is an illegal drug" (Milkman & Sederer, 1990, p. 7).

The 2003 National Survey on Drug Use and Health estimates that 19.5 million Americans are current illicit drug users (SAMSHA, 2003). This means that they had engaged in using an illicit drug at least once during the 30 days prior to the interview. This number represents 8.2 percent of the population 12 years old and older. This is a significant increase from the 1991 survey. The survey results indicated that 33 million of this group engaged in binge drinking, and 12 million were heavy drinkers, meaning they had 5 or more drinks on one occasion 5 or more days during the past 30 days (SAMSHA, 2003).

A National Longitudinal Alcohol Epidemiological Survey conducted by the National Institute on Abuse and Alcoholism and Bureau of the Census (NIAAA, 2000) in 2003 estimates that 4.4 percent of adults were alcohol dependent and another 3 percent were classified as abusing alcohol with the past year. The Executive Office of the President and Office of Drug Control Policy (SAMSHA, 2003) conducted a study in 1996-2002 to evaluate the

136

economic costs of drug abuse in the United States. The study was published in July 2003 and indicates that the overall cost of drug abuse to society increased by a rate of 5.9 percent annually. Thus, by 2002, the societal cost of drug abuse was $143.4 billion. The study estimates that by 2003 the cost would rise to $152.5 billion and by 2004 to $160.7 billion. In the first half of 2002, hospitals in the United States reported 292,098 estimated drug-related emergencies in which illegal drugs were the presenting problem and 535,646 emergency room visits in which drugs were mentioned in the physicians report but were not the presenting problem (SAMSHA, 2001a).

These statistics illustrate the widespread and national problems of substance use and abuse (McNeece & Barbanell, 2005). The statistics seem overwhelming and yet chemical dependency is rarely diagnosed (Doweiko, 2002) and even the experts are still in disagreement as to whether it is a disease or a behavior problem (McNeece & Barbanell, 2005). These issues related to diagnosis are simply one point of consideration. There are additional factors even when the diagnosis is given.

Many issues complicate the process of recognizing an addiction and the individual receiving the necessary treatment. The challenge for families and healthcare providers is that chemical dependency and addiction expresses itself differently from one individual to the next. The addiction may manifest itself differently in an individual depending on the duration of the addiction or use, the individual's overall health, financial situation, social and personal resources (Buelow & Buelow, 1998; Doweiko, 2002; Edwards & Lader, 1994; Wilcox & Erickson, 2005).

Chemical Dependency and Coping

The genesis of substance use and dependence varies from person to person, as do the theories surrounding it. There is not one explanation for why people become addicted to drugs or alcohol (Edwards & Lader, 1994; McNeece & Barbanell, 2005; Milkman & Sederer, 1990). In fact, there are multiple risk factors involved: an individual's psychological state [using the substance to relieve stress, anxiety or tension] (Gottheil, Druley, Pashko & Weinstein, 1987; Wilcox & Erickson, 2005), psychopathology (Doweiko, 2002; Robson, 1999; Wilcox & Erickson, 2005), family history, biology, and genetics (Leonard & Blane, 1999; Wilcox & Erickson, 2005), social and cultural influences (Dodgen & Shea, 2000; Hawkins, 2005), and medical conditions (DiNitto & Webb, 2005; Schuckit, 2000). Due to the many factors influencing the process, numerous theories have been formulated and explored.

Researchers have concluded that biological factors are a crucial component in this phenomenon (McNeece & Barbanell, 2005; Milkmann & Sederer, 1990). However, the genetics and biology have not been the only factors that influence individuals. In the diagnostic criteria, the physiological aspects of chemical dependency are addressed, along with the psychological aspects of dependency and abuse. Researchers (Doweiko, 2002; Wilcox & Erickson, 2005) argue that the use of one model of treatment, merely focusing on the biological aspects of addictions, is not effective treatment. The psychological component is an essential factor in the process of treatment.

Psychiatric Comorbidities

Some research indicates a relationship between chemical dependency and various forms of psychopathology (Vaillant, 1983; Wolkstein, 2002). Researchers report that individuals with a diagnosis of major depression are seven times more likely to also be diagnosed with a drug use disorder (Wise, Cuff & Fisher, 2001). Kessler et al. (1994) found that 41 percent of those with any Axis I mood (affective) disorder, also have some type of addictive disorder. Thirty-eight percent of those diagnosed with an anxiety disorder also have an addictive disorder. And 82 percent of those diagnosed with an Axis II disorder (conduct disorder or adult antisocial behavior also have an addictive disorder. Khantzian (1999) found that addicts often reported sensation seeking and anxiety reduction as reasons why they began daily opiate use.

Edwards and Lader (1994) report there is no evidence that demonstrates that depression leads to dependency on any drug. However, Merikangas, Mehta, Molnar, Walters, Swendsen, Aguilar-Gaziola, Bijl, Borges, Caraveo-Anduaga, DeWitt, Vega, Wittchen, & Kessler (1998) completed an international study based on six countries. They also found strong associations between substance use disorders and mood, anxiety, conduct and antisocial personality disorders across their sites.

The National Council on Child Abuse and Neglect (2001) reports that alcohol and drug-related family violence remains high, with an estimated 826,000 child victims of family violence in 1999. The National Institute for Alcohol Abuse and Alcoholism (NIAAA, 2000) report that as many as 60 percent of male alcoholics were violent toward a woman partner within the last year, and alcohol is also implicated in 30 percent of all child abuse cases. Lieboschutz, Mulvey and Samet (1997) found that 42 percent of the women they sampled who were seeking chemical dependency treatment had been physically or sexually abused at some point in their lives. Windle, Windle, Scheidt and Miller (1995) found that of the individuals undergoing inpatient treatment for alcoholism, 49 percent of the women and 12 percent of the men reported they had been sexually abused.

It is clear from the research that substance use and abuse is linked to mood states, various types of abuse, and psychopathology. The genesis of the addiction is not the only aspect to explore when trying to understand coping and chemical dependency. Quinn, Shepard, and Rose (1973) conducted a National Quality of Employment Survey and the results revealed that a variety of stress indicators including low self-esteem and depression were associated with escapist drinking. Dare (1998) also explored the issue of an individual's utilizing a substance to alter their affect following a particular experience. The model demonstrates how the individual experiences or recalls a painful experience which produces a negative affect or emotion. Khantzian (1999) and Forrest (1985) hypothesized that addicts turn to a chemical in order to regulate their internal life, more specifically their emotional state. The individual does not wish to experience these feelings and uses a substance to alter their affect. The pattern is maintained as the individual continually attempts to escape the negative emotional experiences.

According to the National Household Survey on Drug Abuse, one in ten Americans ages 12 or older had driven under the influence of alcohol at least once in the preceding 12 months (SAMSHA, 2001a). Among young adults between the ages of 18–25, the rate is nearly 20 percent. The Bureau of Justice (1988) report that between 1970 and 1986, arrests for drunk driving increased by 223 percent. According to the United States Department of Justice (1999), the number of individuals under correctional supervision for driving under the influence (DUI) increased from 270,100 in 1986 to 454,500 in 1997. Six percent of prison inmates and 12 percent of jail inmates reported they had previously been sentenced for DUI five or more times (BOJS, 1999). These individuals also reported that they drink to relieve tension, to relax, to be more social, and for comfort.

Many studies that focus on stress and alcohol consumption have reported that the subjects acknowledge they drink in response to stress. The studies indicate that subjects drink as a means of coping with economic or job stress, marital problems and the absence of social support (Jennison, 1992; Kalant, 1990; Kinney, 2000; McNeece & Barbanell, 2005; Sadava & Pak, 1993). Additionally, subjects also reported the more severe or chronic the stressor, the greater the consumption of alcohol (Pohorecky, 1991). However, this response is also dependent upon if the individual perceives a sense of control in the situation, feels adequate social support, type of stressor, and the range of ability to cope (Sadava & Pak, 1993; Volpicelli, 1987). Pohorecky (1991) also reported that alcohol consumption increased by 30 percent in the two years following a flood in Buffalo Creek, West Virginia.

The research also addresses issues of coping following treatment episodes and issues related to relapse. Following treatment for chemical dependency or substance abuse, individuals experience a high relapse rate. Relapse rates vary from one treatment program to another but these rates can be as high as 90 percent (Edwards & Lader, 1994; Wilcox & Erickson, 2005). A considerable amount of research has focused on the reasons for relapse. Cummings, Gordon and Marlatt (1980) found that 71 percent of alcohol relapses were related to three high risk situations. These include: negative emotional states (such as anger and depression), a conflict, argument, or unpleasant encounter with another person and pressures from others.

Situations that an individual in recovery encounter can be the trigger to once again turn to the substance. Relying on the substance or chemical as a method of coping with a situation or mood state is often referred to as "escapism." The individual may be utilizing the substance to escape or avoid the negative emotional state or situation (Kinney, 2000; McNeece & Barbanell, 2005). Rhoads (1983) and Judson, Goldstein and Inturrisi (1983) found that heroin addicts relapsed mainly due to negative emotional states and a lack of social support. Kosten, Kreek, Ragunath, and Kleber (1986) found after a two and a half-year follow-up study, heroin addicts encountered more negative life experiences following treatment, as well as increased levels of depression in subsequent treatment intakes.

The research literature and clinical data demonstrate that individuals often use a substance to cope with stressful life events, psychological traumas, and psychopathology. This is a primary factor of consideration in the treatment process. Whether the substance is utilized to reduce negative affect or gain a more positive affect, essentially the substance is used to alter how one feels. This method of coping may be one pathway to addiction and the research also illustrates that this is also a factor in relapse. It is evident that finding ways to manage these experiences and feelings is essential in the process of treating individuals with a chemical addiction. Without adequately addressing and treating these coping styles, the individual will leave treatment unable to manage stressful life events; thus, simply relying on old, maladaptive patterns and methods of coping.

Essentially, the recovering individual is drawn back into the cycle of use, abuse, and addiction for lack of a better way to manage these life experiences. Individuals frequently engage in using a substance as a means of coping with psychological, emotional, or interpersonal issues they feel ill-equipped to manage. Engaging in substance use to manage these issues does not bring resolution for these issues and often brings to the forefront a variety of other issues.

These may include marital and family problems, work-related issues, increased substance use, chronic health concerns related to substance use, and financial or legal problems. Heiderscheit (2005), developed a conceptual framework (see Appendix B) to address the complex needs of the individual seeking substance abuse treatment. Addressing these issues is a necessary component of treating the addiction and helping the individual change these maladaptive ways of coping. Additionally, tailoring the approach to the individual is a key component of the treatment process, including the implementation of innovative approaches.

Music Therapy

Music is a universal experience in which individuals from all backgrounds and cultures create, experience, perform, and engage in the art form. Everyone has experiences with music and has developed their own specific music preferences (Davis & Gfeller, 1999). Music therapy is the prescriptive use of music to address the needs of an individual or group (Heiderscheit, 2008). In the music therapy process, music is the applied medium which facilitates the achievement of the therapeutic goals in the process of therapy.

A music therapist utilizes music to address physical, emotional, cognitive, and social needs. Music therapy sessions are designed to address the following needs (AMTA, 2006; Heiderscheit, 2008): improve and facilitate communication, manage stress and anxiety, facilitate expression of feelings, explore and resolve emotional issues, improve self-esteem, develop new insights, develop self-acceptance and self-concept, and discover and develop new ways of coping.

Music therapy techniques vary greatly among clinical settings and with clinical populations. Music can be meaningful in a variety of ways to a variety of individuals because it is a flexible art form (Thaut & Gfeller, 1999). Music therapists implement support-oriented interventions that require active engagement in the here and now, insight and process-oriented sessions that facilitate problem solving, self-awareness, and emotional expression, or catalytic experiences that uncover and resolve subconscious conflicts (Houghton, Scovel, Smeltekop, Thaut, Unkefer & Wilson, 2005).

Rationale for Music Therapy

The music therapist employs methods and interventions tailored to meet the presenting needs of the individual. An issue of concern in healthcare today is substance abuse. Medical and health complications may arise as a result of the substance use and consequently the individual may encounter a physical dependence to the substance (APA, 2000).

In chemical dependency treatment, individuals present a variety of needs. The individual faces the stressors that may have led them to using the substance, along with the stressors that have surfaced as a result of the use of the substance. Addressing the issues that lead to the substance use as well as the interpersonal, mental, and physical health issues is imperative for this clinical population. Due to the fact that a myriad of complications and comorbities can accompany an individual in substance abuse treatment, the treatment process must be able to address the wide array of needs. The complexities of each individual and their clinical presentation support and require utilizing a modality that is equally complex and yet easily approachable. This ultimately requires matching the client to the appropriate therapy medium and intervention. The flexibility of music as a therapeutic agent allows the therapist to individualize the process and also meet a wide variety of needs simultaneously.

Music offers a unique means of expression at a time when feelings and emotions may be fragmented, elusive, and inaccessible to language. In the practice of music therapy, music functions as a catalyst for human emotions. Music is able to tap into the deepest of human emotions and provide a release for those feelings that words may not adequately express (Langer, 1967). Parente (1989) suggests that music therapy improvisation allows the client to explore and express emotions in a non-verbal manner and that this act of musical expression serves as a bridge between the conscious mind and the expression of those feelings. Nolan (1989) also states that "improvisation is useful in facilitating psychotherapy because it stimulates the awareness and expression of emotions and ideas on an immediate level" (p.167).

A number of clinicians have described their clinical applications of the Bonny Method of Guided Imagery and Music (GIM) in addictions treatment. Summer (1988) believes that GIM can assist the client in achieving sobriety (letting go), which is the first step in the 12-Step Alcoholics Anonymous (AA) process. Summer further states that GIM brings to light issues that often interfere with the therapy process and sobriety. And furthermore, that "GIM changes the basic addictive formula from tension–alcohol–tension reduction to tension–GIM–tension reduction" (p. 43).

Borling (1992) proposes a rationale for the use of GIM in the recovery process of addictions. He suggests that GIM can assist in dealing with emotions that have long been denied or repressed, often the very emotions that may have fueled the addiction. Confronting these emotions begins the process of changing old behavior patterns. Pickett (1991) described her work with a woman with a dual diagnosis, including addiction to alcohol. She identifies that it was during the course of the GIM sessions that the client began to confront her feelings of rejection, deprivation, and abuse. Pickett purports that the creative process of GIM allows the client to discover their own human potential and ability to heal.

Skaggs (1997) also writes that the music and imagery process is beneficial in the treatment process in that it allows clients to: view their life from various perspectives, develop a sense of inner trust, resolve internal conflicts, alter moods, develop self awareness, experience a healthy model of coping, and create a sense of cohesion with the fragmented parts of one's life. The GIM experience allows the individual to access and confront those parts of themselves that they have utilized the substance to avoid and repress.

Heiderscheit (2005) conducted an experimental study utilizing GIM with adults in inpatient chemical dependency treatment. She found that after an average of nearly six GIM sessions, subjects demonstrated significant decreases in three of the eight subscales on the Inventory of Interpersonal Problems. Experimental subjects reported decreased struggles with domineering, cold, and non-assertive behaviors in the interpersonal relationships. Additionally, experimental subjects demonstrated a significant increase in their ability to better manage life's challenges and demands based on the Sense of Coherence Scale.

Although the literature on the application of music therapy in the chemical dependency treatment is limited, the references and literature are still noteworthy. The illustrations outlined in the previous paragraphs support the clinical implementation of music therapy for adults in chemical dependency treatment. The case examples that follow further demonstrate and clarify how music therapy is an integral component in the recovery process and how music uniquely meets the vast and complex needs of adults in treatment.

Clinical Illustrations

The names of the individuals utilized in the case illustrations have been changed to protect their identity. Additionally, specific identifying details have been altered or deleted to further protect their identity. The details of the therapeutic process have not been altered to illustrate the role of music therapy in the overall treatment process.

The Case of Joe and Song Communication

When a client brings a song into therapy session, they are providing a window into their world. The client is communicating what they are consciously aware of, but also that which has not yet come into conscious awareness. Joe had not yet come to grips with his vulnerability. He wanted to be the strong man that others could rely on. Joe consciously recognized his desire to be reliable, but he was unaware of his weak, vulnerable side that needed someone to rely on.

Joe is a 37-year-old African-American male attending a chemical dependency program for individuals with a dual diagnosis (this included a diagnosis of mental illness and chemical dependency). Joe was struggling to overcome a cocaine addiction while learning to manage his depression. Joe had grown up in an abusive home. His father was an alcoholic and physically abused Joe and his siblings. Joe believed his mother was aware of the abuse, but was powerless to stop it.

Joe attended weekly music therapy sessions at the chemical dependency program day treatment program. The members of the group were asked to bring in a song to the upcoming session. The only guidelines given to the group included that the song be important to them or communicate something about them. Joe came to the next session with a recording of "Count on Me" (1995) written by Babyface and performed by Whitney Houston and CeCe Winans.

> *Count on me through thick and thin, a friendship that will never end.*
> *When you are weak I will be strong, helping you to carry on.*
> *Call on me I will be there, don't be afraid.*
> *Please believe when I say, count on me.*
> *I can see it's hurting you, I can feel the pain.*
> *It's hard to see the sunshine through the rain.*
> *I know sometimes it seems as if it's never gonna end.*
> *But you'll get through it, just don't give in.*

The group listened to the song and afterward, Joe told the group that these were the words he wanted to speak to everyone. He wanted everyone to know that they could count on him. He would be there for them when they needed someone to help. When the music therapist asked Joe, "Is there anyone in your life you want to hear these words from?" Joe became tearful and shared that he wanted to hear his wife speak these words to him. He was afraid she would leave him after all the years of cocaine abuse and he felt he needed her support to recover.

The gender of the vocalist is pivotal in the relationship of the client and the song; two female vocalists perform this song. Since the gender of the vocalist(s) is not the same as the gender of the client, this can be an indication that these may be words the client may wish to hear. If the gender of the vocalist is the same as the gender of the client, it can be an indication that these are words that the client may wish to speak (Heiderscheit, 2008).

In this case, these were not words that Joe wanted to speak, these were words he wanted to hear, but this was outside of his conscious awareness. Two women who project their strength vocally perform this song. This is image that did not describe Joe, but the strength he wanted and needed from the women in his life. He had lacked a strong female presence in his life from childhood. His mother could not stop the abuse by his father. Now that he is working to overcome his cocaine addition and cope with his depression, he wants to know that the significant female in his life has the strength to help him. Joe was projecting onto this song the words he wanted to hear from his wife. Consciously he was not aware of his desire to have someone to lean on, but his subconscious knew the road to sobriety was not to be easy and that he could not go it alone.

The Case of Rose and Song Analysis

Rose was in her mid-fifties when I first met her. She was referred to a chemical dependency program for individuals with a dual diagnosis. In addition to her addiction to alcohol, she suffered from major depression. Rose attended the weekly music therapy session that I lead at this program.

When Rose first began attending the music therapy sessions, she was quiet and often withdrawn. She did not appear to have much hope for herself. She seemed resigned to the fact that her life would always be a complete disaster. She shared in group that her ex-husband was in prison, soon to be out on parole. And she was fearful that he would try to physically harm her. Rose was also experiencing many difficulties with her teenage son. He was refusing to attend school, staying out all night, staying away from home for days at a time, and also drinking.

Rose was currently living with a man who was also an alcoholic. She began to realize that she was supporting him financially, by providing him with food, shelter, alcohol, and bail for jail. The final straw came when he took her car, was arrested for driving without a valid license, which resulted in having the car impounded. This left Rose with the responsibility of appearing in court and paying the court and impound fees.

This experience pushed Rose to begin a process of self-examination. She slowly began to discover how she had allowed others to control her life. She began to get mad and finally decided to stand up for herself and make some changes. It was during this process of discovery and change that Rose brought a song into the music therapy session. She had asked me prior to the session if she could share the song with the group. I agreed to her request and she told the group a friend had given her the recording of this song. The song was "A Rose is Still a Rose" performed by Aretha Franklin.

> *Listen dear, I realize that you've been hurt deeply.*
> *Because I've been there, but regardless to*
> *Who, what, why, when and where*
> *We are all precious in His sight.*
> *And a rose is still and always will be a rose.*
> *There was a Rose I knew I met her once of twice before.*
> *She was a pretty sweet thing, not the least bit insecure.*
> *Then you came with your sticky game and player with her youth,*
> *Unashamed of the way you lied and played with her.*
> *She never knew what hit her. Steal her honey then forget her.*
> *She was awesome, trying to forget about you.*
> *Because a rose is still a rose, Baby you're still a flower.*
> *He can leave you and take you, make you and then break you.*
> *Darling, you hold the power.*

The song begins with Aretha gently speaking the words, softly accompanied by upper strings and free movement on the upper octaves of the piano. This introduction portrays a feeling of empathy and compassion to the listener. Aretha's tender voice gives the listener the sense that she too has had a similar experience. Following the introduction, a strong, steady beat begins while Aretha scats for six measures. She then begins singing her story in a voice full of power and conviction. In this process of telling her story, she demonstrated that she did not succumb to the pain. She survived and thrived.

Rose was struck by how this song seemed to directly address the reality of her life. She shared with the group that despite the fact that she had been used and abused by the men in her life, she was still valuable as a person. Rose received a great deal of feedback and support from her peers. She began to see that her past did not need to control or determine her future. She had not realized until now that she was the one who holds the power in her life. Hearing these words from another woman (Aretha Franklin) was like an epiphany for Rose. She gained strength from hearing these words from a powerful woman who is familiar with pain and suffering. Rose was able to see herself in Aretha.

Shortly after this session, she began to make some major changes in her life. She finally ended her relationship with the man she was living with and took steps to protect herself from her ex-husband. She chose to eliminate other unhealthy relationships in her life and refused to let others use her again. She began to look at her priorities in life and not let others determine them for her. She placed her children and grandchildren as a top priority. Rose discovered that she was valuable and worthwhile and that she could take back the power in her life.

Case Illustration of Group Songwriting

The process of writing a song can feel like an overwhelming task for an individual or group, especially for a group of women that have encountered constant struggle, disappointment, and failure in life. However, when it is incorporated into the therapeutic process under the guidance of a music therapist, the experience can be empowering. The following is a song written by a group of women at a halfway house undergoing addictions treatment and integrating back into the community following incarceration. This group of eight women ranged in ages from their mid-twenties to mid-fifties.

These women attended weekly music therapy sessions during their time at the halfway house. These women had been abused in childhood and in their adult lives, been in jail and prison, been abandoned by their families, and in some cases had their children removed from their care. They had been involved in codependent relationships and had been involved in dealing drugs or engaged in prostitution to support their addiction. These were disempowered women, they felt unsure of themselves, and felt capable of little in their lives.

Following several weeks of music therapy, the concept of writing a song as a group was broached by the music therapist. The group shared they did not feel capable of this type of endeavor and that they did not have the skills to be able to complete the task. The music therapist asked the group to trust the process would be structured to successfully take the group through this endeavor. The group timidly agreed to trust the music therapist, the process and each other. The song that follows is what the group wrote within one music therapy session, entitled "Sisters of Sobriety."

Sisters of Sobriety

Sisters of sobriety that's who we are.
Livin' by the 12 steps and going far.
Livin' everyday just for today.
Been through hell heaven's on the way

CHORUS
Sisters of sobriety, Sisters in sobriety
Sisters of sobriety, Sisters in sobriety
Sisters of sobriety, Sisters in sobriety
Sisters of sobriety, Sisters in sobriety
Sisters of sobriety, Sisters in sobriety
Sisters of sobriety, Sisters in sobriety

Success is doing my best,
Women of the world.
Don't have a goal if you don't have a plan.
'Cause we're not flexible or a rubber band.
No need for control,
And we don't need a man.

CHORUS
Sisters of sobriety, Sisters in sobriety
Sisters of sobriety, Sisters in sobriety
Sisters of sobriety, Sisters in sobriety
Sisters of sobriety, Sisters in sobriety
Sisters of sobriety, Sisters in sobriety
Sisters of sobriety, Sisters in sobriety

The song is in rap style, this was the musical genre the group selected. The group also decided to create a recording of their song. Utilizing a portable drum machine, the group selected the backbeat to utilize and decided who would sing each line and they unanimously decided to sing in unison on the chorus. The words and their voices in their recording is testament to their sense of achievement and empowerment in this process.

By the end of the recording, they were smiling, laughing, and dancing (some on the furniture). These women were proud of what they had accomplished. They each received a copy of the recording; they even shared their recording with the program director that then shared it with the board of directors. Their song was later published in the annual report, which further contributed to the pride in their work and themselves.

The Case of Songwriting and Active Music-Making

The song "Chronic Craving" was written by a group of adults attending weekly music therapy sessions at a dual diagnoses day treatment program. This program was designed for individuals that were dually diagnosed with mental illness and substance abuse. This group was a mix of men and women and ages ranged from college age to mid-sixties.

The concept of songwriting was introduced to the group by the music therapist. The group decided they would like to work collectively and write a song. They decided the song would have a blues funk style, they felt the blues style was an appropriate genre to discuss the issues related to addiction. They chose to write about the struggles of addiction: grief and loss, powerlessness, being haunted by cravings and desires to use and loss of self and self-worth. As songwriting is a process, the group discussed these issues and experiences in writing the song. The lyrics are comprised of several metaphors that describe life with an addiction.

Chronic Craving

My friend's now riding in a hearse.
Couldn't quench that insatiable thirst.
For the gin, the beer or the rum,
Everybody knew that his day would come

Drunk again just like a fool,
Booze just ain't that cool.

How did he stay so blind,
To the fact that he lost his mind.

The alcohol took him over,
He just could not stay sober.

Unrefundable chips cashed in,
Sold his soul for a bottle of gin

Hittin' the blunt with all his power.
Gettin' stoned at the top of the hour.
Monkeys on his back, been smokin' that crack
Keep lookin' forward, don't step back

Something inside just won't let me be.
My bag is empty, my heart's in misery.
He comes lookin' for an ear to lend,
But he ain't got a nickel to spend.
Everyone around me is searchin'
While the crack bird sits there perchin'

Vultures circle closing in,
Sold his soul for a gram of sin.

Following the writing of the song, the group decided they would like to record the song. There were two individuals in the group that happened to have music experience. One young man, Marty, in his mid-twenties, had confided in the music therapist that he played guitar but not played since his drug use became heavy. He further acknowledged that despite the fact he had hocked many of his belongings to support his habit, he never allowed himself to sell his guitar. He was encouraged by the music therapist and the group to bring his guitar and play on the day of the recording, although he was initially hesitant, he did play on the recording and began to rediscover his passion for music as well as a belief in himself.

Another gentleman, John, that attended the group currently was homeless and came to the program each day from the shelter carrying all of his belongings in his backpack. One day he shared with the music therapist that he played the harmonica which he kept in his backpack with his life's belongings. On the day of the recording, he played blues harmonica on the song and played a soulful riff at the end of the song.

Writing and recording this song allowed the group to discover they could achieve something they had not tried or achieved before. This was a profound realization as it allows an individual or group to succeed at something they had not conceived they could achieve. This can help to quell doubts they may have about achieving or maintaining sobriety. This experience also provided the opportunity for two members of the group to rediscover abilities they had left behind for their addiction.

The Case of Roger and Guided Imagery and Music (GIM)

Roger is a 47-year-old single white male, the youngest of two children. He explained that his childhood was quite normal. He obtained his high school education and was looking forward to building a life with his high school sweetheart. Shortly after graduation, he discovered his girlfriend with another man. He was so distraught that he enlisted in the military the next day. He was soon shipped off to Vietnam and never spoke to his girlfriend again. Shortly after arriving in Vietnam, he was involved in a motor vehicle accident and suffered a brain stem contusion. This resulted in some short-term memory loss and difficulties with balance. Following this accident, Roger was in physical rehabilitation for 13 months. During this time, he became depressed and then continued to experience bouts of depression in the years to follow. He has been unable to maintain any steady employment, develop social or relationships, and is full of regret.

Roger identified that he has been drinking alcohol since high school and that he has been addicted for about 20 years. He sought treatment when a bleeding ulcer developed and he began vomiting blood. This is Roger's sixth time in treatment for his addiction. He reported not wanting to return to drinking as he knows that his health will only continue to decline. Roger was not sure what issues he wanted to address through the GIM sessions, but he knew he was not happy and wanted to change that.

The imagery examples that follow are not full transcripts from the sessions or sessions in their entirety, but only portions of the sessions. The words in parenthesis are the comments/remarks of the guide/therapist, everything outside parenthesis are descriptions given by the subject. The postlude is the time following the session when the subject and guide discuss and process the images and imagery experience.

Session #3:

Program: Relationships
Induction: Incorporated the image of a tree
Segments of imagery transcript:

(What are you experiencing?) a tree in my father's backyard, he planted the tree 35 years ago, it's a big tree (What do you notice?) it was struck by lightning, it is scarred, but it kept growing (Scarred?) He put paint on it to cover it. (How does it feel to see that?) Feel a sense of belonging. I've watched it for so long. I see what I helped my dad build. (What do you notice about your-self?) Feel at peace with myself. (Where do you feel that peace?) In my legs.

Postlude: Roger recognized the metaphor of the tree. How the tree had been struck and scarred and how he could see himself as the tree, injured and wounded. He was able to see that the tree continued to grow despite the damage. Whereas, following his accident, he struggled and often shut people out and closed himself off from others.

The image of the scarred tree remained significant for Roger throughout treatment. Following this session he continued to recognize the similarities between himself and the tree. He felt encouraged that despite the fact the tree was injured, it continued to grow, that being "damaged," did not mean dead. He felt he had been "damaged" in the accident and that no one would want to share a life with him and he was simply drinking himself to death. Through the image of the tree, he began to see hope for his life rather than despair.

Session #6

Program: Pastorale
Induction: Road or path
Segments of imagery transcript:

(What are you experiencing?) I am walking down a road toward the lake. (What do you see?) The trees, the river winds back and forth. I am going down to the lake. (What do you notice?) There is a swing by the lake, a homemade swing. (What do you notice about the swing?) There is a girl on it. She has long brown hair. I am pushing her on the swing. (Pushing her) Now she is slowing down to stop. (Is this familiar?) I tell her I am sorry. (Who is the girl?) It is Debbie. (Is there anything else you want to tell her?) Maybe, it's too hard. (Let yourself be there). Her face is fading. (How do you feel?) There are no words to describe it. (What is happening now?) She is gone.

Postlude: Debbie was Roger's first love. He abruptly joined the military when he saw her with another guy shortly after graduating from high school. Roger recognized that these feelings of regret and leaving this issue unresolved were contributing factors in his addiction. And that expressing these emotions was extremely difficult for him.

This session began to open Roger to recognize the impact of these unre-solved feelings in his life. Seeing Debbie in the image brought him back to that moment and he realized that those feelings were strong and he was not able to fully express them even within the imagery experience. This allowed him to understand how these feelings were still influencing his life even though he thought he had run away from them. He now understood he had only continued to carry those feelings with him and he was trying to drink them away through his addiction. Roger's new insight was important to his recovery. Despite his 20-year addiction and five previous treatment attempts, this was the first time he began to address these deep-seeded feelings.

Drumming and Addictions

Therapeutic drumming and drum circles have gained popularity through-out the world, in mainstream society as well as treatment programs. Music therapists and drumming facilitators find that drumming helps a group develop cohesion, connectedness, and a sense of community (Mikenas, 1999 & 2000; Winkelman, 2003). Mikenas (2000) reports that drumming gives individuals an opportunity to explore and learn leadership skills and discover one's potential. Smith (2000) and Winkelman (2003) utilize drumming to address the physiological, psychological, and social needs of individuals in addictions treatment, as the support and interactions within these groups are of considerable significance to individuals in the process of treatment.

Conclusion

The universality of music lends itself to the therapeutic process in that it can meet each person wherever they are on their journey of recovery. The complexities within music speak to the subconscious, connecting to our emotions, and providing the outlet for those feelings that have been unresolved. The process of music therapy can empower the individual to discover the answers within rather than grasp for answers outside themselves. Music and music therapy can help them recognize what they have not been able to see or hear in any other way before. This process of discovery that takes place within the therapeutic application of music can hold the keys the individual needs to unlock the door to their own recovery.

Appendix A–Terms

Improvisation–An intervention utilized in music therapy that incorporates creating music in the momemnt or spontaneously.

Riff–A spontaneous improvised musical creation with a song or composition. The musician decides in the moment what to play and creative freedom is given to the musician to create and play freely.

Song analysis–Incorporates the use of a song selected by the client or the therapist. The song is utilized as a therapeutic vehicle to examine or explore an issue pertinent to therapy.

Song communication–This is the use of a song selected by the client. The song (music and lyrics included) express that which the client wants, needs or wishes to communicate.

Songwriting–A process where the music therapist engages with the client or clients to create a song relating to therapeutic issues, feelings, experiences, or what the individual or group choose to write about. The complexity of the process is tailored by the music therapist based on the skills and needs of the individual or group.

Appendix B

Conceptual Framework of GIM for Enhanced Psychological Well-being and Immue Function to Persons Undergoing Chemical Dependency Treatment.

<u>Influences</u>

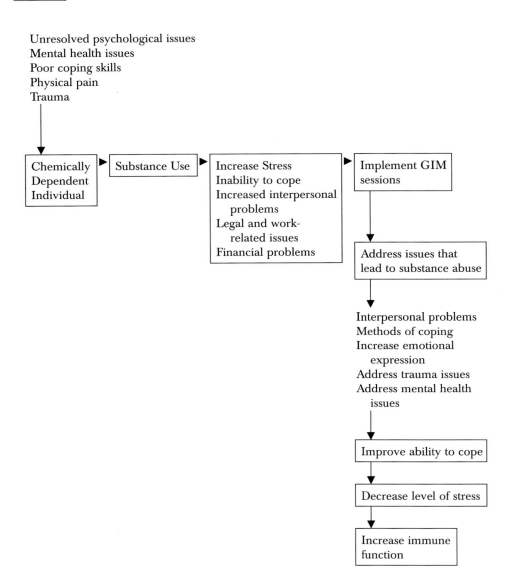

Appendix C

The Bonny Method of Guided Imagery and Music

The Bonny Method of Guided Imagery and Music (GIM) was developed by Dr. Helen Bonny in the early 1970s. Dr. Bonny (1980) was hired as a music therapist at the Maryland Psychiatric Research Center, where a group of therapists were studying the effects of hallucinogenic drugs in the treatment of their patients (Bonny, 1980). It was during this course of research she observed that specifically chosen selections of classical music enhanced the LSD psychotherapy (Bonny & Pahnke, 1972). Bonny found that as patients listened to carefully selected programs of classical music in a relaxed state, powerful feelings and symbolic images were evoked, which led to significant insights into therapeutic issues (Goldberg, 1995).

In time, the use of hallucinogenic drugs in therapy began to decline and Bonny began to experiment with music as the catalyst in psychotherapy (McKinney, 1994). Music has been used in drug research to help the patient relinquish control and enter into an inner-world experience, facilitate the release of intense emotions, contribute to a peak experience, provide continuity in an experience of timelessness, and structure the experience (Bonny, 1980). Bonny reasoned that if the research team was correct in their assumptions, music enhanced the sensory experience and facilitated the action of the drug indicating that music alone may be just as effective (Bonny, 1980). She found that the subjects were able to experience these inner images and emotions of the unconscious with careful selection of classical music and without the drug.

Dr. Bonny developed and refined her method and in the process was influenced by the work of Freud, Jung, Maslow, and the imagery techniques of Assagioli. She was also influenced and encouraged by Carl Han Leuner, who developed the method called "Guided Affective Imagery" (Leuner, 1969). Bonny was particularly influenced by Leuner's ideas regarding imagery in psychotherapy (Goldberg, 1995). Leuner's (1969) premise was that the images experienced during a session were that of a quasi reality, an experience that occurred in an altered state. The feelings and emotions the patient's experienced during this process were the essential component of the psychotherapeutic process.

The Bonny Method of Guided Imagery and Music is distinguished from other methods incorporating music and imagery, in that the music is used to evoke and direct the images, the therapist does not suggest the images. The uniqueness of the experience is that the music allows whatever is important to the imager to emerge during the session. "The multidimensional qualities of musical sound allow it to touch many levels of consciousness both simultaneously and/or in sequence . . . the movement of the music, the rise and fall of dynamics brings about a wide sweep of those levels or layers of consciousness" (Bonny, 1975, p. 130).

The Structure of a GIM session

GIM sessions are often facilitated in individual sessions. The sessions for this study were all individual sessions. An individual session typically lasts from one and a half hours to two hours in length. The sessions are divided into four parts: (1) the pre-session or preliminary conversation, (2) the induction (relaxation and focus), (3) the music listening phase or imagery phase, and (4) the post-session integration (Bonny, 1978a).

Pre-session

The pre-session is the preliminary time during the session in which the imager or traveler shares any relevant information with the guide. The information can include life events, feelings, personal history, or any other information or material the individual feels is significant. This is also a time in which the individual may share insights gained from a previous GIM session. During this time, the guide is listening to what the traveler is sharing, and working to develop rapport with the traveler. The therapist/guide is not only listening to what the traveler is sharing, but also observing non-verbal communication, assessing mood, and energy level. The therapist is drawing upon all of this information, as it is key in the process of selecting the induction and the music for the session.

Induction

Following this period of sharing during the pre-session, the traveler reclines into a comfortable position, usually in a recliner, couch, or on a mat. The guide then leads the traveler through a relaxation exercise to aid the traveler in moving from the conscious state to an altered state of consciousness. The induction helps to physically relax the traveler and focus the mind. The guide uses the information that the traveler shared during pre-session phase to formulate the induction.

The induction typically consists of three parts. The first part focuses on a physical relaxation, the second part focuses on engaging the imagination (focusing on an image, a scene or experience), and the third part is bridging the image to the music. The guide may bridge the image to the music by simply suggesting that the traveler "allow the music to be with you" or "let the music take you wherever you need to go." At this point, the music is initiated into the session and the traveler begins imaging to the music.

Music Listening or Imagery Phase

The music for the session is selected by the therapist/guide. The choice of the music is based on the therapist's assessment of the traveler's therapeutic issues, current emotional state, energy level, and any other issues raised during the pre-session. The music programs are sequences of selected pieces of classical music (see Appendix for the specific selections included in each music program). The music programs have been developed by trained and experienced GIM therapists. These programs have also been tested for their ability to "elicit and support images and to meet a wide range of emotional states and energy levels of the traveler" (McKinney, 1994, p. 262).

While the music is playing, the traveler shares and describes whatever he or she is experiencing. The images that are experienced are not only visual, they can include various sensory experiences such as sound, smells, movement (spinning, walking, floating, flying, sinking, as well as others), memories from the traveler's personal history, this may include unfinished business, body sensations (tingling, tightness, pain or physical discomfort), feelings, perceptions, and emotions. While the traveler experiences the images, the guide listens and supports the experiences, and encourages the traveler to engage deeply in the experience. The guide is completely in tune to the traveler and the music. The guide is observing, listening and verbally reflecting during the imagery process (Goldberg, 1995).

During the imagery phase, the guide writes down the images and experiences that the traveler describes. The information that the guide writes down is referred to as a transcript. The transcript is a way to not only record what the traveler describes, but also a means of recording any non-verbal reactions, such as physical tension, facial expression, and or movement. The transcript provides the guide and traveler with the means to review images, experiences, and recurring images or themes that may occur from session to session.

Post-session

Following the music listening and imagery phase, the therapist/guide works with the traveler to integrate the experience. When the music stops, the therapist guides and assists the traveler in bringing the imagery to a close and returning to a waking, conscious state. During this integration phase, the therapist is following the lead of the traveler. The therapist encourages the traveler to acknowledge and address any images or experiences they feel are significant or stand out. The role of the therapist is not to interpret the images, but assist the traveler in the integration of these images. This integration can take place through verbal discussion, but it can also happen through non-verbal expression. Some therapists utilize mandala drawing, sculpturing clay, or other mediums the traveler may be familiar with and find beneficial. The traveler may also wish to journal, sketch images, or use any combination of these methods (Bonny, 2002). Most travelers have a need or desire to discuss their GIM experience and, "although there is some clinical evidence of behavioral change without verbal processing of the images, cognitive understanding usually plays an important role in the therapeutic process" (Goldberg, 1995, p. 115).

References

American Music Therapy Association. (2006). *2005 Music Therapy Sourcebook.* Washington, D.C.: American Music Therapy Association.

American Psychiatric Association. (1994). *Diagnostic and Statistical Manual of Mental Disorders,* 3rd Edition (DSM-IV). Washington, D.C., American Psychiatric Association.

American Psychiatric Association. (2000). *Diagnostic and Statistical Manual of Mental Disorders,* 4th Edition, Text Revision (DSM-IV-TR). Washington, D.C., American Psychiatric Association.

Babyface. (1995). *Count On Me* from album Waiting to Exhale performed by Whitney Houston and CeCe Winans. Recorded 1995. Compact disc.

BOJS. (1988). Report to the nation on crime and justice (NCJ-105506). Washington, D.C., U.S. Department of Justice.

BOJS. (1999). More than 500,00 drunk drivers on probation or incarcerated in 1997. Washington, D. C., U. S. Department of Justice.

Borling, J. (1992). Perspectives on growth with a victim of abuse: A Guided Imagery and Music (GIM) Case Study. *Journal of the Association for Music and Imagery 1,* 85–98.

Bonny. H. (2002). *Music consciousness: The evolution of guided imagery and music.* Gilsum, NH: Barcelona Publishers.

Bonny, H. (1980). *GIM Monograph #3: GIM therapy: Past, present and future implications.* Salina, KS, The Bonny Foundation.

Bonny, H. (1978a). *The role of taped music programs in the GIM process: GIM monography #2.* Baltimore, ICM Books.

Bonny, H. (1975). Music and consciousness. *Journal of Music Therapy 12*(3), 121–135.

Bonny, H., & Pahnke, W. (1972). The use of music in psychedelic (LSD) psychotherapy. *Journal of Music Therapy 9*(2), 64–87.

Buelow, G., & Buelow, S. (1998). *Psychotherapy in chemical dependence treatment: A practical and integrative approach.* New York, Brooks/Cole Publishing Company.

Census Bureau. (2003). *National Longitudinal Alcohol Epidemiological Survey (NLAES).* Washington, D.C., Department of Health and Human Services.

Cummings, C., Gordon, J. R., & Marlatt, G. A. (1980). Relapse: Prevention and prediction. *The addictive behaviors.* (Ed.) W. R. Miller. New York: Pergamon Press.

Dare, C. (1998). Psychoanalysis and family systems revisited: The old, old story? *Journal of Family Therapy 20*(2), 165–177.

Davis, B., & Gfeller, K. (1999). Clinical practice in music therapy. In Davis,W., Thaut, M., & Gfeller, K. (Eds). *An introduction to music therapy: Theory and practice* (3–15). Boston, MA:

McGraw-Hill.

Doweiko, H. (2002). *Concepts of chemical dependency.* Canada, Brooks/Cole.

DiNitto, D. M., & Webb, D. K. (2005). Substance use disorders and co-occurring disabilities. In D. M. DiNitto & C. A. McNeece (Eds.), *Chemical dependency: A systems approach* (4pp. 23–483). Boston: Pearson.

Dodgen, C. E., & Shea, W. M. (2000). *Substance use disorders: Treatment and assessment.* New York: Academic Press.

Edwards, G., & Lader, M (1994). *Addiction: Processes of change.* New York: Oxford University Press.

Forrest, G. G. (1985). Psychodynamically oriented treatment of alcoholism and substance abuse. *Alcoholism and substance abuse: Strategies for clinical intervention.* T. E. B. G. G. Forrest. New York: The Free Press.

Goldberg, F. (1995). The Bonny Method of Guided Imagery and Music. In T. Wigram, B. Saperston, & R. West (Eds.), *The art & science of music therapy: A handbook* (pp. 112–128). Australia: Harwood Academic Publishers.

Gottheil, E., Druley, K., Pashko, S., & Weinstein, S. (1987). *Stress and addiction.* New York, Brunner Mazel, Inc.

Hawkins, C. A. (2005). Family Systems and Chemical Dependency. *Chemical dependency: A systems approach.* C. A. M. D. M. DiNitto. Boston: Pearson.

Heiderscheit, A. (2005). The Effects of the Bonny Method of Guided Imagery and Music (GIM) on Interpersonal Problems, Sense of Coherence and Salivary Immunoglobulin A of Adults in Chemical Dependency Treatment. Doctoral Dissertation. Minneapolis, MN, University of Minnesota.

Heiderscheit, A. (2008). *Music Therapy.* http://www.takingcharge.csh.umn.edu.

Hill, L. (1998). *A Rose Is Still A Rose* from the album A Rose Is Still A Rose performed by Aretha Franklin. Recorded 1997. Compact disc.

Houghton, B., Scovel, M., Smeltekop, R., Thaut, M., Unkefer, R., & Wilson, B. (2005). Taxonomy of clinical music therapy programs and techniques. In R. Unkefer & M. Thaut (Eds.), *Music therapy in the treatment of adults with mental disorders: Theoretical bases and clinical interventions* (pp. 181–206). Gilsum, NH: Barcelona Publishers.

Jennison, K. M. (1992). The impact of stressful life events and social support on drinking among older adults: A general population survey. *International Journal on Aging and Human Development 35*(2), 99–123.

Judson, B. A., Goldstein, A., & Inturrisi, C. E. (1983). Methadyl acetate (LAAM) in the treatment of heroin addicts. II Double-blind comparison of gradual and abrupt detoxification. *Archives of General Psychiatry 40*(8), 834–840.

Kalant, H. (1990). Stress-related effects of ethanol in mammals. *Critical Reviews in Biotechnology 9*(4), 265–272.

Kessler, R. C., McGonagle, K. A., Zhao, S., Nelson, C. B., Hughes, M., Eshleman, S., Hans-Ulrich, W., & Kendler, K. S. (1994). Lifetime and 12 month prevalance of DSM-III-R psychiatric disorders in the United States. *Archives of General Psychiatry 51,* 8–19.

Khantzian, E. J. (1999). *Treating addiction as a human process.* New York, Aronson.

Kinney, J. (2000). *Loosening the grip: A handbook of alcohol information.* Boston, McGraw-Hill.

Kosten, T. R., Kreek, M. J., Ragunath, J., & Kleber, H. D. (1986). Cortisol levels during chronic naltrexone maintenance treatment in ex-opiate addicts. *Biological Psychiatry 21*(2), 217–220.

Langer, S. K. (1967). *Mind: An essay on human feeling.* Baltimore, Johns Hopkins Press.

Leonard, K. E., & Blane, H. T. (1999). *Physiological theories of drinking and alcoholism* (2nd ed.). New York: Guilford Press.

Leuner, H. (1969). Guided Affective Imagery. *American Journal of Psychotherapy 23*(1), 4–22.

Liebschutz, J. M., Mulvey, K. P., & Samet, J. H. (1997). Victimization among substance-abusing women: Worse health outcomes. *Archives of Internal Medicine 157*(10), 1093–1097.

McKinney, C. (1994). The effect of the Bonny method of guided imagery and music on mood, emotional expression, cortisol, and immunologic control of latent epstein-barr virus in healthy adults. Doctoral Dissertation. Coral Gables, FL: University of Miami.

McNeece, C., & Barbanell, L. (2005). Definitions and Epidemiology of Substance Use, Abuse and Disorders. In A. D. McNeece & D. M. DiNitto (Eds.), *Chemical dependency: A systems approach* (3–21). Boston: Hawthorne Press, Inc.

Merikangas, K. R., Mehta, R. L., Molnar, B. E., Walters, E. E., Swendsen, J. D., Aguilar-Gaziola, S., Bijl, R., Borges, G., Caraveo-Anduaga, J. J., DeWitt, D. J., Vega, W. A., Wittchen, H. U., & Kessler, R. C. (1998). Comorbidity of substance use disorders with mood and anxiety disorders: Results of the International Consortium in Psychiatric Epidemiology. *Addictive Behaviors 23*(6), 893–907.

Mikenas, E. (1999). Drums, not drugs. *Percussive Notes,* April, 62–63.

Mikenas, E. (2000). *Drumming on the edge of leadership: Hand drumming and leadership skills in the new millennium.* Lynchburg, VA: Urban Wilde.

Milkman, H., & Sederer, L. (1990). *Treatment choices for alcoholism and substance abuse.* New York: Lexington Books.

National Council on Child Abuse and Neglect (NCCAN). (2001). *Alcohol and Drug Related Family Violence.* Washington, D.C., Department of Health and Human Services.

National Institute on Alcohol Abuse and Alcoholism (NIAAA). (2000). Tenth special report to the U. S. Congress on alcohol and health. Bethesda, MD, U.S. Department of Health and Human Services.

Nolan, P. (1989). Music therapy improvisation techniques with bulimic patients. In L. M. Hornyak & E. K. Baker (Eds.), *Experiential therapies for eating disorders* (pp. 167–187). New York: Guilford Press.

Parente, A. B. (1989). Music as a therapeutic tool in treating anorexia nervosa. In L. M. Hornyak & E. K. Baker (Eds.), *Experiential therapies for eating disorders* (pp. 305–328). New York: Guilford Press.

Pickett, E. (1991). Guided imagery and music (GIM) with a dually diagnosed woman having multiple addictions. In K. E. Bruscia (Ed.), *Case studies in music therapy* (pp. 497–512). Phoenixville, PA: Barcelona Publishers.

Pohorecky, L. A. (1991). Stress and alcohol interaction: An update of human research. *Alcoholism: Clinical and Experimental Research 15*(3), 438–459.

Quinn, R., Shepard, R. M., & Rose, J. B. (1973). Alcohol. *Texas Medicine, 69*(6), 63–72.

Rhoads, D. L. (1983). A longitudinal study of life stress and social support among drug abusers. *The International Journal of the Addictions 18*(2), 195–222.

Robson, P. (1999). *Forbidden drugs.* Oxford, United Kingdom, Oxford University Press.

Sadava, S. W., & Pak, A. W. (1993). Stress-related problem drinking and alcohol problems: A longitudinal study and extension of Marlatt's model. *Canadian Journal of Behavioral Science 25*(3), 446–464.

SAMSHA. (2001a). Executive Office of the President and Office of Drug Control Policy (ONDCP). Washington, D.C., Department of Health and Human Services.

SAMSHA. (2003). Executive Office of the President and Office of Drug Control Policy (ONDCP). Washington, D.C., Department of Health and Human Services.

SAMSHA. (2003). National Survey on Drug Use and Health (NSDUH). Washington, D.C., Department of Health and Human Services.

SAMSHA. (2003). United States National Probability Sample of Non-institutionalized

Abusers. Washington, D.C., Department of Health and Human Services.

SAMSHA. (2004). Results from the 2003 National Survey on Drug Use and Health: National Findings. Washington, D. C., Department of Health and Human Services.

Schuckit, M. A. (2000). *Drug and alcohol abuse: A clinical guide to diagnosis and treatment* (5th ed.). New York, Plenum Press.

Skaggs, R. (1997). *Finishing strong: Treating chemical addictions with music and imagery.* St. Louis, MO: MMB Music, Inc.

Smith, D. (2000). Shamanism and addictions: The mask of therapeutic containment midwife to mental health. *Spirit Talk, 11,* 8–12.

Summer, L. (1988). *Guided imagery and music in the institutional setting.* St. Louis, MO: MMB Music, Inc.

Thaut, M., & Gfeller, K. (1999). Music therapy in the treatment of mental disorders. In W. Davis, M. Thaut, & K. Gfeller (Eds), *An introduction to music therapy: Theory and practice* (pp. 93–132). Boston, MA: McGraw-Hill.

Vaillant, G. E. (1983). *The natural history of alcoholism: Causes, patterns and paths to recovery.* Cambridge: Harvard University Press.

Volpicelli, J. R. (1987). Uncontrollable events and alcohol drinking. *British Journal of Addiction 82*(4), 381–392.

Wilcox, R., & Erickson, C. (2005). The brain biology of drug abuse and addiction. In C. A. McNeece & D. M. DiNitto (Eds.), *Chemical dependency: A systems approach.* Boston: Pearson.

Wilcox, R., & Erickson, C. (2005). The physiology and behavioral consequences of alcohol and drug abuse. In C. A. McNeece & D. M. DiNitto (Eds.), *Chemical dependency: A systems approach* (pp. 52–61). Boston, MA: Pearson.

Windle, M., Windle, R., Scheidt, D. M., & Miller, G. B. (1995). Physical and sexual abuse and associated mental disorders among alcoholic inpatients. *American Journal of Psychiatry 152*(9), 1322–1328.

Winkelman, M. (2003). Complementary therapy for addiction: Drumming out drugs. *American Journal of Public Health, 93*(4), 647–651.

Wise, B. K., Cuff, S. P., & Fisher, T. (2001). Dual diagnosis and successful participation of adoelscents in substance abuse treatment. *Journal of Substance Abuse Treatment 21,* 161–165.

Wolkstein, E. Second annual conference on substance abuse and co-existing disabilities: Facilitating employment for a hidden population. Conference held March 2002. Retrieved January 20, 2005 from http://www.med.wright.edu/citar/sardi/rrtc_conference.html

Biography

Annie Heiderscheit, Ph.D., MT-BC, FAMI, NMT is a board certified music therapist with 18 years of clinical experience. Dr. Heiderscheit is a graduate faculty member at the University of Minnesota in the Center for Spirituality and Healing. She maintains a private practice in music therapy, specializing in the use of music therapy in medicine and music psychotherapy. She also continues her clinical practice at The Emily Program, an eating disorder treatment program, where she provides music therapy services in the outpatient and residential programs. Dr. Heiderscheit also provides clinical music therapy services at the University of Minnesota Children's Hospital on the Pediatric Bone Marrow Transplant Unit and Pediatric Intensive Care Units. She has worked with adults and adolescents in a variety of inpatient and outpatient substance abuse treatment programs in Kansas, Missouri, Iowa and Minnesota.

Chapter 10

DANCE/MOVEMENT THERAPY AS AN EFFECTIVE CLINICAL INTERVENTION TO DECREASE ANXIETY AND SUPPORT THE RECOVERY PROCESS

MEGHAN DEMPSEY

Introduction

I rang the doorbell.[1] A sign reading "Elopement Precaution" was anchored next to the door. A small head popped up through the little window in the door. The eyes of the person inside peered at me until I presented my badge. The sound of keys broke the chilling silence as the door was unbolted and I entered the unit: Inpatient Psychiatry. The door was quickly shut and bolted behind me as I crossed over a red line marking the place where patients could not walk past. As I wandered apprehensively down the short hall, a few patients appeared in their doorways to see who was allowed onto the unit. Some patients were immediately friendly, joining me, and excitedly talking to me. Others stared at me blankly with a sense of vacancy. I wondered what I was doing here. Immediately, I questioned my ability to work with this population.

As I became more comfortable in speaking with patients in-between groups, I began to notice a difference between them. There were some patients who were delusional, not aware of the reality, while others appeared to be higher functioning. If I were to hold a conversation with them on the street, I would most likely not be aware of the fact that they had a mental ill-

---

1. This chapter was composed of excerpts from *Guided Imagery in Conjunction with Dance/Movement Therapy to Decrease Anxiety in Substance Dependent Adults,* by M. Dampsey, 2006. Adapted with permission of the author.

ness. These patients, referred to as Mentally Ill Chemically Addicted (MICA), carried a second diagnosis of substance dependency. Not psychotic nor delusional, they seemed to be engaged in reality, had the potential to hold jobs, and had families. Outwardly appearing to be the healthiest of this inpatient population, I expected them to actively participate in dance/movement therapy groups. Instead, many sat throughout entire movement sessions, anxiously bouncing a knee while tightly holding their narrowed bodies. Eye contact or interpersonal interactions were rarely made. Those that did participate loosely mimicked the leader of the session. Many times the MICA patients refused to respond during the verbal processing of the movement experiential. I felt they had much more potential than they showed.

In the dance/movement therapy groups with the substance dependent patients, I observed that they often sat in the same position for an entire movement session, refusing to actively participate. Without the tools to regulate the flow of his/her thoughts, emotions, or physical sensations, an addict is ill-equipped to do so (Caldwell, 1996). In order to protect him/herself from being flooded by these uncontrollable emotions, an addict develops self-soothing behaviors. I observed that although these repetitive behaviors appear to protect an addict, they actually disconnect him/her from his/her conscious awareness. The behaviors are drawn upon in a time of need to put one into a trance-like state. I have noticed that one's focus is directed from unwanted emotions to the physical act of bouncing a knee, rocking, or wringing of the hands. By concentrating on this self-soothing behavior, the addict can deny what he/she feels internally. Without turning to this behavior, and not having the coping mechanisms to diffuse the intensity of his/her emotions, an addict is left feeling out of control.

Eventually, the abuse of substances is how these individuals learn to cope with their emotions. An addict may attempt to self-medicate when he/she experiences unbearable psychological angst or suffering (Dodes, 1990; Johnson, 1999; Khantzian, 1985). Johnson (1999) writes that an addict seeks out substances because he/she is unable to endure being alone. Further, the addict does not have the resources to provide him/herself with the tools to help him/her deal with suffering. Lacking sufficient coping mechanisms, he/she begins to search outside him/herself for something to quell the painful feelings and relieve discomfort. He/she turns externally to a substance to fill what is missing internally. Becoming frequently overwhelmed, an addict is left with a sense of helplessness. In addition, the addict appears hopeless as he/she feels he/she lacks the power to initiate action in life. The substance is seen as something that can reduce his/her anxiety by altering his/her internal state.

Throughout the dance/movement therapy sessions and verbal processing, I was left with a general feeling of emptiness from working with this population. They left me perplexed by not sharing what they experienced in the group. They had failed to provide me with any information or a sense of what happened for them during the session. I wondered why, if they were so creative everyday on the streets in order to hide their addictions and to find money to buy drugs, they were not creative in the group. Self-doubt began to creep in as I became frustrated and thought I was unable to see their creativity. I questioned whether they did not experience anything in the group or they prohibited themselves from allowing anything to happen.

Curious, I wanted to know if these substance dependent patients were unable to identify what happened, or, if they simply refused to share what happened. Sensing that nothing happened for them in the group because they did not allow anything to happen, I originally felt these patients failed to fill me with anything. They did not move or speak about what they experienced emotionally. I kept looking for some sign that the change I expected and wanted to see was occurring within these patients. Although it was difficult for me to receive any verbal or visual feedback, I felt something internally. It is exactly what they did not do, they did not fill me, which is the feedback with which I was left. It was in the feeling of emptiness where I could connect with this population. I suspected that the feeling I was left with was the same feeling of emptiness they experienced and wanted to fill or desensitize. The more they left me unfulfilled, the more I wanted to be filled. The harder I pushed to connect, the more resistance I hit. Braatoy and Reich (as cited in Poole & Rossberg-Gempton, 1992) suggest that the physical anxiety of an individual witnessed by a therapist relates to the amount of resistance the therapist might expect to encounter. I realized that they lured me into the essence of their addiction. Perhaps, if I could learn how to be filled by these patients, they too could begin to learn how to fill themselves without the use of substances.

The Role of Anxiety

Kuettel (1982) hypothesizes that one's abrupt need to sit down is a defense mechanism used by anxious individuals. For an addict, feeling his/her body is too intense and frightening so he/she opts to not participate. To begin moving right away is threatening and that inhibits him/her from actively participating for the rest of the session. An addict's anxiety creates resistance, which does not allow him/her to give or receive throughout the movement experience. At a point where the opportunity for progression towards interaction and engagement arises, the addict retreats into his/her perpetual behavior and regresses. What he/she feels is too intense and instead of staying in his/her body to begin to identify these feelings, he/she runs from them. As a result, he/she moves farther away from self so as to be less aware of an inability to adapt and cope. Thomson (1997) notes that if an addict moves spontaneously, which is one goal of dance/movement therapy, he/she risks the chance of possibly losing control over his/her body. Therefore, not wanting to allow the chance for unwanted emotions to expose self, the addict takes a passive role in the group. I observed that when an addict exhibited a resistant attitude at the beginning of a session, there was little chance for it to shift. I wondered how I could start a dance/movement therapy session in a non-threatening way in the hope of gradually bringing these patients to the place where they felt comfortable enough to allow a felt experience to occur.

I quickly began to realize this was not as easy as I would have liked it to be. I could not randomly pick a movement to start with, but I had to use my somatic countertransference to find something within myself that I could connect to within the addicts. My relationship was no longer towards the patients, but with the patients. I began to discover that I had to learn from and work with each patient. Perhaps it was in this desire to connect where I found the capacity to invest myself. To invest in a patient and understand who he/she is, is a requirement of a therapist (Irwin, 1986). I had to not only realize who the patient was, but who he/she was to me. I had to find the meaning of the person within myself. This connection could have possibly been unknown to myself. In the unknown is where I had to be willing to explore, experience, and learn from both the patient and myself in order to create a therapeutic space.

I reflected on my personal relationship with resistance. When connected with my unconscious, my mind can suddenly shut down and draw a blank while processing. This leaves it extremely difficult for me to reconnect with my thoughts. Trying to think about the disconnection creates even more resistance and I am left staring at a black abyss. I thought about how I am able to reopen this connection so I can proceed with my processing. Guided imagery has always drawn me back into myself in a non-threatening, yet creative way.

The Effects of Guided Imagery

Guided imagery is a form of relaxation and meditation that is used to heal physical, mental, and emotional issues. It draws upon one's imagination to consciously focus internally, allowing one the opportunity to create positive images (Dhyansanjivani, 2004). Working with metaphors, an addict is able to safely distance himself from what he/she experiences internally. Being addressed directly, an addict might resist the opportunity to explore his/her mental, emotional, and psychological issues. These issues, too upsetting to face, can be transformed through his/her imagination. When a thought, feeling, or emotion becomes too intense for him/her to tolerate, instead of falling into his/her typical pattern of numbing self, he/she can shift to his/her imagination. The images an addict creates are a safe way for him/her to continue the process of discovering parts about self. The images and internal experience created by a person have been known to bring about healing to the mind and body (Rossman, 2000). I wondered if using guided imagery would also work for the patients.

The substance dependent patients, unfamiliar with dance/movement therapy, would come to groups complaining that they did not know how to dance. According to Anxiety Australia (n.d.), the thought or experience of an anxiety-provoking situation causes muscle tension. When an addict is anxious, his/her muscles are contracted. This not only limits range of movement and mobility, but it also limits the flow of energy through the body. An addict's body and mind has already resisted the experience before it has begun.

By introducing an addict to the dance/movement therapy group through guided imagery, I questioned if he/she would be more open and willing to move. Easing into the physical self through guided imagery slowly can allow an addict to experience his/her body, preparing him/her to handle more intense feelings that might emerge later in the session through active movement. Starting with simple breathing exercises, an addict is able to begin to identify physical sensations. As he/she begins to tolerate what he/she feels, he/she eventually learns to tolerate and regulate affect. I questioned if using breath and guided imagery at the start of a dance/movement therapy group would be a way to engage patients who typically do not move.

When put into practice, as the substance dependent patients began to relax through guided imagery, I saw the change I wanted to see. The few times I used guided imagery as a prelude to a dance/movement therapy session were the only times I noticed furrowed brows diminish, tense bouncing knees become still, and tightly-held chests softened as they rested calmly in their chairs. Bound faces began to relax and the patients drifted deeper into their imagination. Muscle and psychic tension was decreased as a result of relaxation. Being present with them in this state of relaxation, I felt their resistance lessen. For the first time, I felt a sense of peace and tranquility. I too became relaxed. As the patients appeared physically relaxed with lessened resistance, I wondered if they would begin to feel emotions again. I found that using guided imagery safely brought the patients into their bodies and, perhaps, prepared them to begin to identify what they felt. Relaxed through guided imagery, I imagined that these patients would be more available for dance/movement therapy. With their resistance lessened, I hoped they would be more willing and able to communicate and express themselves through movement.

The Study

From these experiences and observations, I hypothesized that guided imagery in conjunction with dance/movement therapy would decrease anxiety in substance dependent adults. I predicted that these combined interventions would have a greater decrease in anxiety than the single intervention of dance/movement therapy. This pilot study consisted of 60 patients that met the Diagnostic and Statistical Manual of Mental Disorders (American Psychiatric Association, 1994) fourth edition criteria for substance dependency. The participants in this study were voluntarily admitted to an inpatient, medically managed detoxification unit for alcohol and/or heroin dependency. Additional substances used by the research participants were cocaine, marijuana, and benzodiazepines. The participant pool consisted of 47 men and 13 women between the ages of 24 and 59. The individuals were in various phases of withdrawal while participating in this study.

The Adult Manifest Anxiety Scale (AMAS) (Lowe, Reynolds & Richmond, 2003) was administered to each participant of this study. The AMAS-A, designed for ages 19-59, was used to evaluate the anxiety level of each participant pre and post-clinical interventions. The questionnaire contained 36 yes/no questions. Three specific scales and one validity scale made up this test. The Physiological Anxiety Scale addressed how one responds physically to anxiety. The Worry/Oversensitivity Scale addressed factors such as how well a person does in certain aspects of his/her life. The Social Concerns/Stress Scale addressed factors that deal with adult issues, such as money and aging. The Lie Scale, which was the validity scale, addressed factors such as model behavior. The Total Anxiety was the summation of the above scores except for the Lie scale scores. This was a standardized test that gave results as "linear T-scores, standardized scores with a mean of 50 and a standard deviation of 10" (Lowe, Reynolds & Richmond, 2003, p. 3).

The first 20 participants to volunteer for this study partook in the clinical intervention involving only dance movement therapy (DMT). This group was made up of 13 men and seven women. Prior to beginning the clinical intervention, each participant was administered an AMAS-A self-assessment. The intervention that followed utilized Chacian DMT techniques to enhance socialization and communication between others and self (Chaiklin, Lohn, & Sandel, 1993). The same techniques were utilized for each session to minimize the variables being evaluated in this study. At the end of the clinical intervention, each participant filled out a new AMAS-A self-assessment. The second group of 20 participants partook in the clinical intervention involving both guided imagery and DMT (GI&DMT). This group consisted of 15 men and five women. Each participant filled out the AMAS-A for the pre-intervention test. The same predetermined guided imagery script was used for each session of this group, again, in order to reduce test variables. A Chacian DMT intervention followed. At the end of the entire session, each participant filled out a new AMAS-A self-assessment. Lastly, the 20 participants who refused to engage in either of the clinical interventions, but agreed to fill out the AMAS-A self-assessment served as the control group. This final group was composed of 19 men and one woman.

The Results

The outcome of this study was that the anxiety level of each group that received a clinical intervention significantly decreased on all scales. The control group, which received no intervention, showed no significant change, and therefore suggests that those who did not desire change did not experience change. Table 10.1 shows t-scores pre and post-clinical intervention for each group that participated in the study.

This study was designed to use guided imagery to relax the participants in the hope that their decreased anxiety would enable them to participate more fully in the dance/movement experiential. Physiological Anxiety, which is restricted to anxiety located in the physical body, was decreased through a guided imagery script that specifically focused on relaxing discrete parts of the body. Guided imagery was successful according to its predicted effectiveness based on previous clinical observations. There was, however, a factor in using dance/movement therapy as a clinical intervention that allowed for a significant decrease of anxiety on the other scales of Worry/Oversensitivity, Social Concerns/Stress, and Total Anxiety as well.

In the beginning of the recovery process, an addict needs encouragement to transition from an internal disconnected state, to an external engaged state. At this point in recovery, when given the chance to retreat internally and disconnect, an addict will revert back to his automatic defenses. This is what he has known for many years and what keeps him/her in the cycle of addiction. The Chacian techniques of dance/movement therapy used in this study did not allow the participants to take a passive role. They took an active role as their defenses were challenged. Each individual who chose to participate in the study chose to participate in his/her recovery.

When an addict is able to express him/herself and connect with others, he/she becomes more conscious and begins to take an active stance towards life. In this pilot study, the traditional Chacian dance/movement therapy sessions formed a space where the addict had to create something from within, allowing him/her to regain a sense of control. This is what is necessary for the recovery process to begin. In the two groups that received clinical interventions, Physiological Anxiety was released from the body by means of creative expression. Worry/Oversensitivity addressed emotional distress, while

TABLE 10.1. RESULTS OF THE AMAS.

		DMT	GI&DMT	Control Group
Physiological Anxiety	t-scores before	65.4	62.25	62.65
	t-scores after	58.4	56.65	61.55
	Significant Difference	.003**	.010*	.389
Worry/Oversensitivity	t-scores before	62.3	61.25	60.6
	t-scores after	57.5	54.5	61
	Sifnificant Difference	.005**	.011*	.727
Social Concerns/Stress	t-scores before	64.75	58.85	61.1
	t-scores after	58.3	53.25	62.15
	Significant Difference	.002**	.03*	.522
Lie Scale	t-scores before	48.65	51.45	48.9
	t-scores after	49.95	53.15	48.45
	Significant Difference	.491	.228	.761
Total Anxiety	t-scores before	65.9	62.35	62.55
	t-scores after	59.05	55.5	62.75
	Significant Difference	.001**	.013*	.866

*$p < .05$ **$p < .01$

Social Concerns/Stress addressed social connection and interpersonal relationships. Participating in dance/movement therapy, the individuals did not have the opportunity to begin in a dependent, passive state. As a result, they were more available to experience social interactions, express emotions, and form connections with others. Through movement, the addicts were presented with the opportunity to change habitual patterns of inherent passivity. The significant decrease on all of the scales demonstrates that interpersonal connections were made and psychotherapeutic change occurred. In this particular study, the interventions containing dance/movement therapy addressed anxiety relating to habitual patterns of affect regulation, relationships, and physical anxiety.

Dance/Movement Therapy as an Effective Treatment Tool

From clinical experience, I have observed that an addict becomes detached from the act of living as his/her search for the next time he/she uses drugs becomes automatic. Unfortunately, an addict never has enough of the substance he/she abuses. He/she needs more and more until his/her whole being, conscious or unconscious, becomes focused solely on obtaining and using the substance. This lack of consciousness, along with the use of substances, helps the addict stay numb (Caldwell, 1996). This eventually depletes his/her authentic pleasure in life. The addict is no longer consciously living and reaching out towards life, but he/she is withdrawn and focused only on his/her addiction and filling the emptiness. Soon, an addict's life involuntarily revolves around the need for a substance, the need to fill his/her internal emptiness, and the need to numb self.

Collier (as cited in Poole & Rossberg-Gempton, 1992) claims that one's internal emotions are expressed externally through movement. Through clinical experience, I have found that it is difficult for an addict to work in dance/movement therapy because, being in an addicted body, he/she has never felt fulfilled. An addict's inability to regulate can be seen through movement. A substance abuser is generally less aware of his/her body. His/her movement, rigid and bound, prohibits the individual from moving and responding spontaneously.

As Milliken (1990) states, and I have observed, an addict's need for control leads to extreme control of his/her movement. When muscles are tense, the availability for flow of movement is blocked. It can also lead to one's having difficulty in coordination (Duffy, as cited in Poole & Rossberg-Gempton, 1992). This reduces the ability to expand and experience his/her full movement repertoire. An addict is often unable to change the flow of his/her movement. When he/she moves too quickly, he/she is unable to sustain his/her quickness and has to slow down. When he/she slows down, he/she begins to feel, so he/she tries to maintain quick movements. The only way an addict knows how to regain control is to get rid of his/her feelings. He/she needs to numb self. This is done though the extremes of movement; either not moving at all or quickly moving. Like drugs, this quick movement numbs the addict to the emotional experience and he/she is left with a physical feeling of exhaustion.

Rose (as cited in Levy, 1995) states that most addicts find it too painful to put into words their feelings of shame, loneliness, and hopelessness. A physical form of expression is sometimes needed to express anxiety because words cannot fully express an addict's feelings. Dance/movement therapy allows addicts to come together without having to verbalize their painful feelings. It gives the addict a chance to communicate non-verbally through bodily self-expression. Since an addict is so disconnected from what occurs internally, movement encourages him/her to begin to identify what he/she is detached from.

As an addict begins to reconnect to his/her body, he/she gains the ability to sense pleasure again. An addict needs to experience the joy that comes from being in his/her body in a healthy way. This is difficult because he/she associates being in his/her body with feelings of helplessness, shame, and guilt. Caldwell (1996) affirms that the foundation of one's recovery is in the ability to feel and express physical experience. By doing this, the addict has taken the first step towards re-entering the house of pain, his/her body. It is challenging for an addict is to stay in this uncomfortable place and not immediately withdraw. When he/she can learn to take a breath and allow the unwanted feelings to be felt, he/she can start to learn to identify what he/she senses. It is not until the addict begins to learn to acknowledge his/her feelings that he/she can take responsibility for them and begin to express them. Gaining control over his/her internal state, an addict will eventually accept his/her feelings. When he/she is able to do that, he/she will no longer need the substance to numb them. The addict will become more spontaneous and able to better emotionally give and receive with others. He/she will also be able to identify stressors and learn to cope with them before they take over and cause another relapse.

Milliken (2002) believes that an addict can be trained to recreate and reform the boundaries that have restrained him/her for so long. Creative expression is a way in which an addict can break free from his/her restraints. When he/she can create, he/she can begin to take back the freedom to choose, which will enable him/her to adapt to the internal and external environments more easily. It is my understanding that we find the ability to create, produce, and actively live in our healthy selves. As a dance/movement therapist, it is my job to aid my patients in finding and tapping into this healthy self. This can help them to begin to discover new ways to express themselves. Through freedom of expression, an addict can begin to transform within movement. Reiland (1990) asserts that through dance/movement therapy, an addict can begin to expand his movement repertoire, develop control over his own body and bodily boundaries, and separate out his/her internal feelings from what occurs externally. As his/her movement repertoire is expanded, he/she creates more room for expression.

Quickly bouncing of the knee or tightly holding his/her body does not allow room for someone to enter into a relationship with an addict in a group. His/her movements often reflect the feelings of self-isolation that distances self from others. Being in a dance/movement therapy group decreases one's sense of isolation and it increases his/her sense of self (Low & Ritter, 1996). Brooks and Stark (as cited in Low & Ritter), found that one-hour of dance/movement therapy significantly decreased anxiety and depression in inpatient psychiatric patients. As the addict begins to express him/herself through movement, Lohn and Stark (1989) affirm he/she will gain a greater identification and connection within the group. Through movement, an addict can observe that others in the group share his/her experience and this supports feelings of connection and validation. Thomson (1997) claims that as the addict begins to relate to others, his/her sense of self is strengthened.

As members of the group connect with the therapist and the rhythm of the music, they, in turn, begin to connect individually (Schmais, 1985). Rhythm is a practice that works towards group cohesion. The therapist, enforcing the rhythm, is connected to the group. A member has the opportunity to engage with others without having to come in direct contact or confrontation with another. With everyone moving and experiencing together, each member of the group feels supported and seen by the others. An addict's preconceptions that relationships are unfulfilling and unsuccessful are reworked in a cohesive, supportive atmosphere (Thomson, 1997). As he/she begins to experience trust of his/her peers, his/her defenses and muscular tension will gradually decrease, allowing room for new ways to connect with others.

The dance/movement therapist begins to support the addict through mirroring and verbal confirmation. The therapist can encourage the addict to authentically move how he/she feels, and not to mimic others. This allows the addict to develop the distinction between self and others. Being seen and accepted by others, in turn, helps him/her accept self. When an addict can learn to move by him/herself, he/she begins to take responsibility for his/her own physical actions. He/she takes ownership of his/her own emotions and feelings as well. It is when he/she can begin to own parts of self and the power that goes along with this acknowledgement and acceptance that he/she can begin the recovery process. As an addict gains a sense of self, he/she can begin to separate from his/her merged relationship with his/her drug of choice. It is the power of the ownership of the self that creates space for further personal discovery and growth (Caldwell, 1996).

Appendix–Terms

Mirroring, as stated in Chaiklin, Lohn, and Sandel (1993), "involves participating in another's total movement experience, i.e., patterns, qualities, emotional tone, etc. . . . Mirroring is often the first step in establishing empathic connections, particularly with patients who are unresponsive to other modes of interpersonal exchange" (p. 100).

The Chacian technique includes "those elements of dance which serve a therapeutic function, and in the development of the interpersonal role of the therapist on a movement level" (Chailkin, Lohn & Sandel 1993, p. 77). The main categories that make up this technique are body action, symbolism, therapeutic movement relationship, and rhythmic group activity (Chailkin, Lohn & Sandel, 1993).

According to the Wikipedia (2008, March), *countertransference* is "a condition where the therapist . . . begins to transfer the therapist's own unconscious feelings to the patient. . . . Countertransference is also sometimes defined as the entire body of feelings that the therapist has toward the patient."

References

American Psychiatric Association. (2000). *Diagnostic and statistical manual of mental disorders* (4th ed.). Washington, DC: Author.

Anxiety Treatment Australia. (n.d.). *Treatment options: Relaxation.* Retrieved July 13, 2006, from http://www.anxietyaustralia.com.au/treatment/relaxation.shtml

Caldwell, C. (1996). *Getting our bodies back.* Boston: Shambahala Publications.

Chaiklin, S., Lohn, A., & Sandel, S. L. (1993). *Foundation of dance/movement therapy: The life and work of Marian Chace.* Columbia, MD: Marian Chace Memorial Fund of the American Dance Therapy Association.

Dempsey, M. (2006). *Guided imagery in conjunction with dance/movement therapy to decrease anxiety in substance dependent adults.* Unpublished master's thesis, Pratt Institute, Brooklyn, New York.

Dhyansanjivani (n.d.). *Guided imagery: What is it?* Retrieved October 26, 2004, from http://www.dhyansanjivani.org/ganral/Guided_Imagery.asp

Dodes, L. M. (1990). Addiction, helplessness, and narcissistic rage. *Psychoanalytic Quarterly, 59,* 398–419.

Irwin, E. (1986). On being and becoming a therapist. *The Arts in Psychotherapy, 13,* 191–195.

Johnson, B. (1999). Three perspectives on addiction. *Journal of the American Psychoanalytic Association, 47*(3), 791–815.

Khantzian, E. J. (1985). The self-medication hypothesis of addictive disorders. *American Journal of Psychiatry, 142,* 1259–1264.

Kuettel, T. J. (1982). Affective change in dance therapy. *American Journal of Dance Therapy, 5,* 56–64.

Levy, F. J. (1995). *Dance and other expressive art therapies: When words are not enough.* New York: Routledge.

Lohn, A. F. & Stark, A. (1989). The use of verbalization in dance/movement therapy. *The Arts in Psychotherapy, 16*(1), 105–113.

Low, K. G. & Ritter, M. (1996). Effects of dance/movement therapy: A meta-analysis. *The Arts in Psychotherapy, 23*(3), 249–260.

Lowe, P., Reynolds, C., & Richmond, B. (2003). *AMAS: Adult manifest anxiety scale.* Los Angeles: Western Psychological Services.

Milliken, R. (1990). Dance/movement therapy with the substance abuser. *The Arts in Psychotherapy, 17,* 309–317.

Milliken, R. (2002). Dance/movement therapy as a creative arts therapy approach in prison to the treatment of violence. *The Arts in Psychotherapy, 29,* 203–206.

Poole, G. & Rossberg-Gempton, I. (1992). The relationship between body movement and affect: From historical and current perspectives. *The Arts in Psychotherapy, 19,* 39–46.

Reiland, J. D. (1990). A preliminary study of dance/movement therapy with field-dependent alcoholic women. *The Arts in Psychotherapy, 17,* 349–353.

Rossman, M. L. (2000). *Guided imagery for self-healing.* Tiburon, CA: H J Kramer.

Schmais, C. (1985). Healing processes in group dance therapy. *American Journal of Dance Therapy, 8*(1), 17–36.

Thomson, D. M. (1997). Dance/movement therapy with dual diagnosed: A vehicle to the self in the service of recovery. *American Journal of Dance Therapy, 10*(1), 63–79.

Wikipedia. (2008, March). *Countertransference.* Retrieved May 17, 2008, from http://en.wikipedia.org/wiki/Countertransference

Biography

Meghan Dempsey currently works as a dance/movement therapist on an inpatient psychiatric unit in Brooklyn, New York. After receiving her Bachelor of Arts from UCLA in World Arts and Cultures with a concentration in dance, she earned a Master of Science in Dance/Movement Therapy from Pratt Institute in Brooklyn, New York. Subsequent to receiving her MS and ADTR, Ms. Dempsey went on to receive her CMA from the Laban/Bartenieff Institute of Movement Studies, where she has had the honor of being a guest teacher. As a member of the New York chapter of the ADTA, Ms. Dempsey is currently working on a public relations film entitled *Moving Stories: Portraits of Dance/Movement Therapy.* Please contact Ms. Dempsey at move2improve@gmail.com for further information.

Chapter 11

USING EXPRESSIVE ARTS THERAPY WITH YOUNG MALE OFFENDERS RECOVERING FROM SUBSTANCE ABUSE IN A DE-ADDICTION SETUP IN INDIA

PRIYADARSHINI SENROY

Introduction

This chapter is an attempt to illustrate the research the author did on using the process of expressive arts therapy with a group of young male offenders recovering from substance abuse. The chapter begins with a very brief introduction of this client group in relation to their abuse and the criminal justice system in India. The introduction also attempts to explore some of the mental health reasons behind the manifestation of their abuse. It then gives information about the hosptial treatment program in the prison, where this research takes place, and the challenges faced by the author while facilitating the group sessions. The chapter continues by explaining the expressive arts therapeutic approach that formed the basis of the therapeutic work. The session vignettes attempt to explain and share the outcomes of this process work the group and the therapist undertook together. The aim of the research was to use the different modalities of expressive arts therapy to assist the client to make contact with his/her authentic self. Dance, drama, music, and visual arts were used to bring special strengths and abilities in bridging the expanse between the literal reality of "here now" and the world of the imagination. It is in this realm where life stories are written in mythic form and life experiences are held in symbols, which provides a therapeutic environment for recovery (Art Therapy, 2008). The chapter finishes with a conclusion followed by a glossary and reference.

The Setting

This research took place in Tihar Jail, the largest prison in South East Asia in 1998–1999. The facility has approximately 14,000 prisoners, eighty percent of whom are under judicial custody, awaiting sentences for different kinds of crimes committed. Young male offenders in the age range of 18–21 years make up approximately 15 percent of this demography. Approximately 40 percent of this group are drug dependent individuals, who are incarcerated for offenses directly or indirectly related to substance abuse and related crimes. They are housed in a de-addiction and rehabilitation facility set up in the young offenders section of the prison (Tihar Prison, 2007).

Substance abuse is becoming a major health problem in India with some estimates indicating that as many as 20 million people in India could become addicts by the end of 2008. A report on India recently compiled by the UN Drug Control programme on Drugs and Crimes, the first of its kind, cites that in Delhi the capital of India, 44.7 percent of treatment seekers were heroin addicts while alcohol abuse accounted for 26.4 percent (Joshi, 2007). A link between drug abuse and crime is well established and recently the association between drug addiction and HIV/AIDS has been a prime concern for health authorities in India (Gupta, 2007).

The problem has now reached the higher echelons of society, along with the lower strata, and includes children and students in urban areas. Daily wage earners/laborers, rag pickers, truck drivers, medical workers, and youths are all equally susceptible to the menace of addiction (Gupta, 2007).

Prepared in collaboration with the Union Ministry of Social Justice and Empowerment, the report says that most addicts are initiated into drug abuse by age 24 (Joshi, 2007). Heroin in urban areas and opium in rural areas have emerged as the two most commonly used drugs. Increasing trend of drug and alcohol, addiction in large cities, especially the metropolitan cities is alarming (Gupta, 2007).

Medical experts have attempted to define factors responsible for driving a person to drug addiction. Case histories compiled by medical experts/psychologists have indicated that many people start using drugs for pleasure, while others do so for a sense of adventure. Other reasons include dejection as a result of medical discomfort, social and psychological maladjustment, and parental neglect. Environmental factors are also, to some extent, responsible for drug dependence. Rapid technological development, associated with the need for extended periods of education, inapplicability of old solutions to modern problems, TV, world trade, and affluence are other factors which encourage drug addiction (Joshi, 2007).

The Ministry of Social Justice and Empowerment as the focal point for drug demand reduction programmes in the country, has been implementing the Scheme for Prohibition and Drug Abuse Prevention since the year 1985–1986. As implementation of programmes for de-addiction and rehabilitation of drug addicts, require sustained and committed/involved effort with a great degree of flexibility and innovation (Ministry of Social Justice and Empowerment, 2007).

There are various substance abuse treatment centers in India based in both private clinics and in government-managed programs operating out of hopitals and prisons. Accordingly, the voluntary organisations provide actual services through the Counselling and Awareness Centers; De-addiction cum Rehabilitation Centres, De-addiction Camps, and Awareness Programs. One of the de-addiction wards, which deals with adolescents and the young adults, houses about 25-30 clients who have been victims of substance abuse. Functioning at a hospital level, the clients are under treatment and stay there until they recover from their withdrawal symptoms. They then go back to the other wards to face the trials and sentences.

The group consists of male members, ranging between 16–23 years of age. They predominantly belong to the low socioeconomic strata of the society and have been arrested for crimes related with substance abuse. Few of them have stable families while most of them live on the streets and are illiterate. Most of them were able to continue with their addiction by committing petty thefts (Aids Awareness Group, 2006). Since they come to de-addiction wards for treatment, the nature of the group is transitory in nature. The stay varies according to the medical treatment, the maximum stay being six months.

The de-addiction ward is based on the *Therapeutic Community* model of dealing with individuals recovering from substance abuse This model entails dividing the prisoners into families with a big brother to oversee the behavior and general progress of the small brothers. This is a method used to substitute the biological family which is on occasion the reason for a person falling prey to drugs (Aids Awareness Group, 2006). The traditional therapeutic community is distinguished from other major drug treatment modalities in several ways, including coordinating a comprehensive range of interventions and services in a single treatment setting. An important feature of the Therapeutic Community model is that the primary therapist and teacher in the Therapeutic Community is the community itself, consisting of peers and staff members who serve as role models, with staff members also serving as authorities and guides in the recovery process (United Nations Office on Drugs and Crime, 2007).

Typically, a new offender joins the family as small brother to be looked after by big brother. The inmates are given a structured schedule of everyday activities in order to promote recovery. This includes counselling, education, meditation, mood-making sessions, sharing one's recovery, concept seminars, family group, community meetings, barrack meetings, anger and brief workouts, educational, and recreational activities. Psychodrama is used effectively. These activities are integral to community building (Tihar Prison, 2007).

The Approach

Creative art therapy, which is psychotherapeutic in nature, is used in several settings. In respect to the prison setting, the therapy serves as a reformatory process in several ways. Firstly and most importantly, it helps to express, channelize and ventilate self. One has to keep in mind that anyone convicted or otherwise exiled from the rest of the world is initially bound to have tremendous anger, aggression, sense of helplessness, hopelessness, and emotional problems (Tihar Prison, 2007). Creative arts therapy can provide a form of expression for feelings that cannot be easily identified or put into words. In the context of using it with clients who have been substance abusers, this modality can help the abuser connect with his/her more authentic self. This can be done by understanding themselves better through the development of a more firmly based self-consciousness (Goldring, 2001). The expressive therapies can help raise self-esteem and provide an opportunity to create new experiences beyond habitual and painful emotional patterns. The creative arts foster a renewed ability to relax without drugs or alcohol (Addiction Recovery Guide, 2007).

In prevention contexts with young people, evaluation studies provide evidence that arts programs can reduce offending behavior and incidents of disruption, help disaffected young people re-engage with education, and sponsor personal and social development (Mountford, 1998). Although the arts in criminal justice sector is not bound together by a coherent set of practices or consistent thinking, it is possible to identify a number of major thematic strands in practice. Arts as therapeutic interventions are one such model of intervention (Mountford, 1998).

The Session Structure

During the short-term pilot project conducted by the author, approximately 50 adolescents attended the drama therapy sessions in groups of 8–10, once a week for an hour and a half. Each session was structured through a warm-up, main event, and grounding. The toolkit included expression, imagination, and metaphor, involving group members in dance and drama, rhythm, and movement. These modalities facilitated access to materials on the borderline of consciousness, even to subconscious materials, and through this, to the therapy and liberation of catharsis. The sessions made use of movement, voice, dramatic games, improvisation, puppets, picture-cards, and masks, any method that in the context of the clients' needs, stimulated verbal or non verbal self-expression (Goldring, 2001).

Verbal feedback was also encouraged to emphasize the importance of expressive language. The therapeutic process engaged by the client and the facilitator was based in a non-threatening and creative space. It was important to have a creative space as it has often been suggested that arts interventions in criminal justice contexts are successful because they offer a non-traditional, non-institutional, social and emotional environment, a non-judgmental and unauthoritarian model of engagement, and an opportunity to participate in a creative process that involves both structure and freedom. At the same time, engagement in the participatory arts requires respect, responsibility, cooperation, and collaboration (Mountford, 1998). This was reiterated by the client never being judged by the quality of their contribution as the work is not geared towards performance. All the work of the session was done within the art form, with no attempt at "interpretation" of personal material (Pearson, 1996).

The general aims and objectives of the project were to explore the creative medium with relation to self-discovery, awareness and growth, to work on positive self-image, self-trust, and feeling a sense of worth in their life and their surroundings. The session also tried to create opportunities where the clients could experience and value activities that are not compatible with substance abuse thus discovering ways of connecting internalized responses with external behavior and vice versa. The purpose was also to try and develop healthy and meaningful relationships with others including supportive adults and other role models. The specific aims and objectives were to slowly encourage the clients to develop interests and see life beyond substance abuse.

Some of the challenges in working in this environment varied from session to session. The first couple of months were spent trying to establish the work in the de-addiction facility. The prison wardens, the guards, and the doctors were skeptical of the nature and purpose of introducing this project. Some expressed that this was just a way to pass time not only for the inmates but also for the author. Some suggested that trying to invest time and energy with the group who they thought belonged to the lowest echelon of the society would have no positive result at all. The only official who had faith in the process and the project was the superintendent of the juvenile prison, who was an advocate of providing alternate therapeutic intervention modalities for this group. Once the nature and purpose of the group was established, some of the other challenges faced by the author and group were external. Once the session had to be cancelled as the de-addiction facility was locked down as drugs were found on the premises. Also, the group number was sometimes small as the inmates had court dates or were discharged from the facility. As the turnover rate was extremely high in this group, the group had to be open in nature. Several times there was an overlap between new and old clients. The groups had to be catered and planned according to themes and self-contained in one session. The working contract of the sessions and the boundaries had to be clearly defined every session to accommodate new members joining the group. At the same time, sessions had to incorporate therapeutic endings to facilitate smooth transition for members leaving the group.

Session Vignettes

Sessions Using Visual Imagery

The introductory sessions comprised of working with visual imagery in the form of postcards, as 79 percent of the inmates were illiterate (Tihar Prison, 2007). This tool was used as a non-threatening medium of expressing themselves as well as create opportunities for the client to become aware of anomalies in thinking and feeling. It also created and expanded options for viewing, clarifying, and making meaning of their feelings, beliefs, and the events in their past and present lives (Lark, 2001).

The first set of picture postcard images consisted of a wide selection of known and unknown images of people, places, family and so forth, which were introduced for them to select and then share those images. They were selected to give an insight into the personalities of the clients. The following are some of the responses that came up: A picture of skyscrapers in the night represented the feeling of being lost in the crowd during growing up as an adult and a picture of a rickshaw puller (a tricycle to transport people in the urban cities and rural towns) entering a smoke-filled alley which represented childhood, the passenger representing the present and the smoke representing the uncertain future or old age. The second set of postcard images were images about relationships, abstract pictures and images of life in general. The boys were first invited to choose three images which represented their past, present, and future and then share it with the group. Some of the "stories" through the postcards images were:

Q's three images had sky and flight in it. He said that he was still "flying" and would need to fly before settling down. And he mentioned that his story did not have a end because he could not see it.

R's beginning was the image of a old woman, tired, and bent. He said that he is also tired and he would like to move on represented by a second image of a camel caravan in a desert. The final picture was that of a farmhouse, which represented his wish to find a new place where he could farm and raise his family.

S's picture had a mother and a child in the first image, a small boy holding a bird in the second one, and the third one was of a scene in a desert, with lots of children being entertained by a magician. He said that his life had become like the desert after a life he has lived full of drugs and felony.

The discussion that followed was that most of them felt that they had wasted their life being under the influence of a substance. They felt alone despite having a family. The group was able to process these images and feelings together. They were able to give each other feedback and the discussion continued as to how someone is not alone because they have themselves and need to respect their own individuality, taking the setbacks in their strides in order to make them stronger. One of the clients was able to reflect on how the substance abuse had destroyed him and now it was time to create again. According to him, this destruction was necessary in order to create a healthy self. He ended his statement by saying that the more one suffers as a result of destruction, the joy of the next creation is sweeter.

Session on Aspirations and Desires

The emphasis of the session was to talk about the aspirations and desires that the clients might have and to express them through visual imagery. Some of them found it challenging to express their emotions or talk about them, but found it easier to draw simple pictures to share them. The drawings helped them to explain what they were feeling and thinking when they did not have words to do it. For inmates, art therapy is a chance to work through anger, traumatic pasts, and stress (Spring, 2007). They can be as angry or deviant as they want in their art and it cannot be transcribed. Many inmates do not want to talk about something that makes them very emotional, but they can draw that in the picture (Spring, 2007).

The session structure was to invite each person to choose a memorable dream that they saw for themselves in the future, and to focus on it. They were then encouraged to make a drawing of their dream sequence and were reassured that it was okay not to be perfect at drawing. The purpose of this exercise was to let the emotion of the dream make the images onto the paper and slowly let it take form and shape in front of them. After the drawing, the group was invited to show their picture as they described their dream with the others. The group was also advised that they could give feedback on the dream and mention anything positive that they could relate to. Once the dreams were shared, the group was invited to enact each dream. Each dreamer was a director for his piece and was invited to use the other clients in the group as characters and dramatize the dream. They were also invited they could make changes as they went along in making this dream sequence.

Once the dreams were dramatized, there was a discussion held about how the dreamer felt having his dream played out and any insight others may share. Some of the drawings of dreams were:

E's dream was to have a "mansion" but he did not know how to draw it. Instead he drew a colorful peacock. His interpretation was that he felt like a bird who wanted to fly but often fell down but flew again. He hoped that in the future, like the bird, failure would not stop him from flying.

A's painting had a human form. Lines represented legs and hands and did not have a torso. The face had spiky hair, no eyebrows, ferocious teeth, and pockmarks on the face. He used the colors blue, orange, and red on a yellow background paper. He interpreted that the face represented his fear of the unknown and that he was anxious as to what would happen to him once he was back on the streets. He was not able to come up with coping strategies. During feedback session, *E* suggested that maybe *A* would be like his peacock and not give up if he was faced with the temptations of abusing drugs again.

B's picture had a sun with a face, stars, and two human forms. Two "blobs" represented children. The "man" had hair all around his face. The "woman" had a pair of braids. Both the human forms only had hands and legs with five digits. He mentioned he hoped that he would be well enough to go back to his family and take care of them.

C's dream had a house in a picturesque setting—with a river, date trees, mountains, and birds. He drew a profile of a man near the house. There was a balloon lying on the the bank of the river. *C* interpreted that he would like to be alone in a big house in the future and he would like to rest and not always fly aimlessly like a balloon.

D's drew a portrait with spiky hair, no mouth, no body, lines for limbs with a flower beside it. He said the words "I see my mother in the flower." And he mentioned that he missed his mother and was looking forward to going back to her.

The enactments were done in silence and some of the feedback was that they had never thought of having hopes and aspirations again. Some of them said that they had aspirations but always thought that they would not come true, but drawing and dramatizing it helped them to visualize what it might look like. The drawings were able to help them explain what they were feeling and thinking when they did not have words to do it. Most inmates do not want to talk about something that makes them very emotional, but they can draw that in the picture (Spring, 2007). Spring further elaborates that clients are often surprised by what they draw and they do not always realize what they are thinking about until it is drawn. For instance, the symbolism and meaning behind what an inmate paints can often show a new part of the psyche (Spring, 2007).

Session on Mask

Using masks and other theatrical metaphors in a prison setup are inspired in part by cognitive behavioral theory and research into criminal thinking and behavior. For example, a mask can represent the front or persona performed by an offender in a specific context. Within workshops and performances, participants are challenged to lift the mask and say what they think and feel at a deeper level. This develops an awareness of destructive patterns of thought and feelings and offers the possibility of changing behavior. Theatrically, the mask allows the actor to represent dynamically the "inner voice" (the thought process)—emphasizing thoughts, beliefs, rules, values, and their effect on behavior (Mountford, 1998).

To introduce working with masks, different kinds of animal and face masks were brought in to generate interest and begin a discussion of using masks as a tool for expressing the inner self to the outside world without exposing the real person behind it. The sessions gave an opportunity to the individual to process their inner feelings. To stimulate a discussion, some of the questions addressed were:

What is a mask?
Answer: Another face that we wear on top of our real face.
What happens when we wear masks?
Answer: People cannot see the real person but only what is shown (projected) through the mask.
Why do we need to wear masks?
Answer: To hide ourselves or to save ourselves from being vulnerable in front of others.
When does one feel the need to wear a mask?
Answer: When we don't want the world to know of our true identity or true feeling.
Can we wear more than one mask and if so what can they be?
Answer: Intoxication, anger, love, jealousy, thoughtfulness, and honesty.
Who then is the real person behind the mask?
Answer: The human being.
Why does one feel the need to wear a mask?
Answer: Everybody—to protect ourselves from being "burnt."

Once the discussions were over, all the group members were given plain templates and colors to make masks for themselves. The theme was making a mask that represented their lives before addiction and after addiction. Colors relating to emotions and feelings used primarily were red for anger, green for jealousy, black for loss, and yellow for shame. Once the masks were made, they were then invited to share them within the group. Some of the individuals chose to interpret their masks and share how their lives were before and after addiction.

Once the masks were shared with an audience, they were invited to share any thoughts or feelings about the sharing. Some of the comments were that, "I have forgottten who I am really"; "My whole life has been wearing one mask or the other"; "I think I need to do something about the masks I wear"; " I feel that my life has been a lie"; and "I let my addiction become a mask and rob my inner identity."

The facilitator at this point reflected back to the whole group about the entire process and explained that when it came to a way of expressing deep emotions, masks have always been used as perfect medium. Masks are worn for various reasons and are sometimes worn in order to survive to get along in the world. The aims of becoming aware and recognizing all the different social and emotional personas is not to get rid of them but to use them to explore which of the personas they would really like to explore or which ones they want to get rid of or which ones they would really like to pay more attention to. The whole process of working with masks can be very pure (Trenshaw, 2007).

Conclusion

Over the course of the project, the group seemed to have responded positively to the activities. Depending on their history of substance abuse, emotional, and educational background, they were able to relate to the psychological content of the sessions in various levels. It is hoped that the project was able to convey to the group as well as to the prison officials that arts, music, dance, and drama are not only for entertainment purposes, but also provide opportunities to explore and solve their emotional and social problems without direct confrontation. As the project ended, recommendations were made on introducing similar projects in the future to include several different prison sites, providing the opportunity to administer the assessment tools and creative art therapy sessions to inmates who have never been exposed to these procedures. As of 2003–2005, the Tihar Prison has been using creative arts therapy as an expressive therapy as well as a fundraising project where in the inmates' paintings were exhibited and sold to the general public (Tihar Prison, 2007).

Appendix–Terms

Catharsis is an emotional release. According to psychodynamic theory, this emotional release is linked to a need to release unconscious conflicts. For example, experiencing stress over a work-related situation may cause feelings of frustration and tension. Rather than vent these feelings inappropriately, the individual may instead release these feelings in another way, such as through physical activity or another stress-relieving activity.

Expressive Arts Therapy uses five art disciplines to assist the client/artist to make contact with his/her authentic self. We use dance, drama, music, visual arts, and poetry. Each discipline brings special strengths and abilities in bridging the expanse between the literal reality of "here now" and the world of the imagination, where life stories are written in mythic form and life experiences are held in symbols.

Metaphor is a Greek word which means "to transfer." A figure of speech in which one thing is spoken as if it were another, i.e., a house is the dreamer. In a dream, "the house on fire" would symbolize the psychological condition of the dreamer and the metaphor would be "the house," which would represent the dreamer. The fire would symbolize an emotion, attitude or complex, such as anger, destruction, passion, desire, illumination, transformation, and so forth.

Therapeutic Community Model of dealing with drug addicts is the program which is used in Tihar Jail. This entails dividing the prisoners into families with a big brother to oversee the behavior and general progress of the small brothers. This is a method used to substitute the biological family which is occasionally the reason for a person falling prey to drugs.

Persona in the word's everyday usage is a social role or a character played by an actor. The word derives from the Latin for "mask" or "character." The persona is also the mask or appearance one presents to the world. It may appear in dreams under various guises. The persona, used in this sense, is not a pose or some other intentional misrepresentation of the self to others. Rather, it is the self as self-construed and may change according to situation and context.

References

The Addiction Recovery Guide. (2007). *Creative arts therapy.* In The Addiction Recovery Guide. Retrieved June 24, 2007, from http://www.addictionrecoveryguide.org/holistic/arts.html

Aids Awareness Group, India. (2006). *De-addiction Ward Report–In Aids awareness group.* Retrieved June 24, 2007, from http://www.aagindia.org

Goldring, N. (2001). *Drama therapy in Hermon Prison.* In State of Israel, Ministry of Public Security, Retrieved June 24, 2007, from www.mops.gov.il/nr/exeres/7A23C5F0-1F61-4D8D-A50F- 43C66FDF70D1.htm

Gupta, A. (2007). *Drug/alcohol addiction in India, disturbing trends–In Gateway For India.* Retrieved June24, 2007, from http://www.gatewayforindia.com/articles/addiction.htm

Joshi, U. (2007). *Law has failed in fighting drug abuse–In Daily Excelsior* Retrieved June 24, 2007, from http://www.dailyexcelsior.com/web1/03july06/edit.htm#3

Lark, C. (2001). Art Therapy Overview: An informal background paper–The Art Therapy Center. In *Art Therapy*. Retrieved June 24, 2007, from http://www.arttherapy.com/ArtTherapyOverview.htm

Ministry of Social Justice and Empowerment, Government of India. (2007). Drug demand reduction and preventive policies: Government of India's approach a synopsis. In *Ministry of Social Justice and Empowerment*. Retrieved June 24,2007, from http://www. socialjustice.nic.in/social/welcome.htm

Mountford, A. (1998). Doing the arts justice. A Review of research literature, practice and theory researched and written by Jenny Hughes. In A. Miles and A. McLewin (Ed). *The unit for the arts and OffendersCentre for Applied Theatre Research Department of Culture, Media and Sport* (pp. 10–11, p. 112). Government of UK.

Pearson, J. (1996). (Ed.), *Discovering the self through drama and movement–The Sesame Approach.* London: Jessica Kingsley Publishers.

Spring, D. (2007). Art in Treatment. Treatment hues. In interview with S. Etter. In *Corrections.* Retrieved June 24, 2007, from http://www..corrections.com/news/article?articleid=15308

Tihar Prison Reformation. (2007). Creative arts therapy. *In Tihar Prisons.* Retrieved June 24, 2007, from http://www.tiharprisons.nic.in/html/reform.htm

Tihar Prison Profile. (2007). Prison ctatistics & classification of prison population. *In Tihar Prisons.* Retrieved June 24, 2007, from http://www.tiharprisons.nic.in/html/profile.htm

Tihar Prison Infrastructure. (2007). Hospital and medical facilities. *In Tihar Prison.* Retrieved June 24, 2007, from http://www.tiharprisons.nic.in/html/infra.htm

Trenshaw, K. (2007). Breaking the Silence, Healing is having to understand the masks that we have worn to survive. In interview by S. Kumar. *In Resurgence.* Retrieved June 24, 2007, from http:// www.resurgence.org/resurgence/articles/trenshaw.htm

United Nations Office on Drugs and Crime. (2007). Module for Prison Intervention: South Asia. In *United Nations Office on Drugs and Crime.* Retrieved June 24, 2007, http://www.unodc.org/india/en/publications.html

Biography

Priyadarshini Senroy, MA, DMT, CCC is a Drama and Movement Therapist residing in Toronto, Canada. She works with children and women with special needs and mental health issues. She is also on the board of the Creative Arts in Counseling Chapter of the Canadian Counseling Association. She has worked in various clinical settings including prison and psychiatric day centres in India and England. She has presented her multicultural work using Drama and Movement Therapy at conferences and has contributed to books, newsletters, and journals all over the world.

Chapter 12

MOVING INTO ACTION: A CASE STUDY OF DANCE/MOVEMENT THERAPY WITH THE DUALLY DIAGNOSIED IN A METHADONE TREATMENT PROGRAM

Opiate addiction levels in NYC are amongst the highest in the country. Heroin addiction is related to high levels of crime (National Institute of Justice, 1998), the spread of disease such as Hepatitus-C and HIV (Marsch, 1998; Mehta et al., 2005; Moore & Dusheiko, 2005), and homelessness (Abelson et al., 2006). Recently the national government has explored the usefulness of "alternative therapy" in engaging addicted individuals in treatment and has listed dance/movement therapy (DMT) on the SAMSHA (2008) web site. Herein the author argues that DMT is a powerful medium in the addiction treatment palette, specifically in the recovery of individuals addicted to opiates maintained on methadone with their concomitant issues of polysubstance abuse, criminality, trauma, physical disease, and mental illness. The author shares her experience, giving case examples from nine years working as a dance/movement therapist working in a Methadone Maintenance Program (MTP) implementing the Transtheoretical Model of Change (TTM) ((Prochaskas, DiClemente & Norcross, 1992).

Dance/Movement Therapy Research in Substance Abuse Treatment

Addiction is a dynamic process, something that moves, progresses and retreats, and develops its own rhythm, form, and meaning (Perlmutter, 1992). The dance of recovery is: "A dance of loss, shame, remorse, sadness, fear, insecurity, emptiness, resentment, frustration, denial, anger, manipulation, perversions of sexuality, power plays, embarrassment, humiliation–on and on–into the darkness. The dance out of the darkness must first retrace the steps that were made going in" (Perlmutter, 1992, p. 46).

Whereas addiction leads individuals to experience a loss of control, DMT helps them regain control by reclaiming their bodies (selves) via movement (Milliken, 1990; Perlmutter, 1992; Plevin, 1996; Thompson, 1997). In order to accomplish this feat, dance/movement therapists have to empathize with and contain clients' feelings, encourage clients' exploration of healthier behaviors and coping mechanisms, while being a good role model, encouraging a "long-term connection to the recovery process and the individuals and groups which support it" (Perlmutter, 1992, p. 46).

The author has found that dance/movement therapists must be able to move with and reign in chaos when they work with addictions. Patients' defenses can overwhelm dance/movement therapists, particularly projective identification (Plevin, 1996), as they can evoke powerfully charged visceral countertransferences in the therapist. The dance/movement therapist and her interns in the MTP often feel what the patients cannot speak, cry when the patients cannot, and feel like a failure when patients do not succeed. Denial, splitting, rationalization, projection, projective identification, minimizing, and blaming are the most common defense mechanisms utilized by substance abusers. These can lead therapists to reject clients, to join clients' denial, or at times lead to burnout. If dance/movement therapists can effectively manage their countertransferential responses, they can decrease and contain these defenses, increasing patients' motivation to engage in treatment (Milliken, 1990; Perlmutter, 1992; Plevin, 1996; Thompson, 1997).

Drama therapists (Johnson, 1990), art therapists (Matto, Corcoran & Fassler, 2003), and dance/movement therapists (Milliken, 1990; Perlmutter, 1992; Plevin, 1996; Rose, 1995; Thompson, 1997) working in addiction treatment speak to the importance of creating aesthetic distance. Metaphor and creative expression allows for a healthy detachment from the problem and can help clients gain a more objective perspective, which gives space for solutions to emerge.

Experiencing the body can be quite scary for substance-abusing clients thus it can be more difficult to obtain aesthetic distance in DMT, especially for dually diagnosed clients (Thompson, 1997) and clients who have been physically and sexually abused (Fisher, 1990) as it is the body that moves, feels, and expresses. In DMT, there is no object (artwork, musical instrument, or role) to hide behind, unless props are used. However, the author finds that a skilled dance/movement therapist, who engenders trust, can create this safe distance by fully engaging the group in the synchronous rhythmic movement and in meaningful exploration of imagery and symbolism through movement metaphor (Rose, 1995).

"It is only by learning how to identify, tolerate, and process feelings and how to manage stressful life situations that the chemically addicted person can successfully recover" (Rose 1995, p. 108). In addition to aesthetic distance, group catharsis, which can be obtained through "the spontaneous creation of an imaginary domain" (Johnson, 1990, p. 303), is a key component in this process. People use chemicals to medicate or modulate their emotional pain (Khantzian, 1999; Milliken, 1990; Rose, 1995). DMT provides emotional catharsis by allowing group members to unite around a common movement theme without necessarily verbalizing their pain. Creative processes, movement-based or other, contain and reframe the addictive craving by increasing the client's ability to access creative power to fulfill emotional needs rather than depending upon substances to provide an externally-induced experience (Milliken, 1990; Rose, 1995; Shoshensky, 2001).

While the author has seen DMT produce emotionally cathartic effects in the MTP and create feelings of connectedness, belonging, and self affirmation, as Rose (1995) found with other substance abusers, the methadone population may differ from other clients in SA treatment in that they are still ingesting a substance that abolishes physiological cravings. It is not clear how medicated assisted therapy impacts client's unverbalized emotional needs. Some MTP clients have verbalized that they feel numb to their emotions on methadone. However, it is clear DMT helps increase clients' expressive range.

One of the main emotional issues to be addressed in the treatment of addictions is shame (Johnson, 1990). Extreme shame is shown in the movement characteristics of patients who are dually diagnosed, in their "difficulty to claim space, avoid eye contact or any other mutual acknowledgement of being seen" (Thompson, 1997, p. 71). This is even more exaggerated in clients in the MTP as society has stigmatized methadone treatment.

Several dance/movement therapists have embraced the 12 Steps in their work (Fisher, 1990; Perlmutter, 1992; Rose, 1995; Thompson, 1997) as they are widely accepted as a self-help tool in overcoming addiction and as a means of getting in touch with one's spirituality. However, MTP clients are reluctant to embrace the 12 Steps as they often report that they have difficulty finding 12-Step meetings that allow them to speak because of the stigma against methadone.

Fortunately, Creative Arts Therapy (CAT) can heal shame by helping discover the "true self," by fostering a connection with one's spirituality (Johnson, 1990). The most profound way to contact one's spirit is to go deeper into the body. Clients in the MTP have noted "God's presence in the room" during DMT. Providing clients with a "natural high," the feeling they sought when they first started to use drugs (Perlmutter, 1992, p. 47), is a unique capability of DMT and addresses the spiritual needs of those in recovery.

Understanding the drive for one's self to be whole, to recover lost parts of one self–including one's spirit, is important in working with addicted individuals (Fisher, 1990; Lewis, 1993; Perlmutter, 1992; Johnson, 1990). MTP clients often say that without drugs they do not know who they are. Creative self-expression fulfills this drive to know oneself, to be whole (Johnson, 1990). Supporting a state of receptiveness in patients; helping patients find a different mode of expression; providing a nurturing environment to allow for reconstruction of the patients' egos; helping patients' use insight to promote honesty; supporting a healthier ego structure through the use of spontaneity, immediate response, and exploring options; and helping patients feel like they fit in through self and interactional synchrony are all part of this process in DMT (Fisher, 1990).

While no published research specifically addresses DMT with people on methadone maintenance, two interns wrote their unpublished Master's theses (Daly 2002; Oktay, 2004) about DMT with this population under the author's tutelage in the Bellevue MTP. Both reinforce several of the findings from above. First, they both incorporated working towards finding "the true self" (Johnson, 1990) in their theoretical approach to DMT. Oktay did this through video and by addressing the first psychosocial stages of development, trust versus mistrust, via group process. Daly accomplished this through combining movement metaphor, symbolism, and the balancing of opposites by using Hatha Yoga. Secondly, both researchers used non-Chacian approaches and demonstrated that it is possible for MTP clients to reconnect the body mind and increase awareness of themselves via movement. Thirdly, they both facilitated expression of emotion: Daly by helping clients identify where feeling was located in their bodies and Oktay via video use/ analysis of group interaction and dance. Lastly, Daly's movement group addressed the clients' spiritual needs as Hatha Yoga is a spiritual practice.

Case Description: Setting, Context, & Patients

The author has been working in New York City at Bellevue Methadone Treatment Program (MTP) from 1999 to present (2008), which services a maximum of 350 clients and has over 30 professionals on staff. Only adults who have a verifiable dependence on opiates are accepted into the program. One-third of the clients maintain abstinence from all illicit substances, one-third use drugs sporadically, and the last third uses drugs regularly.

The clients who self-select to come to CAT groups usually are dually diagnosed (1/3 of all clients receive psychiatric care; however, the true percentage of mental illness is not known as many clients subvert treatment), multiply diagnosed (85% of all clients have Hepatitis C, 25% are HIV + and 10% have Diabetes), and/or have suffered trauma. As with most substance abusers (Heffernan et al., 2000), 85 to 90 percent of all patients in the MTP have suffered severe forms of physical or sexual abuse. When a client with just substance dependence does come to CAT groups, the individual usually has served a long-term incarceration and needs help re-acclimating to society.

It is easy to understand how these individuals are lured to use opiates and become addicted. Opiates create a sense of euphoria and are analgesic, putting the individual in a drowsy state where all of their cares are forgotten (Kuhn, Swartzwelder & Wilson, 2003). "People under the influence of opiates will often say that they just don't worry about their troubles anymore: they are in a special, safe place where cares are forgotten" (p. 182).

Criminality, trauma, and mental illness make it difficult to engage this population in treatment as they have difficulty trusting (themselves and others), expressing feelings, and feeling shame. Due to social stigma, patients often feel they have to keep their participation in methadone treatment a secret. Shame, it seems, prevents people on methadone from showing themselves, from engaging in treatment or once in treatment from coming to group, and then once in group from opening up. Clients' "not showing up" is the greatest hurdle in doing group therapy in the methadone clinic. This can demoralize group leaders; thus, support and supervision for the creative arts therapist working in this setting is of the utmost importance.

Bellevue's MTP is located within the Addiction Psychiatry Department. The integration of this clinic within a hospital is different as most MTPs are operated as freestanding dispensaries. Clients often call these types of clinics, "Cop and go" or "Cop and bop." Bellevue clients get a strong message that they are expected to engage in treatment but group participation is voluntary. Contingency management is used to engage clients in group treatment. Patients are offered holistic treatment via medical treatment, individual counseling, verbal groups, and creative arts therapy in keeping with the disease model of addiction that views addiction as a biopsychosocial phenomenon. The dance/movement therapist is part of an interdisciplinary treatment team consisting of a medical doctor, a psychiatrist, a psychiatric fellow, counselors, nurses, social workers, addiction counselors, a vocational rehabilitation counselor, support/clerical staff, and interns.

DMT, Motivational Interviewing and the Transtheoretical Model of Change

The author's experience validates Johnson's (1990) claim that Chace technique works well with addicted individuals. In this approach to DMT, the group is structured through the phases of warm-up, theme development, and closure (Sandel, Chaiklin & Lohn, 1993). It is based on a humanistic approach to psychotherapy and utilizes the dance and improvisational skills of the group leader. Movements are elicited from the patients and developed further by the dance/movement therapist to explore group themes using metaphor and symbolism. The four main areas of focus are body action, expression, symbolism, and the therapeutic relationship.

Given the patient characteristics in the MTP, their unpredictability, their difficulty making commitments, their tendency to socially isolate and engage in criminal behavior, bringing a DMT group to a cohesive state, to get to the working stage of the group development in a Chacian session can be an arduous task. At times choreography, yoga, modern dance, butoh, improvisation, body-mind centering exercises, or variations in authentic movement are used instead. This generally occurs when the conditions are not right for a Chacian session, i.e., the group is not large/cohesive enough, or if clients are completely resistant to moving in an expressive and spontaneous way thus cannot work on the symbolic level. As in Thomson's (1997) work, sometimes more familiar or structured approaches to movement are used to initially engage these clients to begin to introduce them to their bodies and their movement. The client's cultural values are important to consider here. Several Hispanic male clients have reported that it is not acceptable in their culture to dance with other men. As 72 percent of the Bellevue MTP clients are male, and 46 percent are Hispanic (29% are Caucasian, 17% are African American), it is often difficult to obtain a good ratio of male to female clients in DMT groups. At these times, more individually-focused movement is utilized.

Motivational interviewing (MI) and non-confrontational methods, increases the quality of care in substance abuse (SA) treatment for "people with various profiles of singular, dual and multiple disorders" as it develops trust, respect, empathy, and empowerment (Sciacca, 1997, p. 46). MI is defined as a "client-centered, directive method for enhancing intrinsic motivation to change by exploring and resolving ambivalence" (Miller & Rollnick, 2002, p. 25). Research has shown that MI helps individuals in SA treatment move through the first two stages of change (Miller & Rollnick, 2002). Chacian DMT does what motivational interviewing does on a body-based level. Comparing SA counseling to wrestling, Miller and Rollnick wrote: "Motivational interviewing is more like dancing: rather than struggling against each other, the partners move together smoothly. The fact that one of them is leading is subtle and is not necessarily apparent to an observer. Good leading is gentle, responsive, and imaginative" (p. 22). Similar to Chacian DMT (Lewis, 1993), MI emphasizes the importance of having the clinician meet the client at whatever phase the client is at (Miller & Rollnick, 2002). The author believes both DMT and MI are "fundamentally a way of being with and for people" (Miller & Rollnick, 2002, p. 25). MI states the therapeutic relationship should embody "accurate empathy, nonpossessive warmth, and genuineness" (p. 6). The Chace approach assumes, "the relationship (that which demands affective movement presence by the therapist for attunement and trust to develop) and the movement responses that emerge from such attunement become the keys to the effectiveness of treatment" (Fischer & Chaiklin, 1993, p. 141).

The TTM, also known as "The Stages of Change," proposes that the pathway to recovery (with or without professional help) is not linear but spiral (Connors, Donovan & DiClemente, 2001). People often cycle back and forth through five distinct stages before sustaining permanent behavior change. These stages are precontemplation, contemplation, preparation, action, and maintenance. In the first stage, *precontemplation,* a person does not consider his or her behavior a problem or may acknowledge it is a problem but does not want to do anything to change because the benefits outweigh the costs. In the second stage, *contemplation,* the person knows he or she has a problem and is starting to think about what to do about it. In the third stage, *preparation,* the person is starting to make efforts to start to change his or her behavior. In the fourth stage, *action,* the person is actively changing his or her behavior. In *maintenance,* the last stage, the behavior change has been sustained and the individual is working to fortify it. The time frame for each stage varies and is unique to each person. However, it has been found that a person usually sustains change for six months in the action phase before moving to maintenance.

In treatment planning, each target behavior the client is trying to change is "staged," i.e., a person may be willing to stop using opiates but not alcohol. Process of change activities are used to help people move through each stage (Prochaskas, DiClemente & Norcross, 1992) as treatment objectives. As the Chace approach to DMT "works with where the client is at," it is useful for organically implementing TTM process of change activities on an experiential level.

Clinical Vignettes

Abstain from opiates and secondary substances, maintain optimal mental health, and improve social interaction/create a sober social network are common long-term goals the dance/movement therapist helps dually diagnosed clients in the MTP work towards. Below are clinical vignettes of how each of the process of change activities have been implemented in DMT sessions and how they helped clients move toward these treatment goals. The word leader is used to refer to the dance/movement therapist (author) who is a LCAT, ADTR, and CASAC.

Many of the process of change activities can be used in multiple stages in the TTM. However, consciousness raising is specific to the precontemplator. This process of change activity involves increasing self-awareness. Body awareness is self-awareness and is a fundamental goal in DMT with every population. Realizing and accepting the negative effects of the drugs can be overwhelming for some clients but can be cushioned by aesthetic distance in CAT and by the comfort of rhythmic group synchronistic movement in DMT.

A middle-aged African American mother of two with a diagnosis of schizoaffective disorder came to one morning DMT session. Her methadone helped her stop using opiates but she continued to drink alcohol and take ben-zodiazapines. This particular DMT group had already become quite cohesive with the same members attending regularly. On this day, the members encouraged Gail to "join the dance group" instead of "going back out there" to get high. As the group proceeded through the warm-up phase, it became clear that Gail had started her day off by drinking wine coolers as her inebri-ated state became more and more obvious in her unsteady gait, difficulty find-ing balance, her slumped posture, and her desire to keep her eyes closed. The leader decided to work with the client instead of throwing her out of the group. The group did not judge Gail, instead as members broke away from the circle creating dyads and triads, two others were encouraged to join Gail, at her level of readiness, in a simple rhythmic rocking movement side to side. They asked her "What's going on that you need to drink so early in the morn-ing?" She said, "I just want to feel good–I don't want to feel pain," engaging further in the pleasurable, rhythmic movement. As members organically came back to the circle and held hands, Gail began to struggle with the con-tact, pulling her neighbors' arms roughly, so much so one member expressed feeling scared and uncomfortable. The leader changed positions to be by Gail's side and went with the struggle she was presenting in her arm move-ment, which led the group into tying itself into knots with each other's arms. When Gail and the group could not figure out how to unknot itself from the tangle, everyone paused. The leader encouraged the group to stay with this feeling of being stuck. Here, tears began to well in Gail's eyes and the entire group mood shifted from struggle, anger and fear, to sadness. Gail then spon-taneously said to the group, "I don't want to use anymore–I want to stop" and her tears began to fall. Group members let go of the tangle as the leader encouraged them to form a small circle and they immediately moved into a group hug while another female member allowed Gail to embrace her and rest her head on her shoulder. The static hug transformed into a soothing, swaying movement while Gail began to list all she could lose if she did not stop, most importantly the custody of her daughters. The group assured her she could get help if she came to group on a daily basis.

DMT helped Gail feel her ambivalence literally in her body, symbolically in the movement metaphor (knot) in the safety of an empathic group. Gail shared her struggle of wanting to medicate her pain–to "feel good" but also not wanting to give up her daughters. This was the start of Gail's movement out of the precontemplation stage.

Dramatic relief involves having a person experience the strong feelings associated with the risky behavior he/she wants to change. Catharsis and connecting feeling with movement is a mainstay of all DMT in the MTP. Repeated movement themes and images have emerged organically in DMT groups over the years with the fighting efforts, i.e., stomping, punching, kicking, while screaming at the drug or personified addiction, such as "I'm not going to take it anymore!" "I've had enough!" These often bring up feelings of rage, helplessness and being out of control. Burying, flushing, throwing away the drugs are other repeated themes.

In one particular group, a middle-aged lesbian African American client personified the drug as her seductress and lover, casting the leader in this role. The client moved in a sexualized manner towards the leader then away, which the leader turned into a pas de deux, allowing the client to sense her intense physical sensation of desire, temptation, and struggle. The leader then helped the client practice rejecting the drug/lover. She embodied her ambivalence in movement and verbalized, "I want you but I hate you, I need you but you will only hurt me, I love you but I have to let you go," eventually leaving the leader to dance by herself. This helped solidify the client's commitment to her new behavior as she was already in the action stage.

Self re-evaluation occurs when a person can experience how engaging in the risky behavior is not consistent with his or her self-image. In most sessions, individual members are given the opportunity to lead the group in movement. In one session, the group was moving inside a buddy band, expressing feeling "safe" and "contained." When it came time for a Caucasian borderline client in her thirties to take over the lead, she decided to get rid of the buddy band. The way she abruptly grabbed the band out of one man's hands led him to retreat from her and the circle. When the leader focused on this interaction, he was able to tell the woman, "I'm scared of you–your actions." Still actively using opiates and cocaine (in contemplation regarding her drug use), she often bragged about the aggressive behavior in her interpersonal relationships. Others in the group then admitted that her unpredictable movements made them feel unsafe around her, beginning to increase the space around her as the leader directed them to move to a more comfortable distance. Finally, able to see and feel this feedback in movement and in spatial relationship, the woman began to cry. She sincerely said, "I don't want anyone to be scared of me. I know how it feels." This created a significant shift in her social interactions and in her drug use. She realized that her heroin and cocaine use increased her tendency to be out of control, act impulsively, and thus scare others. Here she realized that she did not want to be like this and thus began to change her behavior and decrease her drug use.

Environmental reevaluation allows members to explore how the high-risk behavior they are trying to change affects others around them. After the group felt safe and got into the working phase, a new African American client in his late sixties began to move with the group theme of exploring love. He stretched out his arms as wide as he could and told the group how he loves to be surrounded by his grandchildren. He told the group how being a patriarch is important to him and how his drug use had caused him to lose that role and separate from his family. The leader further guided the group into a movement exploration of isolation and desire for love, which helped this client commit to regaining this role, which further motivated him to abstain from drugs, as he was new in treatment and in the preparation stage.

Decisional balance involves looking at pros and cons of remaining in old behavior or engaging in new behavior and is used from the precontemplation to the preparation stage. In DMT, polarities are often explored in movement, which brings out the essence of this decision-making process. Climbing to heights of the drug-induced high by moving into the vertical space overhead and then falling, literally to the floor and collapsing, or moving through space at an excitedly dangerous pace then slowing down to a painfully stunted pace, has often helped group members physically explore the pros and cons of their drug use and help them decide where they want to be, which the leader usually follows by exploring movement in the middle of these two states.

The group dynamic of the moving in a line through space often has brought up images of "a recovery train," "marching off to war," or "getting on the right track." The line usually starts when someone takes initiative to lead and others follow. When the group begins to work on the symbolic level by fully engaging in the movement metaphor and owning the images, i.e., by announcing to everyone "Let's get on the recovery train," the leader asks members to decide whether or not they want to join the movement. Inherent in this is being ready to let go of the drug use. Here members have to make a choice in their minds and movement whether or not they are ready to join, sometimes staying out of the line and deciding to move on one's own.

Self-liberation takes place when an individual is focused on his or her commitment to change–not the actual skill. A repeated dynamic in group DMT occurs when members realize they want to or have started to stop their drug use (at the end of the preparation or in the beginning of action) and want to celebrate this feeling, this new way of being. When the group gets into this mode, members cheer each other on while each dance solos in the center of the circle as others move along on the periphery, and/or clap their hands in rhythmic support.

On one occasion a patient who had not fully stopped his opiate (in contemplation) use began to feel, "I can do this." The leader asked him to express this newfound confidence with a movement. As he stepped into the center of the circle to show his move, the group began a loud call and response, "Can Larry do it? Yes he can!" as Larry chanted, "Yes I can!" in time with the others. They repeated the chant for each member who felt ready to step into the center and experience his self-confidence while receiving group encouragement, focusing each member's sense of self-liberation.

In self-efficacy, the individual is focused on his/her skill to successfully change the behavior. It is useful from the contemplation stage onward. Over the years, MTP clients have rehearsed and performed dances, which have been self-affirming experiences. Rehearsing movements to perform gives one a sense of mastery over one self, a sense of self-efficacy. Mastering new behaviors, i.e., creating choreography, rehearsing and performing it, can boost one's reliance on one's body and skills. In Chacian sessions as well, clients have often begun to build their sense of self-efficacy by spontaneously creating role plays to practice saying no to drugs, assessing their ability, level of comfort, and confidence to repeat this out on the streets.

Stimulus control involves a person restructuring his or her environment so that temptation to engage in the behavior is minimized, used in the preparation stage and onward. Just the act of coming to group and staying for its duration instead of hanging out in the street or at a place where drug use is rampant is one way of restructuring one's environment. Planning one's schedule and time is crucial during this phase. When dually diagnosed clients in the MTP feel good about coming to group, as they often do after they experience the vitalization and sense of togetherness that occurs in DMT, they often become more committed to attend groups for the entire day, helping restructure their lives.

Counter-conditioning consists of helping clients learn how to replace problem behavior with a more positive behavior and is useful from the preparation stage onward. Teaching clients body-based relaxation exercises, doing meditative/contemplative movements, or doing yoga in DMT sessions can provide counter-conditioning for clients. These activities, which they can then practice at home, can give them an internal sense of control to help them cope with living in a world without drugs and with symptoms of mental illness. Connecting with one's life force through movement and dance is an amazing counter-conditioning activity and inherently motivating. Many MTP clients have verbalized in DMT in amazement, "I never thought I could feel this good without drugs."

Helping relationships emphasizes how supportive people can assist someone in making a behavioral change and are used after preparation. This is an inherent part of group therapy as it provides support and encouragement. Several of the vignettes above clearly demonstrate how DMT helps dually diagnosed clients have more meaningful social interactions and relationships.

In the action and maintenance stages, reinforcement management is used to reward the desired behavior change. The leader praises all creative efforts clients make during group as they signify movement towards health and sobriety. The MTP clients seem to have a great need to praise each other's creative efforts as well. Once, an elderly African American man in the action phase of his recovery, who had organic brain damage from over 50 years of alcohol and substance abuse, performed in a dance the DMT group rehearsed for the clinic's December holiday celebration. Hearing people in the audience excitedly call his name as he danced made him smile and later say, "I never felt so important before," which further solidified his commitment to reap the rewards of his recovery.

In social liberation, the individual engages in behaviors that help empower others and is used in the maintenance stage. Giving back to one's recovery community reinforces the changes clients have made. Allowing clients to take on the leadership role in DMT does this. In one session, a client who was drug-free for over six months, engaged her peers—with the leaders encouragement—by dancing duets with them, encouraging them to explore their relationships to their specific triggers and practice saying "No," in movement. Encouraging clients to speak about how DMT has helped them also fosters social liberation. Individuals in the maintenance stage help explain and define DMT to newcomers to the group.

Summary

As no published research, articles, or book chapters exist on DMT in methadone treatment, this chapter is just the beginning of the process to record and describe how DMT can address the needs of individuals who are dually diagnosed and maintained on methadone. More research is needed, especially to look at the efficacy of DMT in SA treatment. This case study validates several of the findings from previous qualitative DMT studies in addiction, that DMT can help SA clients: Regain control over their bodies, decrease their sense of shame, decrease their defenses, embrace their spirituality, become whole, safely experience their emotions, and receive social support. This case study further demonstrates how DMT is an effective means of experientially implementing process of change activities to help dually diagnosed MTP clients increase their motivation to stop using drugs and attain treatment goals–to obtain and maintain abstinence from drugs, to cope with symptoms of mental illness, obtain optimal level of mental health, and to improve social relatedness. Along with the client-centered approaches of motivational interviewing and Chacian DMT, an understanding of the Transtheoretical Model of Change and the underlying issues and dynamics of this unique patient population can help the dance/movement therapist work more effectively in methadone maintenance.

Appendix–Terms

Action: In the Transtheoretical Model of change, it is the stage of change where the person has stopped the targeted behavior.

ADTR: Academy of Dance Therapists Registered; the highest credential given by the American Dance Therapy Association. This signifies a professional dance/movement therapist with enough experience and education to teach dance/movement therapy, supervise dance/movement therapists, and practice dance/movement therapy with individuals.

Aesthetic distance: Term coined by drama therapist Robert Landy. It is the psychic distance obtained when a balance is found between too much distance, overdistancing, which is the same as denial, and underdistancing which is when one gets overwhelmed by their emotions.

Authentic movement: A movement practice often used by dance/movement therapists created by Mary Whitehouse. It can be done with two individuals or with a group and involves taking on two roles, a witness and a mover, with the goal of having the mover, move from the authentic self.

Body action: Is one of the four main therapeutic areas of focus in Chacian dance/movement therapy that emphasizes facilitating movement of the body.

Body-mind centering: A movement practice started by Bonnie Brainbridge Cohen that focuses on connecting sensing, feeling, and action via movement and touch.

Butoh: A dance form started in Japan in the 1950s by Tatsumi Hijikata and Kazuo Ohno, which seeks to get back to natural roots of movement and focuses on transformation of energy.

CASAC: Certified Alcoholism and Substance Abuse Counselor: Credential given to professionals who meet the requirements dictated by the Office of Alcoholism and Substance Abuse Services in New York State to practice substance abuse counseling.

Chace Technique: An approach to dance/movement therapy based on the work of Marion Chace who was a pioneer in the field and the first president of the American Dance Therapy Association.

Closure: The final phase of a dance/movement therapy session where the group reviews the process which has occurred in movement and says good-bye in movement.

Contemplation: In the Transtheoretical Model of change, it is the stage of change where the person is thinking about changing the targeted behavior but has not yet taken any action to do so.

Contingency management: A method, started and researched by Scott Kellogg, which uses incentives to motivate people to engage in treatment or engage in new behaviors.

Dispensaries: Methadone clinics that only focus on dispensing medication and not on the other biopsychosocial aspects of substance abuse treatment such a counseling or group therapy.

Dually diagnosed: Treatment jargon signifying a person who has both mental illness and substance dependence.

Expression: One of the main focus areas in Chacian dance/movement therapy, which includes helping a client produce evocative movements, sounds, and verbalizations that release emotions.

Fighting efforts: A Laban Movement Analysis term, which refers to the way weight, time, and space are used in movement.

LCAT: Licensed Creative Arts Therapist: A license to practice psychotherapy utilizing the creative arts given by the State Education Department in New York State.

Maintenance: In the Transtheoretical Model of change, it is the stage of change where the person is working on sustaining the targeted behavior change. In regard to substance use this involves making plans to avoid relapse.

Modern dance: A form of dance created at the turn of the nineteenth century that was a revolt against classical forms of dance and focused on freedom of expression. Dance/movement therapy is predicated on modern dance principles. All the dance/movement therapy pioneers were modern dancers.

Multiply diagnosed: Treatment jargon signifying a person who has mental illness, substance dependence, and a physical illness.

Precontemplation: In the Transtheoretical Model of change, it is the stage of change where a person may not have any awareness that his or her behavior is a problem or who may know the behavior is a problem but the benefits of keeping the behavior outweigh the disadvantages thus is not ready to even consider changing it.

Precontemplator: An individual in the precontemplation stage of the Transtheoretical Model of change.

Preparation: In the Transtheoretical Model of change, it is the stage of change where the person starts to make plans to change the targeted behavior and may even begin to take some action.

Process of change activities: Activities that can be used as treatment objectives/interventions to help people move through the stages of change. They include consciousness raising, dramatic relief, self-re-evaluation, environmental reevaluation, decisional balance, self-efficacy, self-liberation, stimulus control, counter-conditioning, helping relationships, reinforcement management, and social liberation. In order to be most useful, it is important that these activities be paired with the right stages.

SAMSHA: Substance Abuse and Mental Health Services Administration of the United States federal government.

Symbolism: One of the four main therapeutic areas of focus in Chacian dance/movement therapy that emphasizes the importance of developing and exploring images, metaphors, and symbols in movement.

Theme development: Middle stage of Chacian dance/movement therapy group development, which focuses on exploring movement themes, images, and symbols.

Therapeutic relationship: One of the four main therapeutic areas of focus in Chacian dance/movement therapy. It emphasizes the importance of the empathic relationship between the dance/movement therapist and the client.

Warm-up: The beginning stage of Chacian dance/movement therapy group development which focuses on physically, socially, and emotionally preparing people to move together expressively.

References

Abelson, J., Treloar, C., Crawford, J., Kippax, S., van Beek, I., & Howard, J. (2006). Some characteristics of early-onset injection drug users prior to and at the time of their first injection. *Addiction, 101*(4), 548–555.

Arrestee Drug Abuse Monitoring Program. (1998). *National Institute of Justice research report: 1998 Annual report on opiate use among arrestees.* Washington DC: United States Department of Justice.

Connors, G. J., Donovan, D. M., & DiClemente, C. C. (2001). *Substance abuse treatement and the stages of change: Selecting and planning interventions.* New York: Guilford Press.

Daly, L. (2002). *Discovering the self: Connections between dance/movement therapy and Hatha yoga.* Unpublished Masters Thesis. Pratt Institute. Brooklyn, NY.

Fischer, J., & Chaiklin, S. (1993). Meeting in movement: The work of the therapist and the client. In S. Sandel, S. Chaiklin, & A. Lohn (Eds). *Foundations of dance/movement therapy: The life and work of Marian Chace.* Columbia, MD: The Marian Chace Memorial Fund of the American Dance Therapy Association.

Fisher, B. (1990). Dance/movement therapy: Its use in a 28-day substance abuse program. *The Arts in Psychotherapy, 17,* 325–331.

Heffernan, K., Cloitre, M., Tardiff, K., Marzuk, P. M., Portera, L., & Leon A. C. (2000). Childhood trauma as a correlate of lifetime opiate use in psychiatric patients. *Addictive Behaviors, 25*(5), 797–803.

Johnson, L. (1990). Creative therapies in the treatment of addictions: The art of transforming shame. *The Arts in Psychotherapy, 17*(4), 299–308.

Khantzian, E. J. (1999). *Treating addiction as a human process.* Lanham, MD: Rowman & Littlefield.

Kuhn, C., Swartzwelder, S. , & Wilson, W. (2003). *Buzzed: The straight facts about the most used and abused drugs from alcohol to ecstasy.* NY: W. W. Norton & Co.

Lewis, P. (1993). The use of Chace techniques in the depth dance therapy process of recovery, healing and spiritual consciousness. In S. Sandel, S. Chaiklin, & A. Lohn (Eds.), *Foundations of dance/movement therapy: The life and work of Marian Chace* (pp. 154–168). Columbia, MD: The Marian Chace Memorial Fund of the American Dance Therapy Association.

Matto, H., Corcoran, J., & Fassler, A. (2003). Integrating solution-focused and art therapies for substance abuse treatment: Guidelines for practice. *The Arts in Psychotherapy, 30*(5), 265–272.

Marsch, L. (1998). The efficacy of methadone maintenance interventions in reducing illicit opiate use, HIV risk behavior and criminality: A meta-analysis. *Addiction, 93*(4), 515–532.

Mehta, S. H., Thomas, D. L., Sulkowski, M. S., Safaein, M., Vlahov, D., & Strathdee, S. A. (2005). A framework for understanding factors that affect access and utilization of treatment for hepatitis C virus infection among HCV-mono-infected and HIV/HCV-co-infected injection drug users. *AIDS, 19:* suppl 3.

Milliken, R. (1990). Dance/movement therapy with the substance abuser. *The Arts in Psychotherapy, 17*(40), 309–17.

Miller, W. R., & Rollnick, S. (2002). *Motivational interviewing: Preparing people for change.* NY: Guilford.

Moore, K., & Dusheiko G. (2005). Opiate abuse and viral replication in Hepatitis C. *American Journal of Pathology, 167*(5): 1189–1191.

Oktay, D. (2004). *Using video and dance therapy to treat clients in a methadone clinic.* Unpublished Masters Thesis. Pratt Institute. Brooklyn, NY.

Prochaska, J. O., DiClemente, C. C., & Norcross, J. C. (1992). In search of how people change: Applications to addictive behaviors. *American Psychologist, 47,* 1102–1114.

Perlmutter, M. (1992). The dance of addiction. *The American Journal of Dance Therapy, 14*(1) 41–48.

Plevin, M. (1996). Shape shifting from anthropomorphic to human form: Conscious body ego development in a recovering substance abuser. *The Arts in Psychotherapy, 23*(2), 1211–129.

Rose, S. (1995). Movement as metaphor: Treating chemical addiction. In F. Levy, J. P. Fried, & F. Leventhal (Eds.), *Dance and other expressive art therapies: When words are not enough* (pp. 101–108). New York: Routledge.

Sandel, S., Chaiklin, S., & Lohn, A. (1993). *Foundations of dance/movement therapy: The life and work of Marian Chace.* Columbia, MD: The Marian Chace Memorial Fund of the American Dance Therapy Association.

Sciacca, K. (1997). Removing barriers. *Professional Counselor,* pp. 41–46.

Shoshensky, (2001). Music therapy and addiction. *Music Therapy Perspectives, 19*(1), 22–39.

Thompson, D. (1997). Dance/movement therapy with the dual-diagnosed: A vehicle to the self in the service of recovery. *American Journal of Dance Therapy, 19*(1), 63–79.

United State Department of Health and Human Services-Substance Abuse and Mental Health Services Administration. (2008). *Alternative approaches to mental health care.* Retrieved February 25, 2008 from http://mentalhealth.samhsa.gov/publications/allpubs/ken98-0044/default.asp

Biography

Corinna Brown MA, MS, ADTR, CASAC, LCAT graduated from The Hunter College Dance Therapy Program in 1996. She practices dance/movement therapy at Bellevue Hospital in Addiction Psychiatry and in private practice. She teaches research methods at Pratt Institute's Graduate Creative Arts Therapy Program and supervises professional dance/movement therapists. She has also supervised undergraduate and graduate DMT students from Goucher College, Pratt Institute and Antioch New England Graduate School. She is the Vice President of the NYS Chapter of The American Dance Therapy Association (ADTA) and has been on the Research Subcommittee of the ADTA for over five years. She has co-edited the Research Poster Sessions Abstract from the Annual Conference of the American Dance Therapy Association in the *American Journal of Dance Therapy* since 2005. Her recent research, "The Importance of Making Art for the Creative Arts Therapist: An Artistic Inquiry," will soon be published in *The Arts in Psychotherapy.*

Chapter 13

RECOVERING IDENTITY AND STIMULATING GROWTH THROUGH DRAMA THERAPY

Sally Bailey

Introduction

D rama therapy uses all of the processes and products of drama and theatre to help clients get to know themselves better, make peace with their
pasts, envision their futures, and develop the skills to get along better with
others in their present (NADT Brochure, 1997). This provides a drama therapist a wide array of tools for guiding clients toward their goals. These goals
could include self-acceptance, self-empowerment, learning clear communication skills, improving social interaction abilities, or resolving ongoing conflicts in their lives.

From 1988 through 1999, I worked as a drama therapist at Second
Genesis, a non-profit mental health organization that ran six long-term residential substance abuse treatment facilities in the Washington, DC area. For
a long time, I was the itinerant drama therapist, traveling from house-to-
house to run a weekly two-hour drama therapy group. Later, I became a full-
time substance abuse counselor at Melwood House, a facility that focused on
treatment for women addicts and their children.

Second Genesis's program was based on the Daytop model of Therapeutic
Communities (TC), using confrontation, structure, and tough-love to teach
the skills needed to live a sober, drug-free life. In a TC group, relations the-
ory is applied to the whole treatment milieu, not just therapy groups, to
ensure that every interaction in the environment is safe and therapeutic
(Winship in Waller & Mahony, 1999). The three Cardinal Rules at all Second
Genesis facilities were: No Drugs, No Sex, and No Violence. Breaking a
Cardinal Rule was grounds for immediate termination. If a minor rule was

broken or a direction given by a staff member or a resident with authority was not followed, the disobedient resident received what was called a "consequence" or "learning experience." This could include losing a privilege, wearing a sign that advertised what you were at fault for or listed what you were not working on in treatment, wearing a stocking cap (symbolic of the "old days" in TCs when people's heads were permitted to be literally shaved), sitting on the bench by the front door (reminding the resident that they were one step away from being kicked out), or having to do some kind of unpleasant cleaning task in the facility (like cleaning the grease trap in the kitchen or scrubbing the floor with a toothbrush). If the infringement was serious, the resident could be put "on contract," which meant that he/she lost all privileges and had a number of tasks to complete before he/she got them back. Behavior was also dealt with in weekly encounter groups in which residents were expected to confront each other verbally on their negative behaviors.

Besides the structure of a traditional TC, Second Genesis utilized the treatment philosophy of the Twelve Steps of Alcoholics Anonymous (AA, 1976) and Narcotics Anonymous (NA,1988) and, like both self-help organizations, put emphasis on the role of group support for recovery. Residents worked through three phases that related to specific recovery tasks, the AA/NA Steps, re-entry into the workforce, and re-unification with their families and the community. Anyone who did not have a high school diploma was eligible for classes preparing them for their General Education Diploma (GED). For example, the primary goal of Phase One, Level One—Orientation and Accepting the Need to Change—was based on the first step of AA and NA: We admitted we were powerless over alcohol (our addiction)—that our lives had become unmanageable (Alcoholics Anonymous, 1976, p. 59; Narcotics Anonymous, 1988, p. 19). AA and NA meetings were brought into the facility and once residents had earned the privilege of a "pass" to the outside, they were required to attend AA or NA meetings while out "on pass." Shortly after I began working there, Second Genesis began incorporating Relapse Prevention Training as articulated by Terrence Gorski into required groups (Gorski & Miller, 1986).

Substances that had been abused by residents ran the gamut: Alcohol, cocaine, heroin, inhalants, prescription drugs, stimulants—you name it, they had done it. Most people were addicted to more than one substance and everyone was a practicing nicotine addict. Many of the clients were remanded from prison for treatment or sentenced to treatment by drug court. They lived at the facility for six months to a year and learned how to live without drugs and alcohol, eventually transitioning back to their jobs and families in the community.

A great many addicts—both male and female—were survivors of childhood sexual, physical, and/or emotional abuse and neglect. Some were children of alcoholics or addicts. They had experienced so much trauma and upheaval while young that the only way to cope with the pain, shame, self-hatred, and blame was to numb out their feelings with drugs. Getting high was the only way they could function—to get on with life—until, as inevitably happens with addictive substances, the substances overpowered their lives and led them into prostitution, dope dealing, theft, and robbery in order to feed their habit. Their families fell apart. Their health failed. Most people arrived for treatment so thin they looked like concentration camp survivors.

Emotional Implications of Addiction

Whenever one starts doing drugs, emotional development stops. Someone who starts getting high at fourteen will not mature socially or emotionally beyond that age because the drugs allow the addict to avoid working through problems whether they are personal, interpersonal, financial, or educational. When the addict stops doing drugs, he/she is emotionally right back where he/she was when he/she started doing drugs: He/she returns to his/her previous developmental level of emotional maturity and progresses from there (Gorski & Miller, 1988).

One new drama therapy intern turned to me after her first session with a newly-formed drama therapy group and asked, "How *old* are these women?" I said, "Between 20 and 45—most of them are in their '30s." "Really?" was her response, "They act like teenagers!" And sure enough, when I asked them at the beginning of the next group to share how old they were when they first started getting high, the answers ranged from six to 16. The behavior of recovering addicts in treatment resembles that of rude, unruly, insecure teenagers complete with an unending series of nasty putdowns, snide remarks, and games of one-upmanship. Before any therapeutic progress can be made on either an individual or group level, the drama therapist has to teach basic group skills and how to interact respectfully.

Establishing a Drama Therapy Group

I found the best way to create an environment of respect was through theatre games. Games had to be challenging and fun, but not competitive. Some groups could handle cooperative games at the beginning, but most had not yet reached the stage of cooperative play. Most groups had to start with parallel or associative games (Garvey, 1990). Examples of successful early associative games are "The Winds Are Blowing," "Magic Tube," or "Making an Entrance" (see List of Drama Games at the end of this chapter for descriptions of these and other games).

Once a basic respect was established, I could move on to games where two people had to work together like "Mirroring," "Balances and Leans," or "Open Scenes," working slowly toward more complex cooperative games like "Environments," "Transportation" or "Trust Circles." Group interaction skills slowly improved and group members began to develop trust in the group and respect for each other while they were also developing their basic drama skills. As a result, when we moved into improvisation and role play, they understood how to create dialogue, how to listen to their acting partner, and how to build a dramatic scene through give and take. This parallels Renee Emunah's Integrative Five Phase Model of Drama Therapy in which the group proceeds progressively through more difficult sets of activities over time as they are ready. The Five Phases are Dramatic Play, Scene Work, Role Play, Culminating Enactment, and Dramatic Ritual (Emunah, 1994).

In truth, addicts come into a drama group with many highly developed acting skills: They were acting in order to survive all the way through their addiction. Each time I began an orientation on the first day of a new group, I would tell them that the purpose of drama therapy was not to make them into actors or to put on a play, but to take the negative skills they had developed for manipulating and conning others and transform them into positive skills for living a clean and sober life. I would say, "If you think back to when you were out on the street getting high, you were doing a lot of acting!" They would laugh in recognition.

Using the Process Communications Model

Introducing drama therapy this way made a big difference in whether I was met with resistance or willingness. In addition, I always made sure that in the first several sessions, we had lots of fun. This is easy to do when you are playing drama games. Quickly, I realized that the fun aspect was very important for the "buy in" and later, I discovered why: Drug addicts are all rebels!

There is a wonderful interaction assessment and training tool called Process Communications Model or PCM developed by Taibi Kahler, a clinical psychologist (Pauley, Bradley & Pauley, 2002). It focuses on how people send and receive messages. If you want someone to understand you, you should communicate to them in their preferred communication style, not yours. In other words, you need to learn to speak their language. Another important concept is that before someone will listen to you, they need to have their psychological needs met. In PCM terms, they need to be "stroked."

One of the six communication styles in PCM is Rebel. How are rebels stroked? Rebels need to play! If you can engage a rebel in play, he/she will then be willing to listen to whatever message you have to share because he/she has had his/her "fun-quotient" met. If you do not play with a rebel, you will be met with resistance and sometimes outright rebellion. Through theatre games, I bypassed all the resistance that other therapists faced in their groups and individual sessions. No matter what phase of drama therapy we were in, I always included a warm-up game at the beginning of the session to let everyone release "steam" and have fun.

Identifying Feelings and Trusting Oneself

Drama therapy group was often the first time that many residents explored their feelings or even learned to identify the names of the emotions that they experienced. Because addiction involves numbing out feelings, residents were in the habit of being disconnected from their bodies and intellectualizing their experiences (Browne-Miller, 1993; Gorski & Miller, 1988; Waller & Mahony, 1999). When I would ask during our check-in at the beginning of group what people were feeling, I would get generalities like "OK," "Good," or "Bad"; none of which are feelings. I started requiring group members to identify a specific feeling. I even brought in cards with names of emotions and acted them out for them (they really enjoyed my dramatic performances). Or I asked them to express their feelings through a metaphor like a color, an animal, or a weather report, which gave them some distance from admitting to the feeling, but also allowed them to be creative and explore the multiple layers of complexity available through the connotations attached to a metaphorical image.

I had to get group members to start to trust their bodies and feel their feelings again. To help with this, we followed each check-in with a physical warm-up where we shook out tension, stretched, bounced, and breathed slowly and deeply. Often, I would ask them to report how they felt after the warm-up in contrast with before. This facilitated learning that both physical and emotional sensations can be transformed after a short intervention. This focus on developing awareness of the individual's physical presence was introduced to me by my drama therapy mentor Jan Goodrich, RDT, who had created the drama therapy program at Second Genesis, and was reinforced by my subsequent mentor, Rudy Bauer, Ph.D., at the Washington Gestalt Therapy Training Center.

Once we got "into" our bodies and acknowledged our emotions, pleasant and unpleasant, we moved on to playing a warm-up game. This was another good way to begin to practice experiencing feelings in a non-threatening way. In the course of playing games, most of the emotions that were generated were pleasant, but sometimes unpleasant ones cropped up because someone was not playing fairly or was in a bad mood. We learned how to name and work with all of these emotions, because they are all part of life.

Case Example: Althea, Part One

One day Althea, a very intense, intimidating resident, came into group in a very belligerent mood. Her infant was sick and she wanted to stay with him down in the nursery; however, staff had said she needed to attend her groups. Althea had a lot of trust issues and felt that no one other than herself could take adequate care of her baby. Like most addicts, she only wanted to do what she wanted to do when she wanted to do it; she did not like to follow directions from authority figures. Yes, she was a rebel. She came into drama group and announced that she did not want to be there and she was not going to stay.

I said, "Listen, I can tell that you are really upset and worried and you want to be with your baby, but if you go down to the nursery the way you are acting right now, you are going to get in trouble and there will be serious consequences."

"I don't care," she said.

"Well, I do," I said. "I'll tell you what—I'll make a deal with you. [Drug addicts also tend to be Promoters—another PCM communication style—and Promoters like to make deals!] You stay for check-in and warm-up and play the first game I have planned for today, and then, if you still want to, I'll let you go back downstairs to check on the baby."

She agreed. We did our check-in: We went around the circle and everyone said how they felt (needless to say, Althea was "angry, worried, and stressed out"). We did our physical warm-up to get everyone alert, relaxed, and connected with their bodies. Then we played Machines. First we made Imaginary Machines where one person started with a sound and a movement and another person added on another sound and movement and then another and another until everyone was involved in a gigantic Rube Goldberg contraption. Next, we segued into Emotion Machines. In this version, every part of the Machine (and, therefore, every person) has to express the same emotion with their sound and movement. This version of Machines is very cathartic. There is nothing like a good Anger Machine to get your frustration out. And there is nothing like a Tenderness Machine to get you in touch with your gentle, loving side.

When we finished, I turned to Althea and said, "OK, we're done with our warm-up game. If you want, you can go back down to the nursery."

By that time, she was completely calm and in a state of emotional balance. "No," she said, "I don't have to go now. I'm fine. And staff was right. They will take care of my baby. I should be here in group." Then she pointed her finger at me and said, "You! You did this on purpose! Oh, you're so smart,

Miss Sally. You knew I wouldn't want to leave group after I played that game because you knew I wouldn't be angry anymore!"

"Well," I said, "I didn't know that would happen, but I hoped it would."

"I understand now," she said, "You are teaching us about life in this group! I'm going to pay close attention to what you have us do from now on!" She had discovered what I love all my clients to discover: That I do not just play games to have fun but I also play games to teach impulse control, flexibility, spontaneity, and all the other many skills that they need to live their lives successfully.

Moving into More Serious Therapeutic Work

Once a drama group developed the necessary level of respect and group interaction skills, we could start moving into more serious therapeutic work: Using sociodrama to practice the skills they would need to stay clean and sober, using psychodrama to explore painful personal issues in an honest but playful way, and creating and performing short original plays that metaphorically allowed them to rehearse actions they wanted to take or envision goals they wanted to achieve.

Art was often a very effective intervention because it preempted the verbal rationalizing that addicts so skillfully use as a defense mechanism by funneling their ideas into non-verbal images first (Bailey, 2007). Maps to Recovery, drawn to show the obstacles and the supports on each individual's life journey, were perfect jumping-off points for dramatic enactments. Social atoms, which symbolically depict relationships with family, friends, and (sometimes) enemies, also served as excellent segues into scenes of personal exploration.

One of the most effective exercises I used with many groups was the creation of masks from plaster of Paris bandages. We painted the masks to depict the metaphorical behavioral masks they put on to hide their true feelings. Sometimes, we made half masks and performed in them. Other times, we made full face masks which were painted on the outside and the inside. When each mask was finished, the maker sat in front of it and imagined what the mask would say to him or her if it could come alive and speak. The maker would write down what the outside of the mask said and what the inside said in whatever form the words came to him/her: Poetry, story, or monologue. These therapeutic products were extremely important to each individual because they expressed what they had come to understand were "the games they played as an addict" and "the real person they hid underneath." We talked in group about the necessity of taking off the Mask of Addiction (or of The Victim or of Shame or of whatever it was that they habitually wore) in order to live and breathe and grow out in the open.

Case Example: Althea, Part Two

By the time Althea made her mask, she had humbled herself, accepted the need to change her behaviors, given up intimidation, learned how to work with others flexibly, and allowed the vulnerable person she really was inside out into the world. When she sat down to paint the outside of her mask, at first she hesitated because "The Mask of the Bully," the mask she wore when I first met her, was not one she wore anymore. But, she said, if she were ever to relapse, she knew it was the mask she would put back on. She decided she needed to memorialize that behavior, so she would never forget her addiction and, consequently, never go back to it. The outside of her mask was truly frightening. This is what it said to her:

> Anger is my name.
> Bullying is my game.
> Don't put me in a corner,
> For I will spit fire.
> I don't care what you think,
> Because I just want to get higher.
> If you look into my eyes,
> They will lead you the wrong way.
> Because I don't give a fuck
> What you may say.
> So if my game don't make you jump,
> I'll just move on until I find another punk.
> "I DON'T NEED YOU!!"

She cried every time she looked at it.

Inside was "The Real Me":

> I have this huge concern about being neglected.
> I am afraid you won't like me or just care for me the way I like.
> I am scared you will use me and my body -
> Say you love me, but you don't really care.
> This side of me I am very happy, very affectionate, and soft,
> Very giving, loving, and caring.
> I love to laugh and feel secure,
> But am afraid of being abused.
> I am very vulnerable and will believe your words,
> Because I long for my dreams –
> A dream that may never come true.

So please don't lie to me.
I would appreciate it if you just let me be.

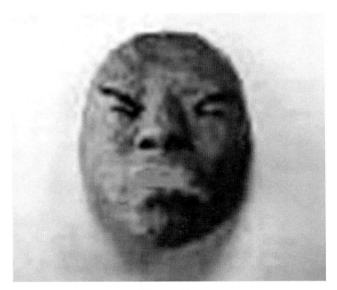

Figure 13.1.

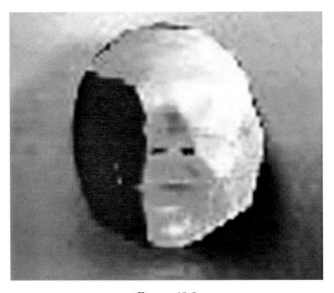

Figure 13.2.

After graduating from the program, Althea got a job in the main adminis-
trative office of Second Genesis. I often saw her at various functions and she
would come back to the facility to talk to new residents. Every time I saw her,
she said, "Miss Sally, I still have my mask. It's sitting on the table in my living room on the stand you gave me. Every time I get angry or frustrated and
think about 'picking up' [getting high] again, I go over, look at it, take it in
my hands, and I cry because I remember what it was like before I found my
recovery. It's kept me honest and it's kept me sober more than once. Nothing
is worth going back to that life. Nothing."

Conclusion

Until the advent of Alcoholics Anonymous in the 1930s, most experts
believed that addiction was untreatable (Alcoholics Anonymous, 1976;
Cantopher in Waller & Mahony, 1999; Diamond, 2000). Once the 12-Step
self-help process was accepted as the treatment of choice, experts believed
that only intervention by other addicts was useful in addressing the problem.
In the late '50s, Therapeutic Communities came into acceptance as a treatment of choice for a certain set of entrenched addicts (Winship in Waller &
Mahony, 1999). Not until the 1960s did the Medical Model gain general
acceptance (Gorski & Miller, 1998). This was followed in the late 1980s and
early 1990s with belief that addiction could be treated through psychotherapy or counseling (Diamond, 2000; Gorski & Miller, 1998; Groterath in
Waller & Mahony, 1999).

Each of these treatment paradigms sees addiction through a different lens:
As a spiritual disconnection, a social disorder, a biological disease, or a psychological condition. In the case of systems therapists, like social workers
and marriage and family therapists, it is seen as a biopsychosocial condition.
Drama therapy and the other creative arts therapies come out of the biopsychosocial tradition, but bring in addition a holistic approach to the treatment
of addiction that emphasizes creativity and health. Jacob Moreno, the
founder of psychodrama, saw every human being as creative and capable of
discovering their creative resources through interaction with others
(Groterath in Waller & Mahony, 1999). Other founders and developers of
creative arts therapy methods subscribe to similar beliefs. By focusing first on
what is healthy within all the group members, nurturing that health through
creative interactions within the group, and using these creative abilities to
work through internal and external problems, clients begin to recover not
only their sobriety, but also their sense of self, their power to act for positive
goals as the protagonists in their own lives, and their ability to make a difference in the lives of others. Because of this unique strength-based and
health-based approach which incorporates reparative interventions to heal

the trauma and disconnects created by family of origin and addiction issues, it is my belief that the creative arts therapies should be offered as the first line of treatment offered to addicts.

Appendix–Terms

Associative Play–The stage of play in which children are able to acknowledge each other and begin to interact, but cannot yet truly interact and cooperate (Garvey, 1990).

Check-in–The initial part of a drama therapy group in which each member "checks in" or reports through words, sounds, and/or actions how he or she is feeling at the moment.

Cooperative Play–The stage of play in which children are able to interact, work together, and cooperate (Garvey, 1990).

Distance–A term that relates to the client's sense of closeness to or alienation from his/her feelings, thoughts and physical self-image (Landy, 1996). When a client feels overwhelmed or too close to his/her feelings and/or body, he/she is said to be "underdistanced" and when too far away, he/she is said to be "overdistanced." Little therapeutic work can be accomplished if a client is under- or overdistanced because his connection to self is incomplete or unbalanced. To be able to heal on an emotional, cognitive, and physical level simultaneously, a client needs to find a place of balance called "aesthetic distance." This is a state in which one can feel and think and experience being connected to one's body/mind/emotions all at once. This "intrapsychic place" is where healing and meaning-making can happen (Bailey, in press).

Improvisation–Acting that is done spontaneously, without a script, by making up the words to a scene on the spur of the moment.

Integrative Five Phase Model–Approach to drama therapy developed by Renee Emunah which comprehensively structures how to safely incorporate many different drama therapy methods in a progression that parallels group dynamics and development. Early phases build trust and basic drama skills. Middle phases deepen the therapeutic work. The final phase focuses on therapeutic closure (Emunah, 1994).

Map to Recovery–A drawing of a "road" (usually from above as in a road map) from the Land of Addiction to the Land of Recovery. Obstacles to the journey and supports which help the traveler stay on the path might be in the middle of the road or at the side of the road.

Parallel Play–Stage of play in which children can play in proximity to each other, but do not have the social skills to interact, share, or work together (Garvey, 1990).

Psychodrama–A specific method of drama therapy, developed by Jacob L.

Moreno, which focuses on the enactment of scenes (past, present, or future) from one group member's life. That group member is called the protagonist. Other members of the group can be chosen by the protagonist to act out the roles of other people in the scenes of his or her life (Fox, 1987).

Relapse Prevention Training–A method of addiction treatment, developed by Terence Gorski, which focuses on identifying the symptoms of impending relapse and implementing specific plans to prevent relapse or minimize its destructive potential (Gorski & Miller, 1986).

Role Play–A general term used for all improvisational scene-creating in which an actor takes on a role in order to explore the aspects of that persona.

Sociodrama–A specific method of drama therapy, developed by Jacob L. Moreno, which focuses on the enactment of scenes about problems the group as a whole have in common and have chosen to explore dramatically. Many of the techniques used in psychodrama are used in sociodrama; the main difference is that psychodrama is most often non-fictional and socio-drama is most often fictional (Sternberg & Garcia, 2000).

Social atom–A sociometric diagram, developed by Jacob L. Moreno, which uses the metaphorical structure of an atom with a nucleus (the self) in the middle and electrons (significant others) at various distances from the nucleus. A social atom can be used as a diagnostic tool, an assessment tool, or as a starting point from which scenes can be developed (Fox, 1987).

Warm-up–A warm-up is an activity that focuses group members physically, emotionally, and cognitively. A warm-up could be a drama game, physical stretching, singing, dancing, or another simple activity that allows each member of the group to connect to him/herself and others in the present moment and let go of worries from whatever happened before the group began.

Drama Therapy Games

Balances and Leans–Partners find different ways to balance together: Leaning away from each other face-to-face while holding wrists, sitting down and standing back up together while face-to-face and holding wrists, sitting down and standing back up together while back-to-back with elbows linked, carrying the other on one's back, etc.

Environments–The group is divided into subgroups of three to six people. Each subgroup decides on a place or environment they will act out for the other groups. Actors can be people, objects, or animals in these places. Actors can speak or they may pantomime. The individuals watching guess by joining in the scene: If a "joiner" is correct, he/she is incorporated into the scene; if he/she is not correct, he/she is ignored.

Machines–All machines are made out of moving parts. In order to play the

Machine game, each person becomes one moving part in a larger machine. To build a machine, one person starts doing a sound and a movement, then another person adds a sound and movement in relationship to the first, and so on until everyone is involved or the machine is built.

Magic Tube–The group stands or sits in a circle. Each person, in turn, transforms a paper towel roll into different objects by pantomiming how it is used. The rest of the group guesses what it is.

Making an Entrance–One person enters the room, acting out an emotion, and everyone else guesses what she is feeling.

Mirroring–Two partners stand face-to-face making eye contact with each other. One is the "mirror" and one is "the person looking into the mirror." The "person" moves slowly while the "mirror" copies his/her movements. The goal is to move together so well that an outside observer cannot tell who is leading and who is following. Often, when a pair is working well together, they begin to make a strong non-verbal connection and find that they can communicate without speaking.

Open Scenes–Simple scenes of six to eight short lines between two actors that are written in such a way that if the actors change their tone of voice or the entire meaning of the scene changes. This provides practice in non-verbal communication based on tone of voice.

Transportation–The group is divided into subgroups of four to six people. Each subgroup must one by one transport each member across the room safely using a different configuration or way to move the person. All group members must be used in each "transportation method."

Trust Circles–The group (no more than 12 people for safety) stands in a tight circle around one person who stands as stiff as a board with arms crossed across his/her chest and head bent. The group keeps their hands out ready to catch the middle person who falls backwards into the circle and is passed around from person to person.

The Winds Are Blowing–The group sits on chairs in a circle with the Leader (who does not have a chair) standing in the center. The Leader calls out commonalities people in the circle have and everyone with that attribute must change places. The Leader is also looking for a chair so one person is left standing at the end of the round and he or she becomes the next Leader.

References

Alcoholics Anonymous. (1976). *Alcoholics Anonymous: The story of how many thousands of men and women have recovered from alcoholism.* New York: Alcoholics Anonymous World Services, Inc.

Bailey, S. D. (2007). Art as an initial approach to the treatment of sexual trauma. In S. L. Brooke (Ed.), *Creative arts therapies in the treatment of sexual abuse* (pp. 59–72). Springfield, IL: Charles C Thomas, Publisher.

Bailey, S. D. (in press). Playwriting with the Group in Drama Therapy. In R. Emunah & D. L.

Johnson (Eds.). *Current approaches to drama therapy,* 2nd ed. Springfield, IL: Charles C Thomas Publisher.

Browne-Miller, A. (1993). *Gestalting addiction: The addiction-focused group psychotherapy of Dr. Richard Louis Miller.* Norwood, NJ: Ablex Publishing Company.

Diamond, J. (2000). *Narrative means to sober ends: Treating addiction and its aftermath.* New York: Guilford Press.

Emunah, R. (1994). *Acting for real: Drama therapy process, technique, and performance.* NY: Brunner/Mazel.

Fox, J. (Ed.). (1987). *The essential Moreno: Writings on psychodrama, group method, and spontaneity by J. L. Moreno, M.D.* NY: Springer Publishing.

Garvey, C. (1990). *Play.* Cambridge, MA: Harvard University Press.

Gorski, T. T., & Miller, M. (1986). *Staying sober: A guide for relapse prevention.* Independence, MO: Herald House/Independence Press.

Landy, R. (1996). The use of distancing in drama therapy. *Essays in drama therapy: The double life.* London: Jessica Kingsley Publishers.

Narcotics Anonymous (1988). *Narcotics Anonymous,* 5th ed. Van Nuys, CA: World Service Office, Inc.

Pauley, J. A., Bradley, D. F., & Pauley, J. F. (2002). *Here's how to reach me: Matching instruction to personality types in your classroom.* Baltimore: Paul H. Brookes Publishing.

Sternberg, P., & Garcia, A. (2000). *Sociodrama: Who's in your shoes?,* 2nd ed. Westport, CT: Praeger.

Waller, D., & Mahony, J. (1999). *Treatment of addiction: Current issues for arts therapies.* London: Routledge.

Biography

Sally Bailey, MFA, MSW, RDT/BCT, is associate professor of theater, director of the drama therapy program and director of graduate studies in theater at Kansas State University in Manhattan, Kansas. She is author of *Wings to Fly: Bringing Theatre Arts to Students with Special Needs* and co-author of *Dreams to Sign,* a manual for creating theatre with deaf and hearing actors for deaf and hearing audiences. A past president of the National Association for Drama Therapy, she is the recipient of the 2005 NADT Service Award, the 2006 Gertrud Schattner Award for contributions to the field of drama therapy in education, publications, practice, and service, and the 2007 Distinguished Service in Arts and Disabilities presented by Accessible Arts and the Kansas Board of Education. Visit her website at www.dramatherapycentral.com

Chapter 14

"I JUST NEED FOUR WEEKS"–INDIVIDUAL DRAMA THERAPY AND THE ALCOHOLIC

LINDA M. DUNNE

Introduction

The proof of the shift of roles can be seen in the ability to live with role ambivalence without undue distress and to discover new possibilities of being with oneself and others. (Landy, 1993, p. 54)

The transition from one role to another can be an enlightening period of welcomed growth and development but if the individual is not aware that a major role shift has occurred, he/she may find him/herself with little or no tools to tolerate the unexpected metamorphosis. Such is frequently the case after living and functioning for more than half your life primarily in one role, in this case that of an alcoholic. Imagine the disquieting jolt you would feel arriving late for a rehearsal only to discover that all the roles have been recast and no one informed you. It is a bitter downgrade to be mercilessly torn from the lead role and expected to sweep the stage when you have never lifted a broom in your life.

This chapter discusses the journey of a man who had never discovered nor enjoyed the benefits of engaging with his many roles without the chemical partnership of alcohol and how working through the medium of drama therapy changed his self-perception and that of others giving him more breathing space to reflect, heal, and grow. "I just need four sessions" he announced, head held high, arms braided across his chest peering down at me over his thickened moustache twirled ever so slightly upward on both ends as he stood in the doorway of my office. This is a man used to his independence I

218

thought, exuding an unctuous though not entirely convincing air of self-confidence, not exactly the sort of patient I was used to having appear at my door. I suspected that this request was costing him a great deal of pride. I wondered for a brief moment where this forthcoming journey would take us.

Oddly enough, it had never occurred to me before sitting down to write this chapter that this patient's proclamation of needing only four weekly sessions of drama therapy is also the equivalent to 28 days. It is commonly thought that 28 days is a sufficient amount of time to provide an addict with ample tools to effectively change habits and break out of the addictive cycle of using, behaving, thinking, and living (Doyle Pita, 2004). And yet 14 months later, we continued to carry out our weekly ritual of sauntering down the hall, coffee in hand with a slight reluctance hanging in the air preparing to enter the drama therapy room. Did I fail in my role as a therapist or was there just a little too much woven into 30-plus years of alcoholism to be dealt with in four sessions? I began to make peace with this when after three months this patient announced "Ok, I have come to the conclusion that I trust you now so I am ready to start." He had decided that he needed to slow down his unrealistic expectations of getting well and erase his expectations of me being a magician.

I work at a treatment institution for addiction in The Netherlands whose main goal is to assist patients with detoxification, rehabilitation, and re-socialization in preparation for eventual reintegration back into society. The institution possesses a vision of addiction as being a chronic psychiatric illness which often leads to and in some cases causes a permanent loss of autonomy in the areas of emotion, thinking, and functioning. As a result of this vision, the word "patient" is used instead of client when referring to the individuals admitted for treatment. The hospital's treatment modality finds its roots in a biopsychosocial model and my work comes at the end phase of the treatment program following detoxification and partial rehabilitation. The patients who come to us have been clean for a period of 4–9 months and are ready to start working on other aspects of rehabilitation such as housing, work, regaining financial stability, and rebuilding family relationships. Many have had and continue to have relapses during this phase of treatment and this is most often due to the initial confrontation with life outside the hospital coupled with the first challenges of implementing new coping skills. The focus on reducing the severity of the relapses and increasing the time period between remains an integral part of treatment at every phase. Not every patient can imagine a life void of drug or alcohol use in which case the staff works with the individual to see which goals are realistic in combination with the chemical dependency history as well as the current psychological and somatic state of the patient. After the rehabilitation phase, patients will enter one of several housing options: Protected living, working and living, independent living, or return to their previous home or family. Patients are advised to continue on with the re-socialization program on a part-time basis in the event that they encounter societal obstacles and challenges after the initial discharge.

In this chapter, I will outline the choices and phases characteristic of individual drama therapy at the rehabilitation phase of addiction treatment. The main focus will be on the introductory phase of treatment: Establishing safety, boundaries (psychological and emotional) as well as the creation of a working metaphor for later stages of treatment. The emphasis is placed on the past, present, and future role repertoire of the individual. To illustrate this process, I will discuss an individual drama therapy case that extended over a period of 14 months with a recovering alcoholic male. Since the entire treatment period is too extensive to discuss within the scope of this chapter, I have chosen to highlight specific aspects of the treatment process. In addition, I will outline a number of exercises that have proved effective for both patient and therapist in structuring and facilitating individual drama therapy sessions with this patient population. Details of the patient's history and family have been changed to protect his identity. The execution and intervention of drama therapy methods used as well as the patients reactions and progress are accurately reported as they occurred.

Way of Working

The initial choice of therapy in our clinic is most often cognitive behavioral therapy (CBT) and in the event that this may prove ineffective, the patient can be referred for individual drama therapy. It is often suggested as an additional or complimentary therapy to CBT or as some would say we need to find another "way in." The process always begins with a structured intake which involves giving the patient a chance to formulate his goals in his own words. This gives me the opportunity to explain what drama therapy is and how I work as a therapist. This is a crucial factor for the patient since trust at this point is hovering at the perimeter of the therapeutic relationship and though enthusiasm is visible apprehension, tends to run high. Giving the patient the opportunity to ask questions helps reduce a great deal of anxiety about what is "expected and required" and erases the misconception that one must perform or relive their life story in order to induce catharsis and eventually be freed from the past. In addition, I use this time to explain that the initial two sessions will be observation-based as well as it being an opportunity for the patient and myself to gauge whether or not this is the best therapeutic method. In some cases, despite motivation and will, patients are for a variety of reasons not yet ready to enter drama therapy and this is communicated back to the referring parties. Specific to this patient population, those reasons can be frequent relapses in a short period of time, little or no support group in and outside the clinic, or chronic somatic illnesses that prevent regular attendance.

Setting the Stage

I am most fortunate to have a very large drama therapy space and therefore have divided it into three areas. I keep an open space for enactment and movement and this is what is known to the patients as "the workspace." A second space is reserved for storage and a third is where the sessions find a beginning or as one patient liked to call it "the waiting room." Being consistent with the structure of your space is very important as the patients tend to think of their session as going to their space for one hour. If you make changes without consulting the patient, the disrupted routine for some can be very unsettling. Those with addiction histories tend not to favor unforeseen change. Since extreme chemical dependence has been the "chosen medication" for dealing with painful emotions, most patients are at the first stages of learning how to manage external stimuli and regulate their own emotional state. This coupled with a boundaryless mentality of functioning in the world can lend to uncontrolled flooding of emotions for the newly sober self if they sense expectations from others they are unable to fulfill. It is therefore useful to have visible physical boundaries and consistent space arrangements for the safe containment and expression of emotions and to prevent the onset of another spiral of anxiety and confusion.

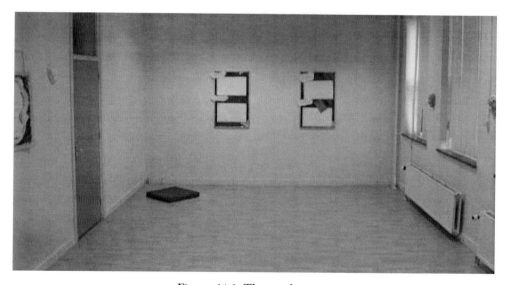

Figure 14.1. The workspace.

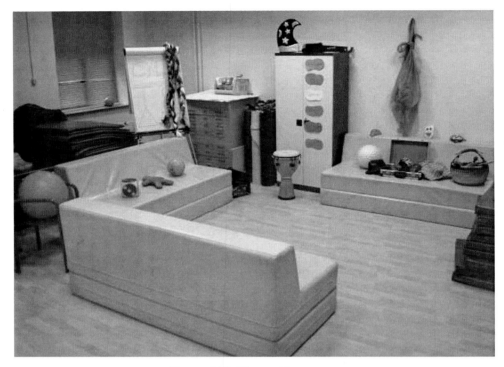

Figure 14.2. The waiting room.

Meet the Player

Hendrik was an intelligent observant man closer to the age of retirement than he cared to mention, slowly exiting a life of adventure including an above-average comfort level of material wealth and prestigious accomplishments. He considered himself vastly different from the other patients in our clinic: They were junkies, ex-prostitutes, and drug addicts of which, according to him, he was neither. According to his self-analysis, which was a favorite pastime of his, he concluded that he already possessed the basic ingredients of normal living and functioning but just needed some "extra tips" for dealing with his emotions. I felt I had been handed my first conundrum and experienced an immediate physical reaction, a pulsating balloon of hyperactive butterflies danced in my abdomen. The butterflies, I thought, were telling me that this man needed more than "a few tips" but who was I to judge? My physical response alerted my perception of what I thought to be his masked fear that I suspected lurked behind a lifelong and very well-constructed wall of emotional armor.

In my session notes after the initial meeting, I had written the words "dichotomous thinking" together with a happy face in the margin of my notebook. All of his responses and reactions to his life events or his own behavior were perceived as either extravagantly superb or devastatingly disastrous. There was absolutely no room for even a sliver of gray possibility. I looked closely at the details of his past and placed them next to the man I saw before me and began formulating how to best move ahead with this seemingly confident, self-assured, worldly man.

Hendrik had been abusing alcohol since the age of 17, which according to his own estimation, rapidly developed into complete dependence six years later. Alcohol played the lead role in his life for more than 30 years. He cannot recall a period in his life when he had what he called a normal relationship with alcohol though he was not sure what that entailed. It was, he stated, simply a way of life. Alcohol was always present and since he could still function without serious problems, there was really no reason to stop until the undeniable signs of the last two years. As Hendrik looks back on his life with a sober eye and sharpened senses, he is of the opinion that his behavior only worsened with time though he thought it normal at the time, until he found himself in a situation where he literally needed to make a choice to live or die.

Since being sober, he reports enormous holes in his memory and a grand frustration at trying to fill them in and make sense of how he lived and even more baffling, how he survived. An image came to mind. This resembles the process of watching a film when you are exhausted and really should go to bed. You see only pieces here and there between dozing spells and if you are questioned later, you try to convince yourself and others that you completely understand the plot but it remains gray, hazy, and in some cases, a collection of large gaping holes supplemented by the odd commercial. Hendrik had innumerable blackouts as a result of his heavy drinking and since being sober, he was constantly plagued by haunting and intrusive fragments of the past. He would often pass along a certain street or park in the city overcome by the penetrating awareness that his body would no longer allow him to suppress the feeling that he had been there in a less than pleasant inebriated state. His heart would pound uncontrollably with his forehead laced in a blanket of sweat and he would have to close his eyes until the bus turned a corner. For a man who was used to being in the governing role, the constant uninvited flooding of memories and the somatic betrayal seemed to be a malicious joke of sobriety that no one had warned him about. He reported this feeling as repeatedly waking up from the same dream only with the added punishment that it was no dream. There were in fact many periods of his life such as weddings, parties, holidays, and vacations of which he had a scant or no recollection.

Though his senses were being revived and as he grew more appreciative of simple pleasures, the protective curtain created by the effects of alcohol had now been lifted. Without warning and entirely unprepared, he found himself center stage with an enthusiastic and expectant audience, which he later discovered included his aging parents, his siblings, children, and wife. He stood under the increasingly warm spotlight and had come to the devastating realization that he had nothing to offer the eager spectators.

In hopes of counteracting this sense of powerlessness and to stimulate immediate involvement in his own healing process, I suggested to Hendrik that he be the one to create the initial rituals for our working relationship. I asked him to think about what he needed to begin therapy and what was important for him to feel comfortable and at ease. I did not mention his earlier reported accounts of feeling powerless or the worry of becoming dependent on a therapist or the therapy itself. I did not want the focus to reside here since these issues could be the first seeds of resistance. I wanted to respect that and simply allow those feelings to be present . Furthermore, starting with the healthy aspects of an individual can generate hope instead of constructing a stage where the patient feels they are standing on the edge of an emotional precipice. It was a simple solution with a tremendous impact.

Hendrik decided he wanted to begin every session with coffee. He would often drink his coffee before I arrived in the lobby and he always seemed to nonchalantly stretch the contents of that little paper cup to an admirable 20 minutes long. I suspected holding that cup was a familiar and trusted way of expending that extra energy leaking from his hands, a subtle somatic sedition with the potential of revealing his true internal state. It served as an important symbol ensuring a safe and gradual transition from the world outside the therapy room to the inner world of Hendrik's emotional state. In the sessions that followed, I left a few small neutral objects yearning to be squeezed at the back of the couch where he always sat. When the coffee cup was empty, he inevitably reached for a small squishy object of some sort. His favorite was a blue faceless form that regardless of harsh external pulls and pinches, always sprung back to its normal state. In the period of his treatment, I have had to replace it twice and interestingly enough, it never seemed necessary to discuss or analyze this meaningful ritual.

Hendrik's life was marked by multiple depressive episodes alongside severe health problems including a series of mild heart attacks, stomach ulcers, high blood pressure, and the beginning stages of poly-neuropathy, as well as occasionally, experiencing some mild autonomic dysfunction. He frequently feels defenseless over the decreased functioning of his body and this feeling intermittently arises unfortunately resulting in him grossly overstepping his physical boundaries. He often deliberately disregards medical advice such as leaving a hospital earlier than recommended or reacting stubbornly to physician's suggestions, ignoring the need and importance for self-care.

He was referred for individual drama therapy by his mentor and the head of the treatment team after conveying that he had enormous difficulty feeling and expressing his emotions. He described a feeling of being frozen and having no words to accurately pinpoint how he felt. He had enormous guilt from the past most notably in the roles of father, son, and brother and could not yet accept that his life had unfolded in the manner that it had. He does accept the fact that he is an alcoholic and firmly believes that his complete dependence on alcohol has determined the events of his life to this point. He does not believe, like many alcoholics, that he will be able to occasionally drink after treatment. He repeatedly states that "If I ever take another drink, then I will be consciously committing suicide." He does not wish to take as his says "the easy way out" by blaming chemical dependence for his past actions. It simply cannot be that easy he claims.

At the onset of treatment, I perceived Hendrik as a willing; yet, hesitant participator and simultaneously one who was completely driven to achieve his goal of overcoming what he then deemed his last obstacle to getting better. He had participated in group drama therapy several weeks before being referred for individual sessions, where he generally preferred the safe confines of sideline participation–occasional verbal contributions or otherwise requesting a time-out and leaving the group early.

What's Behind Door Number One?

The initial meeting of the new and old self, in this case the user self and the clean self, can be a disturbing and confrontational moment for an individual whose life has been primarily driven by the user self. The absence of identity and the emerging guilt surrounding past self-destructive behaviors can have a harrowing effect on the last remnants of self-worth and identity. Patients often wonder, as did Hendrik, "Am I more me when I'm drunk or sober? And if I have been drinking for more than half my life, have I masked the real me or was that indeed the real me?"

At the start of individual drama therapy, many patients find it a challenge to clearly articulate what exactly the problem is and to enter into the transitional space of change through the medium of drama. Therefore, we start with a simple exercise that is concrete, invites immediate participation, and allows the patient ample time to reflect. There is sufficient room for creative expression and it very quickly becomes clear that the end result is patient-specific with no expectation of "right" answers thereby eliminating the "I did it wrong or I didn't do it very well" reaction.

Here, I ask the patient to divide the drama therapy space into three "rooms": The past, the present, and the future. I may have stolen this concept from Charles Dickens' *A Christmas Carol* where Scrooge visits his former, current, and future selves, in which case I am most grateful since this creative yet cognitively and emotionally engaging process serves as a solid foundation on which to build potential for change. Though I did not expect instant overnight transformations, I did wonder if Hendrik would allow himself, as did Scrooge, a profound experience of redemption. I have found this exercise to be a source of great relief for the patient because it gets the complex tangled cognitions out of the head and creates breathing space within the physical self while safely acknowledging the truth of the present moment.

This exercise is usually accompanied by a lot of heavy sighing and responses of "I don't know" since the past and future for an alcoholic or drug addict are the ever-looming demons they would rather avoid or have buried with years of using. It is however important to know and understand the beginning points: "Where am I now," the reasons an individual is impelled to travel a new path, and of course the desired end goal. Though a painful process, it is often the first and necessary realization of what effects chemical dependency has had on a human life.

It is also a good idea to suggest to the patient that they give each room a name alongside the titles of past, present, and future. Robert Landy (1993) writes of roles that "Names are loaded with implication, as any expectant parent about to decide upon a name for the new baby knows" (p. 48). I believe this to be true not only when naming roles but of all symbolic aspects of the self or one's life experiences. As we shall see, this was evident in Hendrik's choices.

If the patient uses broad terms such as the possibility room, I ask them to be more specific and to concretize what exactly it is that they hope will be possible. An ambiguous goal makes it difficult for the patient to realize the strengths they already have since the vague intentions tend to inadvertently assist the patient in dancing around the issue, perpetuates procrastination and postpones significant decision-making. Thus, early established tangible intentions requires the chemically dependent individual to be responsible for their choices, become acquainted with that role, and prepare for the countless rehearsals ahead.

The patient has the option of creating these rooms in any way he chooses. Most often patients choose a combination of mats, scarves, masks, wooden and cardboard boxes, and musical instruments. There should be ample time for construction and reflection so that the patient does not feel hurried or compelled to make choices as a result of time limitations. After the rooms have been created and furnished, I ask the patient to choose which one he would like to visit first. It is not always necessary to actually "sit inside" the room; however, the preferred distance should be first discussed with the patient. I encourage the patient to carry a notebook in the event that they wish to record any feelings or additional thoughts that may arise. In preparation for the role work that will follow, it is helpful at this time if prominent roles for each room are recorded. I always have a list of roles on hand in the drama therapy room if it is not immediately clear what is meant by roles. The list need not be overly extensive as too many options can be overwhelming and invite confusion. Once the three rooms are constructed, I keep the contents in three separate boxes in the event that they need to be quickly recreated for use in a later session.

An additional advantage from this exercise is that the patient immediately enters into the role of architect or designer and slowly begins to acknowledge that the past may have been ruled by the addiction but that they have the choice to construct a different future. Having three concrete metaphors to view and scrutinize can be confrontational, instigating feelings of guilt and regret, which is why it is important to ensure that you also have a neutral space as a container. Sometimes we leave the rooms and go back to the "waiting room" for reflection and in addition, two rooms are always covered so that we only view one room at a time. It is not the intention here that you go into details of all the contents of the rooms since excessive verbal processing and premature analysis can undermine the healing nature of the creative process or even be potentially damaging if new coping mechanisms have not yet been formed.

"If they are encouraged to get in touch with their anger or pain, having no way to handle the feelings, the clients will respond as they always have, by drowning the feelings with alcohol" (Doyle Pita, 2004, p. 128). The very act of creating these life stages can serve as an emotional release, or as one patient once called, "putting it all out there." Aristotle claimed that catharsis and emotional purging were the effects of drama and within the safe confines of these rooms, I witness the beginning stages of that emotional and psychological purification.

Since symbolic representations, in this case the contents of the rooms and the rooms themselves as emotional tableaux, can be very powerful in accessing the emotional energy of an event, the physical sensations the patient feels serve as emphatic reminders of why they have chosen to get clean, rid themselves of the self-deprecating cobwebs of the past, and openly embrace the complex multiplicity of the newly developing roles. It is a common occurrence that people with chemical dependency problems quickly forget why they chose to quit and embark on a new life especially when the road ahead seems riddled with one challenge after another. The embodied reminders are therefore effective devices in reminding the patient what it literally felt like to be or in some cases more importantly not to be in those spaces.

Power and Guilt

Hendrik announced in his first room, which he labeled as the power/guilt room, that this was the room that made him sick. He defined sick as mentally and physically incapable of normal functioning only at the time he was completely unaware that his dependence on alcohol was steering his life path down a steep cliff. This was a practical room with sparse furnishings: A chair, some paper, and a clock He drew a dice as a symbol for this period since he had recently discovered that he did not have as much power and confidence as he thought. Looking back from the present perspective this period of his life was for him a gamble, continually casting the dice with every decision he made, and every drink he took. He described this room as cold but convenient. What he also realized looking at the "Power Guilt" room was despite the severity of the alcoholism, it was in some ways a productive period and "easy" and even when he felt most powerful. "I never worried about hurting people's feelings when having to make tough decisions because I didn't really care and I never took no for an answer so I accomplished a great deal."

The "Power Guilt" past for Hendrik was a room (period) where things were done, not felt or as he liked to say to it "I was a do-er not a feeler and I didn't stop until the goal was reached." He now found himself feeling without warning and relating to others in a way that was both exciting and unsettling. "I don't want to feel these things, I don't care about the next door neighbor, all this makes me insecure. I don't want to care and yet I do and I hate that!" An interesting and challenging path stretched before us. A challenge emerged—releasing the cognitive grip and embracing the affect. It was clear that Hendrik was prepared for just about anything so long as it did not involve connecting to his emotions. Muriel Schiffman's (1971) observation could not be more appropriate for Hendrik: " The hardest feat in therapy is the leap from the conscious to the unconscious, from the apparent to the hidden feeling. It is easy to think about your case history, to theorize about your unconscious motivation, the origin of your neurotic patterns, but it takes courage to let yourself feel the secret stuff" (p. 108).

Feeling the physicality of his emotions and letting them be visible to others was for Hendrik the most difficult undertaking of his life. And while he never wanted to permanently inhabit the Power-Guilt room again, he admitted regularly that the laissez-faire manner of living and being in the world at that time still remained attractive to him, evoking what he experienced as a strange mix of comfort and fear. He chose the following roles for this room: Master controller, James Bond 007, manager, leader, unprepared father, and son. Looking at these roles, he let out a small chuckle that the "unprepared father and son" role did not seem to belong since the others exuded power and control. He recalled a memory of a photograph of himself standing in front of his first apartment, just arriving home from the hospital with his daughter awkwardly held in his arms, preparing for his first important role as a 17-year-old father. He said, "I could not have been more unsure and frightened."

Sober Chaos

Brightly colored braided garlands twisted together in a gigantic knot was the centerpiece of the sober chaos room. Sober because it represented the here and now for Hendrik and chaos because at this point, emotional anarchy and mental disarray were the only ways he could describe his entry into sobriety. He compared it to being at the center of a tornado with nothing but a blurring wind enveloping his senses. He sat in stillness and did not want to enter this room. He was about to write when he looked up and said, "Is this all there is here? The only thing I am here is unsure." I was not sure at first what he meant.

"It scares me that I have no craving to drink, when will that come, and will I be able to handle it? How could I not have known what I was doing to myself and everyone around me?" He then chose anger and depression from the emotion cards to place next to the clump of his colored chaos. He chose alcoholic, partner, and patient as the most prominent roles here. He gestured toward the role of alcoholic, "That is what I must never forget. That is what I am." When he started individual drama therapy, Hendrik had been sober for five months and initially thought he was halfway there though not really knowing where there was. He was slowly beginning to discover himself, a very different self was emerging in these early stages of sobriety. This new emerging self was clad in an unfamiliar insecurity that was challenging his very decision to stop drinking. Everyone was telling him how fantastic it was that he was sober; yet, his own feeling was signaling the slow expansion of a disturbing intrapsychic conflict. This was and still is the most emotionally demanding room for Hendrik because he knows in order to get where he wants to go, he must invest in this room, in the here and now.

Insecure Fear

This room took the longest time to furnish and yet, the end result was a completely empty space squared off with four mats. It was quite large and according to Hendrik, must remain empty since he had no idea what the future would bring. He was frightened by the future and angry at himself for feeling that way since a better future was precisely his goal. His greatest longing had become his greatest fear. He had great difficulty accepting his current situation as it was and being fully present in a sober state of awareness without sufficient access to his internal world. He described his presence in this room as being a distant observer: He could see what he was experiencing, a colossal emotional storm passing over and through him. Not allowing himself to truly feel what he experienced–extreme anger and sadness, which repeatedly bubbled to the surface of his consciousness made him feel weak and "emotionally handicapped." The longer the period of sobriety, the more intense the emotions.

Tian Dayton (2000) writes, "When the self-medicating substance wears off, the person is again overwhelmed by the pain, which now has further isolation, shame and unresolved pain added to it" (p. 18). Hendrik could not at this point imagine what he would like to have in this room. He thought it premature to place his goals here at this point since he had much to discover from himself. He chose the roles of *alcoholic* which must never be too far from his critical eye, *son* because he anticipated the rigorous inquisition from his aging parents that he was sure would come, and lastly *father* though not entirely sure what he must do with this role.

Back to the Waiting Room

Since this initial phase can be quite intense and sometimes even confusing for the patient, it is important to take a step back and process what happened, how is it now, and where do we go from here? To do this, we went back to the neutral territory of the "waiting room." Visits to all three rooms crystallized the very real presence of uncertainty and diffidence in Hendrik and permeated his current emotional and psychological state. He began at this time making a case to return to his old ways of drinking, citing that this therapeutic process was the most difficult task he had ever undertaken. It was also the first time he was aware of how afraid and unsure he had been as he moved through the world, for his true emotions were continually blanketed in alcohol creating artificial boundaries between him and the outside world. The tool he had known as the ruler of his emotions with the power to lessen the intensity of those emotions too intense to feel was now gone and he began a process of grieving.

In the period that followed, Hendrik had repeated nightmares filled with snippets of past events: The loved ones he had hurt, the death of his first wife which he had never mourned, and his own aggressive outbursts haunted him continually. He would awake in a cold sweat and wonder again why he was consciously choosing to go through this. He struggled at that time to acknowledge any benefit of being sober. There were also sessions when he grew angry at me claiming that I was supposed to "make him better" and instead more past memories were returning making him angry and distressed. "For example, clients often feel hurt and angry when they discover we are not going to satisfy their dependency needs" (Doyle Pita, 2004, p. 129). The anger turned out to be quite positive and once we had given it space to be present, in walked Mickey Mouse.

Enter King Kong and Mickey Mouse

Landy (1993) writes that "Much of the actual therapy concerns a working through of the issues embedded in a particular role (or related roles)" (p. 49). As part of the treatment program and to stimulate employment preparation, patients are strongly encouraged to do volunteer work. Though he despised the very thought of it claiming he had not one philanthropic fiber in his body and no desire to spend his valuable time between all those "do-gooders," the day had finally come for Hendrik. "So I started playing Mickey Mouse today," he announced one afternoon plopping down on the couch grinning uncontrollably. I imagined this former head of corporate mergers and maker of policies with two big black ears atop his head. One day a week, he assisted former psychiatric patients with odd jobs around the house and in social activities. He described that giving freely of his time was at times painful and had to be forced. His motivation was not to help others, he emphasized, but was more for himself as he was trying out a new role. He shook his head laughing,

"No that role is not for me."

"What do you mean?" I asked, "Everyone loves Mickey Mouse."

"Then you can be Mickey Mouse."

Working with the role of Mickey Mouse gave Hendrik another opinion of the normally cheery, personable mouse, and later of himself. For Hendrik, Mickey Mouse had a conniving and duplicitous side, with many complex layers.

"I know what you're thinking and I am not playing a mouse."

"Which role can you play today?"

"Myself, I have enough trouble playing that."

I was unable to convince Hendrik to further fictionalize his role as Landy (1993) suggests and since he did not want another name nor his own, he simply chose "man." He provided the details of the scene as follows: Man loses child at Disneyland, child was last seen by Mickey Mouse, man confronts Mickey Mouse. He gave me the role of Mickey Mouse with great pleasure. I playfully greeted the supposedly excited group of children and was then approached by Hendrik.

"Have you seen my child, she was just standing here, she is about this tall with brown hair,"

I looked at him with a big silly grim pasted across my face shaking my head and shoulders. He began to laugh.

"Do you realize how ridiculous you look?" he asked, addressing me out of role "and people are supposed to come to you for help. I'm not talking to a non-verbal mouse."

"Oh sorry sir, I can't hear you over these screaming children." He sighed, hands deep in his pockets, stepping in and out of role.

"You're not so powerful now, prancing around like that. Anyway, (back in role) I've lost my child, have you seen her?" I felt some leakages of his true feeling seeping through, the feeling of being in the hands of another person seemingly having more power than him. More deep sighs.

"No, sorry I haven't seen your child." Again he laughed, harder and harder.

"You're a fake, do you know that?" It was difficult to discern if he meant me or Mickey.

"Hiding behind your big stupid mask and ears." I sensed him getting angry.

"Sir, I'm sorry your lost your child but I can't help you, you should go to security."

"This is stupid, I would never go to Mickey Mouse for help, he's a fraud."

I could see him searching trying to make sense of what he was feeling untangling the sadness and the anger. My instinct told me to bring the scene to a close.

"Is that your little girl sir, over there?" He grinned and mumbled something inaudible.

"Yes, yeah that's her." He sat down on the couch in the "waiting room" with his head resting in his hands, face flushed, staring at the floor. There was a heavy stillness and then he shared his thoughts. Hendrik described that he saw and heard himself talking to himself, strongly identifying with Mickey Mouse. The role that at first seemed the farthest from Hendrik, turned out to be the one with which he shared the most. He also saw himself as a fraud, hiding behind the alcoholic mask for most of life, presenting in his mind, a false image of self to the outside world. I asked him if there were other associations with Mickey Mouse and he told for the first time of his complicated relationship with his father in whom he also saw aspects of Mickey Mouse. His conclusion was that they were a lot alike and that both puzzled and aggravated him since Hendrik had always thought he had set out with the intention of not being the same man and father as his father was. He talked a great deal about his father in the weeks following, emphasizing that I couldn't possibly understand the power and presence this man possessed. You do not ask questions, you just listen he said and if you are *asked* a question, you better know the answer.

When Hendrik spoke of his father, he drew his body inward making himself small and defenseless. I saw a young boy before me, worried of what his father might think of him. He once commented that it would have been easier had his father beat him since that would have at least been clear. His experience of his father was cemented in uncertainty, fear, and rehearsed respect. As a child he had asked for help with his homework and went away feeling so stupid and belittled that he vowed never to ask anyone for anything again in his life. Therefore, being in treatment and therapy and especially drama therapy of which he knew nothing, was a monumental turning point for Hendrik.

A short time after the "birth" of Mickey Mouse, a recurring theme emerged on a weekly basis, one of power and strength and the complexity of mourning the loss of status that power and strength bring. This power and strength found expression through the image of King Kong. After several short scenes with King Kong, I asked Hendrik to do a character sketch of him. He uncovered that King Kong was both dangerous but in a very appealing and adventurous way. He did not have to compete with anyone, rely on anyone, ask for anything nor answer to anyone. But at the same time, he did not really fit in anywhere, was alone, and could also be seen as an overgrown idiot or a gigantic bumbling buffoon with no common sense or understanding of his or others' boundaries. The most startling discovery for Hendrik was the realization that the mighty King Kong became weak and vulnerable when he fell in love. These were more disturbing similarities. He did what interested him with no regard for those around, destroying everything in his path. The role of "arrogant bastard" emerged here which was used in later sessions.

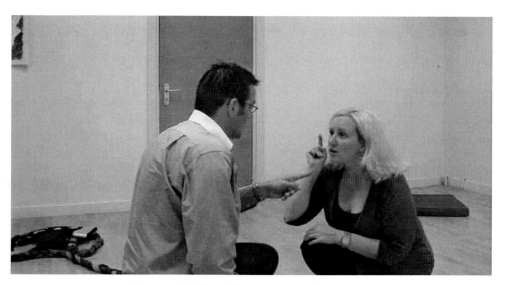

Figure 14.3. King Kong asserting his power.

This way of working proved most effective for Hendrik as it provided him with enough distance for the safe expression of emotions and awakened in him the crucial connection between his more familiar cognitive ways of functioning in the world and the less familiar and somewhat threatening emotional side of himself. Landy (2008) writes, "When working through role method, clients often experience catharsis especially when they become aware of the connection between the fiction and the reality. This awareness can occur unconsciously in the enactment, or more consciously in the reflection. However, the form of catharsis is unique in that it integrates both affect and cognition" (p. 125).

My own images of King Kong and experiences with Hendrik sprung forth. I recalled from the film that the natives on the island were forced out of fear and concern for safety to build enormous walls to keep the beast out and periodically offered a member of the tribe as a sacrifice. Yet, the King Kong that was entering the drama room every week was also building walls and searching for ways to offer himself up as self-sacrifice for an emotionally imprinted past. King Kong initially offered little hope for Hendrik since his life ended in a dreadful demise with everyone against him. I was worried Hendrik would sink back into hopelessness and depression or tangentially

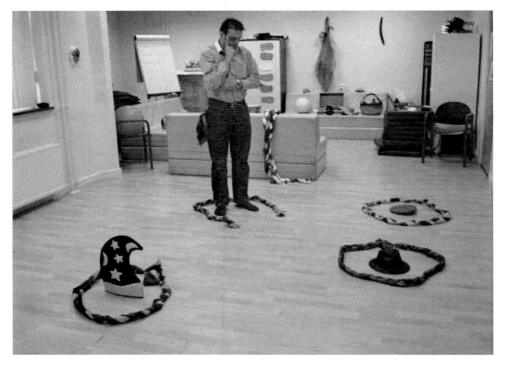

Figure 14.4. Choosing a new path.

disconnect from his emotions again. I wanted him to see that there was space and time for new choices. I suggested we make two life paths one of Hendrik and a fictional one of King Kong. While there were innumerable and not entirely favorable similarities, the breakthrough at a pivotal point came when I had " interviewed" Hendrik in the role of King Kong. He was getting ready to leave the jungle and go to the city and when questioned of his preparations and expectations, he had none. He did not have to prepare. He was after all King Kong, what could possibly go wrong?

During the reflection, we discussed the consequences of rigorously rooting yourself in one role regardless of changing circumstances, environments, and intentions, attempting to move forward while clinging to the past, resisting the necessity of development and opportunity. King Kong could not behave and interact with others in the city as he did in the jungle, there were countless unforeseen obstacles such as the modern metropolitan way of life, and the new and changing roles of those around him. As a gigantic, clumsy gorilla moving through such a world, this meant potential danger for both himself and the world around him. There was little space and his need to utilize so much of it brought him quickly in conflict with others. To make this aspect of Hendrik's King Kong more tangible, we brought the role into the body through body sculpting and movement. In adapting the physical characteristics of King Kong into his own body, it immediately became clear how restraining and demanding this role was on his physical being. Hendrik would often comment that it cost him a great deal of energy and he often felt as if he continually had to blow himself up, to appear larger, than he was and more importantly than he felt. "We have seen how a psychological progression from one state to another is expressed in actual physical movement from one position to another and this is one of the unique properties of drama" (Duggan & Grainger, 1997, p. 135). As Hendrik assumed the physical statue of a fictitious gorilla and attempted to move through the space as a human being, it was at times, difficult to witness. He seemed helpless and discouraged and yet as Duggan and Grainger point out, it is here that a psychological progression becomes evident. Duggan and Grainger go on to write that "When we move, we change our perspective, we can move closer or farther away. We alter our point of view" (p. 135). Metaphors of movement became an important feature in Hendrik's sessions.

Hendrik had made assumptions about getting sober and moving forward into a new way of living and functioning in the world. He assumed he just had to stop drinking and everything would take care of itself. He too was accustomed to charging forth with a blind confidence that everything would turn out as he wanted, only now he was moving through a sober world with sober eyes, and a physical self that was no longer willing to dangerously tread the boundaries of health and illness. He has uncovered many past and present roles during this often painstaking journey and even some new roles for the future have gained some attention. He is slowly beginning to let go of past roles that no longer have a function. He is working on releasing the "arrogant bastard" that grew out of King Kong. Also, he is searching for a balance and yet seems more aware of the pitfalls in thinking that achieving balance is a static state. Further, he can laugh at himself and no longer has the strength for building walls nor does he desire this from others around him. He occasionally revisits his rooms, but peers gingerly through the window just enough to assess the current state of events.

The powerful primitiveness of this beast that loomed above everyone and everything, a gigantic innocence lacking insight, standing at a distance from his own feelings, attempts to make time for Mickey Mouse. Mickey Mouse and King Kong were frequent visitors during Hendrik's therapy; however, they gradually lost their status as being the two most prominent roles for Hendrik. At this point, he is concentrating on being more present in the role of husband and slowly reentering the latent roles of son and brother through this time with a whole new script under his arm.

In the Absence of Alcohol–Challenges and Celebrations

We who lived in concentration camps can remember the men who walked through the huts comforting others, giving away their last piece of bread. They may have been few in number, but they offer sufficient proof that everything can be taken from a man but one thing: the last of human freedoms—to choose one's attitude in any given set of circumstances. Viktor Frankl (1984, p. 75)

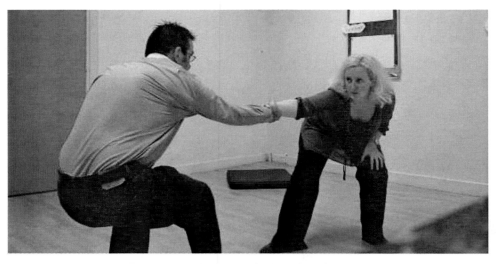

Figure 14.5. Asserting the Newfound Power.

Increased periods of sobriety work very well in highlighting the harsh realities of life for chemical dependents. Confronting this truth can easily and rapidly pave the way back to the tried and trusted pattern of drinking and using. Hendrik had no relapses and was sober for almost 17 months. Just like the men in Frankl's concentration camp, he had to make this choice every single day to maintain sobriety. Though he now recognizes its illusory presence, alcohol was for Hendrik a protective layer that effectively shielded him from external and unwanted turmoil. That the challenges continue long after getting clean is often a confusing concept for dependents. Many will say it gets worse before it gets better and that it is the "getting through the worst of it" that determines if you will make it. They will also tell you that like many chronic illnesses, your dependence will continue to play a crucial role in your life and you must never underestimate that. Hendrik would say that if he makes a choice to take one drink, he is leading himself knowingly to his grave. He still despises the emotional challenges but sees that respecting his boundaries prevents getting stuck in gaps of old patterns and failing to recognize and eventually integrate new creative potentials is an aspect of being human we all miss at one time or another.

The Show Must Go On

Working therapeutically through the medium of drama requires challenging your imagination, engaging in your own spontaneity, and that of the therapist. I am incredibly grateful to Hendrik for allowing me to tell his story and be part of his healing process and for all that his process has helped me to understand. It has been an honor and an unforgettable experience. His strength, vulnerability, and honesty remind me why I choose to do this work and its value and impact on the human mind and spirit. And while King Kong and Mickey Mouse may never marry or even become best friends, I think an occasional visit might just be the right ingredient to give Hendrik the flow and balance he has been searching for.

My experiences in individual drama therapy with patients suffering from addiction problems have sharpened both my senses and awareness of the needs human beings possess as they fight their way to a safe healing place. There is an intense drive to be seen and have an opportunity to tell their story, an often painful ache to be understood and a chance to find a new and safe place among those of us deemed "well." When I think of Hendrik today, long past his one year anniversary of sobriety and still not proud of himself, I think of an inquisitive, charismatic figure occasionally submerged in a mild universal innocence.

References

Dayton, T. (2000). *Trauma and addiction: Ending the cycle of pain through emotional literacy.* Florida: Health Communciations Inc.

Doyle Pita, D. (2004). *Addictions counseling: A practical and comprehensive guide for counseling people with addictions.* New York: Crossroad Publishing Company.

Duggan, M., & Grainger, R. (1997). *Imagination, identification and catharsis in theatre and therapy.* London: Jessica Kingsley Publishers Ltd.

Frankl, V. E. (1984). *Man's search for meaning.* New York: Simon & Schuster.

Landy, R. J. (1993). *Persona and performance: The meaning of role in drama, therapy, and everyday life.* New York: Guilford Press.

Landy, R. J. (2008). *The couch and the stage: Integrating words and action in psychotherapy.* Maryland: Rowman & Littlefield Publishing Group, Inc.

Schiffman, M. (1971). *Gestalt self therapy & further techniques for personal growth.* California: Wingbow Press.

Biography

Linda M. Dunne is a registered drama therapist originally from Canada who now makes her home in the Netherlands. She is a member of the National Association for Drama Therapy, the Nederlandse Vereniging voor Drama Therapie (NVDT), Federatie Vaktherapeutische Beroepen, (FVB), and the Dutch training group for Developmental Transformations and the Association of Traumatic Stress Specialists. She holds a Bachelor of Arts degree from Memorial University of Newfoundland and a Master of Arts from Kansas State University and is currently training in Jungian Analysis and Sandplay Therapy. She has developed and runs a drama therapy program for groups and individuals recovering from chemical dependency and counsels recovering addicts. She is expanding into private practice using the creative arts therapies to foster personal growth and development. She can be contacted at info@indi-goopties.nl

Chapter 15

SURVIVING THE FREEDOM OF CHOOSING OUR FEELINGS: EXISTENTIAL DRAMA THERAPY AND ADDICTIVE BEHAVIOR

COSMIN GHEORGHE

Introduction

S ubstance dependence and addiction have been studied from different perspectives and have generated a variety of theoretical approaches and treatment techniques. Many of these approaches focus on the individual only, as an isolated being who exhibits a weird behavior produced by an illness, for which he/she is not necessarily responsible. The following chapter will underline the importance and necessity of a multidisciplinary and systemic approach. It is the author's strong opinion that addiction and addictive behavior are directly related to the social, political, and cultural environment. Therefore, a complete understanding of addiction requires an approach that goes beyond reductionist statements ("I am an addict, because I drink too much. But why do I drink too much? Evidently, because I am an addict"). Existential Drama Therapy provides the opportunity for the deconstruction and analysis of the subtle mechanisms (intentional and non-intentional) created and maintained by a specific sociocultural environment.

In order to establish a relationship between the processes facilitated by drama therapy and existential therapy, and their role in the treatment of addiction, the following chapter will start by taking a look at some of the most common psychological denominators that build the foundation of and create the conditions for the addictive behavior that accompanies them. Then we will see why and how existential drama therapy is appropriate for describing, understanding, and treating the addiction.

Definition of Terms

Existential Drama Therapy is a multidisciplinary and systemic approach and uses elements of drama therapy (defined as the "intentional and systematic use of drama/theatre processes to achieve psychological growth" (Emunah, 1994, p. 3) and concepts of existential philosophy. Rollo May defines existentialism as "the endeavor to understand man by cutting below the cleavage between subject and object which has bedeviled Western thought and science since shortly after the Renaissance" (May in Yalom 1980, pp. 22–23). Yalom goes further and states that by cutting below that schism, the individual is regarded not as a subject able to perceive reality, but as a "consciousness who participates in the construction of reality" (Yalom, 1980, p. 23). According to Yalom, existential psychotherapy is a dynamic approach to therapy which focuses on (1) four ultimate concerns that are rooted in the individual's existence (death, freedom, isolation, and meaninglessness), as well as on (2) the conflict that flows from the individual's confrontation with the givens of existence (Yalom, 1980, pp. 5–8).

Addiction and Substance Abuse

Most of the theoretical approaches to addiction intend to isolate a specific factor and declare it responsible for creating the addiction. In this chapter, addiction is described as being the result of the concomitant action of three categories of factors: Sociocultural, biochemical, and psychological, which influence each other on one hand and create and are shaped by addictive behavior on the other hand. It is obvious that the biochemical group of factors is the most acknowledged and promoted in the Western cultures and especially in the United States, for reasons that are determined, interestingly enough, by the social, political, economical, cultural, and moral factors. For this reason, I decided to use a different approach in this chapter, using concepts from theater, existential philosophy, and mythology.

The word addict is the individual who habituates or abandons himself or herself to something compulsively or obsessively and comes from the Latin *addictus*, which means assigned, surrendered (Random House, 2000). In the same way abuse comes from the Latin *abusus* = Ab – usus = to mis-use = to use wrongly or improperly; to treat in a harmful or injurious way; to speak harshly or insultingly to or about; to deceive or mislead (Random House, 2000). There are several observations that devolve from the above definition of terms. First, addiction can be related to both a substance that is ingested, and with an activity (a practice, a habit). The addiction to a substance is more visible and has more dramatic consequences, as it is usually morally and legally unacceptable. However, in terms of origin and purpose of addiction, as well as from an existential drama therapeutic point of view, this chapter does not differentiate between individuals who are addicted to alcohol, work, shopping, cocaine, gambling, marijuana, internet and TV, mushrooms, therapy, sex, food, and so forth. The purpose of this chapter is to identify some of the mechanisms created in a given psychosocio-cultural environment, which create and maintain individuals who indulge in their actions with sufficient abandon, leading to the addicted state (Peele, 1989).

> People seek specific, essential human experiences from their addictive involvement, no matter whether it is drinking, eating, smoking, loving, shopping or gambling. . . . Nonetheless, even in cases where addicts die from their excesses, an addiction must be understood as a human response that is motivated by the addict's desires and principles. All addictions accomplish something for the addict. They are ways of coping with feelings and situations with which addicts cannot otherwise cope. . . . Addicts seek experiences that satisfy needs they cannot otherwise fulfill. (Peele 1989, p. 146)

There are only two main categories of reasons for the individuals who become addicted: To avoid or alleviate pain (physical and/or emotional) and to obtain pleasure without struggle (Carrere, 2001, personal communication). Peele (1989) notices that all the experiences that facilitates addiction offer people a sense of power or control, of security or calm, of intimacy, or of being valued by others; or on the other hand, the potential addictive experiences block out negative sensations like pain and discomfort.

A second observation related to the definition above, refers to the addicts as being individuals who abandon and surrender themselves, in a compulsive or obsessive manner, to some entity. One of the main theses of this chapter is that human beings permanently experience anxiety, which increases or decreases in intensity according to a variety of factors, created, and supported by the social, cultural, political, and economical environment. Consequently, the addictive behavior represents an extreme of the attempt to manage this background anxiety, for which the modern human beings seem to have less and less tolerance and almost no capacity (internal wisdom) or education to understand and integrate. Pascal noticed that people devoted a great part of their activities to avoid "'thoughts of themselves,' for if they should pause for self-contemplation, they would be miserable and anxious" (Pascal in May, 1977, p. 30). It is interesting to notice that the 12-Steps philosophy implies also a surrender (i.e., addictus), just that is represented by a higher power. From this point of view, it might be argued that the AA/NA philosophy is based on replacing a destructive surrender with a spiritual one, which at a first glance makes sense, as it might be understood as a reorganization and restructuration around a different, non-destructive core belief. In reality though, the 12-Step approach seems to work at the same superficial level like drugs, alcohol, TV, weight loss programs, etc., feeding into the same behavior and simply replacing the focus and object of one's anxiety. Later in this chapter, we will see how Existential Drama Therapy (EDT) approaches addiction in a systemic and multidisciplinary way. EDT aims to: (1) stimulate the individual to look for meaning and solidly grounding his/her life axis; and (2) teach the individual to accept and learn to tolerate discomfort and non-structure, without having to act on the "perpetual restlessness in which men pass their lives" (Pascal in May, 1977, p. 30). As it will be presented later in this chapter, Existential Drama Therapy realizes the translation from harmful to non-harmful in a systemic way, by replacing a broken, vicious circle, with a complete cycle that includes transition as an essential phase, necessary to link two main existential stages: Separation (individualization/loneliness) and integration (togetherness/ engulfment).

The Purpose of Addictive Behavior

There are three main categories of benefits that reinforce the abuse of a substance or activity, creating addiction. First, the abuse of a practice or substance provides forgetfulness, as a way of dealing with meaninglessness, existential and social loneliness, fear of separation and individuation, and fear of dissolution (death). Later on, we will see how Heidegger's (1962) concepts of Forgetfulness of Being and Mindfulness of Being apply to the addiction, and how existential drama therapy facilitates the transition toward mindfulness.

Second, addiction offers a substitute for relationship. In a world that lacks more and more genuine human relationships, the abuse of a substance or practice offers the superficial and false feeling that the need for togetherness is being satisfied. The type of relationships promoted within a given society or culture are connected directly to the individual's understanding of attachment. The relationships established by the addict have an I-it format, as opposed to the I-You human relationship (Buber, 1965). The I-it relationship between the individual and the object of his/her addiction is an accurate reproduction of the business relationship, which in its fundamentalist form completely eliminates meaning, aesthetics, and moral values, if they result in less profit. The I-it relationship promoted by market fundamentalism has intruded deeper and deeper into the civil society (Soros, 1998), eroding the sociocultural fabric, introducing, and normalizing the idea that one's needs can and should be always and immediately satisfied, and consequently creating a social environment, which justifies the attitude of its members (increased anxiety combined with very low tolerance for it), reinforcing the addictive behavior. The therapist-client relationship is, from that point of view, an I-You relationship, but with elements from the I-it business model, necessary to maintain a structure and create boundaries aimed at avoiding the replacement of togetherness with enmeshment.

Third, a substance or practice abuse provides meaning and structure, defined and described in my existential drama therapy technique as Axis Mundi, which literary can be translated as Center of the World. In a society where aesthetics, art, health, love, friendship, and learning exist mainly as commodities, I-it relationships and social loneliness prevail, leading to a subtle form of alienation, unacknowledged, or even celebrated as just a different way of being. The drug of choice and addiction become the Axis and everything is referred to it. The addict feels the urge to replace the lack of meaning, fills up his/her time with the permanent goal of finding the substance, and/or activity to achieve that state of mind (forgetfulness), which drives him/her away from the inconvenient and uncomfortable reality.

Fear of Death, Fear of Life:
The Absent Angel and the Experience of Loneliness

Kierkegaard distinguishes between fear, characterized by the fact that it has an object and a location, as it is a fear of something; and anxiety, which has no particular source and therefore cannot be precisely located: It is a fear of no thing (Kierkegaard, in Yalom, 1980). There is not always a clear boundary between the objective fear and anxiety (the subjective fear).

All our fears and anxieties appear to lead to four ultimate concerns: Death, Freedom, Loneliness (isolation), and Meaninglessness (Yalom, 1980). I believe there is a combination of social and existential determinant factors that play a crucial role in most of substance/practice abuse cases. Performing an action and/or ingesting a substance in a compulsive and obsessive manner are aimed at managing fear and anxiety. Yalom describes two major sources of anxiety: the fear of life (fear of existing as a separate individual, fear of separation, individuation anxiety) and the fear of death (fear of fusion, of engulfment) (Yalom, 1980).

The fear of separation is perceived by clients as fear of loss of connection with a greater whole, fear of having to face life as an isolated being, fear of not belonging, and of not having the protection conferred by that belonging (Yalom, 1980). Often, those who experience this existential loneliness translate it into their social milieu, perceiving it as social loneliness and trying to "treat" it as such. The sociocultural structure in the United States, which is based on practicality, fluidity, and disposability, with disregard for mere contemplation, intellectual dialog, and constancy, contributes to a great extent to the achievement and perpetuation of the fear of life stage. Yalom (1980, p. 353) writes: "The decline of intimacy-sponsoring institution – the extended family, the stable residential neighborhood, the church, local merchants, the family doctor—has, in the United States at least, inexorably led to increased interpersonal estrangement." When the anxiety produced by the fear of life achieves a certain level, one will try to eliminate it by moving toward giving oneself to another, and when this move is made out of fear, the result is a fusion with another, a dissolution of oneself into another (Yalom, 1980). "Another" is usually represented by a [potential] partner (boyfriend, girlfriend, spouse, lover, friend), or a social group (friends, family, coworkers, classmates, support groups, church, army, etc.). But what happens when that another is not there? In the absence of another, one will tend to unconsciously assuage one's fear of life by giving oneself to what is available and to what one perceives as being the equivalent of another: a surrogate, a pseudo-other. It happens that in many cases the equivalent of another is a substance: Food, alcohol, legal and illegal drugs; or an activity: Gambling, working, shopping, surfing the internet, watching TV, text messaging, checking the email, physical exercising, going to therapy, workshops and support groups, and so forth. In conclusion, one's surrender and abandonment to a substance, one's "commitment to a habit or practice" (*Random House Webster's College Dictionary*, 2000) is directly related with: (1) an initial absence of another; (2) a fear of existential loneliness, usually translated in, and enmeshed with, social loneliness; and (3) a substance/practice/habit that are chosen to replace the absence or the loss of a known or unknown other.

For practical reasons, related to the existential drama therapeutic techniques, I would like to underline the double quality of the absence that fuels one's addictive behavior. The client can experience a primordial absence, something or somebody who never existed, but whom/which existence has always been desired and yearned for. And on the other hand, we have the absence that manifests itself as a Loss: Something or somebody who, at some point in time, was part of the client's life, in a form or another, but now has disappeared, temporarily or definitive. As part of the existential drama therapy techniques that I use with substance abuse clients, the Absence and/or the Loss are represented by a character called the Absent Angel. From this perspective, a client's Absent Angel represents the symbol and/or the metaphor that describes an unfulfilled dream, a nostalgia, a crucial loss, an unbearable absence. Also, for some clients, the Absent Angel may represent what Almaas calls one's "essence," as the pure, unconditional nature of who we are (Davis, 1999), which has been ignored or buried under layers of forgetfulness.

Anxiety Producing Cultures:
The Confidence of a Consumer's Social Life

What happens when a culture does not promote and does not encourage human social relationships? What happens when within a society, the preferred and encouraged relationship is the I–it (similar to the relationship human-machine), or it-it (like machine-machine relationship (Buber, 1965)? What happens when the members of a culture are educated (intentionally and unintentionally) that the only reason human beings establish relationships is to satisfy their individual needs? What happens when the members of a culture attain such a high level of civilization and prosperity, that in order to maintain it, they do not allow themselves to waste time on human, social interactions, which they reduce to superficial, unauthentic encounters? What happens when these individuals do not create and do not develop anymore material, spiritual, and moral facilities that would stimulate and support authentic, need-free relationships (Yalom, 1980)?

My answer for all of these questions has two parts: (1) people become increasingly fearful and anxious, integrating these feelings in every aspect of their life; and (2) they try to replace what they do not have, they look for and they achieve surrogates. One of the most common ways of avoiding anxiety is to repetitively (and eventually compulsively) effectuate something. Put it in different words, we avoid something by doing something else: Working 12-14 hours a day, spending all the free time jogging or at the gym, surfing the internet, playing video games or watching TV, eating, shopping, looking for and having sex. Like in the DSM IV definition of substance dependency, we end up spending more and more time, energy and money to achieve and to perform recommended activities and assuage or indefinitely postpone the encounter with our anxiety. Thus, we develop a relationship, an intimate and deep relationship with Ms. Job, with Mr. Mall, with Mrs. 24 Hours Fitness, with Madame Junk Food and Mr. Alcohol, with Sir Vicodin and Lady Cocaine. These relationships, all established on an "I–it" format, are nothing more than ways of replacing our desire of belonging, our need of fusion. Christina Grof writes: "Addiction is an attachment amplified. . . . In an attempt to satisfy our genuine, unfulfilled need to be loved and accepted, we attach ourselves to other people, to animals, or to social or professional roles that promise to bring us what we long for" (Grof, 1993, p. 143 and pp. 145–146).

At the other end of the spectrum, the abuse of a substance or of a practice may be also an attempt to avoid or to manage the Fear of Death, manifested as fear of loss of individuality, fear of being dissolved [again] in the Whole. In this state, one perceives stability as stagnation, and fears that stagnation will lead to extinction (Yalom, 1980). Though Fear of Life and Fear of Death seem at opposite ends of a continuum, they share the inescapable confrontation with loneliness: No matter how much physical, political, or social power one has, no matter how many properties and millions of dollars owns, one has to face death only by oneself, i.e., alone.

When life and death are experienced as overwhelming fears, individuali-

ty becomes individualism and loneliness and togetherness becomes enmeshment and dissolution of self. The abuse of a substance or practice might be
seen as an attempt to avoid or manage positive or negative feelings (distress,
anxiety, exuberance, excitement) produced by: (1) the fear of life, fear of
existing and living autonomously; (2) the fear of death, fear of being engulfed
by a greater whole (Yalom, 1980), fear of being totally absorbed by the other
(May, 1977); and (3) the rapid, ceaseless, and exhausting oscillation between
the two stages, individuality/separation and fusion/integration, without realizing it and without ever being satisfied with any of them. The engine of this
rapid and maddening swinging is nothing else but the good, old anxiety, and
the product of it is even more anxiety. Next, we will explore this vicious circle, as well as the solution proposed by the existential drama therapy.

The Three Cycles of Existential Drama Therapy

There are three processes that form the foundation of this chapter. First of
them is represented by the cycle fusion–individuation, which is a basic component of humans' physical and psychological life, and which has been
described from an existential point of view in the previous section of this
chapter. The second one is represented by the classic Rite of Passage, with its
three stages: Separation, Transition, and Integration (Van Gennep in
Grainger, 1995). During these three stages "a threshold of human experience
is approached, crossed and passed, in the sense of being achieved"
(Grainger, 1995, p. 124). The third cycle accompanies the transformations
contained within the Rite of Passage and is represented by the shift from one
mode of existence to a higher one: Forgetfulness of Being and Mindfulness
of Being, in the presence of a Boundary Experience (Heidegger, 1962).
Forgetfulness of being has been described by Heidegger as an "inauthentic"
mode of existence, "in which one is unaware of one's authorship of one's life
and world, in which one 'flees,' 'falls,' and is tranquilized, in which one
avoids choices by being 'carried along by the nobody.'" In this state, "one
surrenders oneself to the everyday world, to a concern about the way things
are" (Yalom, 1980, p. 31). It is important to notice that the permanent abuse
of a substance/practice, with its subsequent addiction, is nothing more than
a way to perpetuate a state of forgetfulness of being, in which the anxiety,
and the discomfort provoked by the awareness of choice, separation, or
engulfment, temporarily disappear. Mindfulness of being is called also the
"ontological mode" (from the Greek ontos, which means "existence"). "Since
it is only in this ontological mode that one is in touch with one's self-creation,
it is only here that one can grasp the power to change oneself" (Yalom, 1980,
p. 31). Later on we will explore how drama therapy introduces Transition
between the fusion and separation stages of the addict, by facilitating the shift

toward mindfulness of being, in which a real, sustainable change can take place.

The Individuation–Fusion Cycle: Creating a Vicious Circle

The creation of a human being starts with a process of fusion: Energies, organs, anxiety, happiness and fears, hopes and disappointments, physical and emotional fluids, ovules and spermatozoids, are combined and the result is what biologists call the zygote, or the primordial cell. Floating for nine months in our mother's amniotic liquid is the first fusion experience we ever have. Similarly, the first separation experience follows immediately after: It is the moment we are born and separated from our mother's womb, which implies the experience—in various degrees and forms—of the feelings of anxiety, separation and loneliness. Again, right after we are pressed, pushed and pulled through a narrow channel, and then exposed to cold, gravitation and powerful light and sounds, warm arms hold us and direct us to a comfort source: The breast. It is time for fusion again, and from now on, we will have to figure out by ourselves how to cope with these endless, confusing successions of separation, and fusion experiences.

Stan Grof (1985) did the most extensive and detailed research (extended over a period of almost three decades) of the way we experience our birth and how these experiences are later translated into our adult life. Using LSD, and later developing holotropic breathwork, Grof identified four Basic Perinatal Matrix (BPM), which describe a succession of processes of fusion and individuation that are re-lived by the clients during the holotropic breathwork session. BPM I corresponds to what I called the first fusion, which is "the experience of the original symbiotic unity of the fetus with the maternal organism at the time of intrauterine existence," and usually it is experienced as a "lack of boundaries and obstructions" (Grof, 1985, p. 102). BPM II is related to the beginning of the biological delivery, when "the fetus is periodically constricted by uterine spasms; the cervix is closed and the way out is not yet available." Grof found that the people who re-live BPM II identify themselves with "archetypal figures symbolizing eternal damnation," such as Sisyphus and Prometheus. Also, "agonizing feelings of metaphysical loneliness, helplessness, hopelessness, inferiority, existential despair, and guilt" are standard constituents of this matrix (Grof, 1985, p. 103). As we will see later, Sisyphus represent, together with the already described Absent Angel, a key character and metaphor in existential drama therapy work with addicts. The third BPM is the expression of the second part of the biological delivery, and it is directly related with the *death-rebirth struggle*. BPM IV is related with the actual birth of the child and is represented by "a sudden relief and relaxation" that follows the previous struggle (Grof, 1985, p. 103).

However, although relief and liberation are the results of the individuation, once by himself/herself, the individual has to face the cold and overstimulating outside world. Therefore, whenever one perceives as unbearable these external stimuli, as well as the internal feelings of loneliness and isolation, one will tend to run toward a fusion experience.

Me And Not Me: Aesthetic Distance
As A Breaker Of The Vicious Circle

As it has been previously shown, one of the easiest ways to achieve a surrogate of fusion experience is by abusing a mood-altering substance or by compulsively executing an act. "Fusion eliminates isolation in a radical fashion–by eliminating self-awareness," when "the lonely 'I' disappears into the 'WE'" (Yalom, 1980, p. 380). In a similar way, one's abuse of a substance or practice can be also seen as one's need and tendency to assuage one's anxiety resulting from either the fear of being alone (separated and individuated) or the fear of being fused (engulfed by a greater whole). It is important to note that the potential addicts put themselves in a double bind, by experiencing at the same time a need and a fear of both fusion and individuation. Therefore, one's addiction can be seen as the result of one's necessity to satisfy one's need for fusion (with a substance, a practice, a person, a group), or one's need of affirming oneself as separate, specific individual. Roger Grainger, in his book *Drama and Healing: The Roots of Drama Therapy* describes this double bind as an "inability to see the other, without homogenization or alienation, as someone else who might be me" (1995, p. 11). The use of drama therapy allows the client to experience and live through both "analogy and homology, metaphor and statement" (1995, p. 12). In other words, by using a dramatic enactment within a therapeutic setting, the client will experience (1) a state of individuation ("me") and a state of fusion, when the individual temporarily disappears (the "not me," the character). Also, the client will develop an understanding and awareness of the distance that exists between fusion and individuation as well as an awareness of where exactly he/she can comfortably place himself or herself, so that none of the above states becomes a source of anxiety. This comfort zone is called in drama therapy Aesthetic Distance. It is actually the source of healing which, as Grainger (1995) put it, "is taken up by an experience which is neither fusion nor separation, but involves both of these things in an oscillation of 'me' and 'not me' (p. 32). Grainger (1995, pp. 23–26) goes on to say:

> The experience of engulfment by, or fusion in, another person or people. . . is as necessary to our relationship with the world as is individuation, the "personal view" which expresses our ability to stand back and draw conclusions. We need

to be perpetually united with a source of being recognized as authoritative in order to have the confidence in ourselves to be ourselves. . . By acting other people I establish myself as a person with regard to them, and consequently as a person for myself. My words and gestures constitute a triumph of individuality over engulfment. . .

Illo Tempore: The Sacred Time of Aesthetic Distance

Addiction can also be considered as the result of one's inability to hold anxiety and ambiguity and to resist to the immediate need to act upon one's impulse. From this point of view, drama therapy provides the tools that facilitate the client's search for his or her personal aesthetic distance, as defined by Robert Landy: The internal state when two roles occur simultaneously— the cognitive observer and the affective actor. "At aesthetic distance one is able to simultaneously play the role of the actor, who relives the past, and of the observer, who remembers the past" (Landy, 1994, pp. 113–114) and this is possible due to the optimal mixture of safety and challenge provided by the drama therapy techniques (Grainger, 1995).

Robert Landy (1994) asserts that "when the individual is at a point midway between the two extremes of overdistance and underdistance, he is at aesthetic distance, where catharsis occurs" (p. 114). In my paper, "The Retrieval of The Lost Time: My Three Steps Toward Aesthetic Distance," I extended Landy's definition by pointing out that aesthetic distance is not necessarily a "midway point," equally distanced from the extremes. Instead, in terms of space, in a given moment of one's life, one's aesthetic distance point can be closer to overdistance or underdistance, according to one's needs for more emotional charge or more cognitive clarity. In terms of time, the moment when the client becomes aware of the aesthetic distance is a suspended one, it is an awareness of escaping out of the biological time. Precisely in that moment, the client finds himself or herself in what Eliade calls "illo tempore," which its literary translation from Latin is that time, and signifies the sacred time, or "the time before the time," the mythic time that existed before the actual, profane time (Eliade, 1991, p. 68). According to Eliade, the myths of numerous cultures describe illo tempore as a very distant age, when there was a direct communication between the gods in the sky and the human beings on the earth. Many ancient healing methods aim to project the ill person to that archaic time, as a required condition for the health to be restored (1991, pp. 69–73). Thus, the healing power of achieving the aesthetic distance within a drama therapy session resides precisely in this dramatic autoprojection in the mythic, sacred time, where the client gets in contact with the archetypes of his or her feelings, needs, desires, behavior. As Eliade writes in his monumental essay, "The Myth of Eternal Return," the constant periodical projection in illo tempore during cultural celebrations and rituals (and which in this case is realized by the drama therapeutic technique), produces a renewal, a regeneration, which is healing in itself (1969). Grainger (1995) is very specific in showing the healing effect of what Jones calls "dramatic projection":

> The effect of involvement in the imaginative world of the theatre is to modify the nature of the emotions caused by events which happen in the real world. Instead of being turned inwards upon the self, painful feelings are projected outwards onto the character of the play. The important thing to realize, however, is that even though they are projected outwards, these feelings of distress are not simply denied or disowned, because of the sympathetic involvement which takes place with the stage characters, who are like ourselves but not ourselves. (p. 129)

Gaining Access To The Sacred Time: Drama Therapy As Axis Mundi

But how is the connection with the mythic time realized? I believe that symbol and metaphor are the main means by which the client gains aesthetic distance and access to the archetypal time that provides healing. C. G. Jung shows how symbols (and by extension, drama therapy, which operates with symbols) gives access to the sacred space and time: "Symbols . . . operate like a healing draught and divert the fatal incursion of the living Godhead into the hallowed space of church" (Jung in Grainger, 1995, p. 133). Making reference to Eliade's concept of Axis Mundi, Grainger writes: "The drama therapy space connects two kinds of reality, acting like that meeting place between earth and heaven which Eliade identifies as an original religious symbol" (Grainger, 1995, p. 125).

The axis mundi (Latin) is translated by the axis of the world, and it represent a core, a center around which things are organized. The fruits start to develop from, and are organized around, their pith. The embryos start to grow from and around what later will be the belly button, which is the center of the body. Similarly, the cells organize their elements around the nucleus. In numerous traditions the world, the Universe has been created and expanded from a central point, and the first human being has being created in the Center of the World, as a replica of the cosmogony (Eliade, 1969, p. 22). Scientists also consider the Big Bang as the birth of the physical Universe, which continues to expand itself ever since.

Axis mundi is considered in a huge number of cultures as the connection between, and the meeting point for Heaven, Earth, and Inferno. Eliade writes that the most common axis mundi are represented by [sacred] mountains and tall trees, and then by temples and churches, towers, pyramids, and so forth. (Eliade, 1991, p. 19). Reiterating Eliade's words, Penny Lewis talks about the relationship to the axis mundi as a way to "connect the initiate to the center of the universe" (Lewis, 1988, p. 309). "In our attached, addicted existence, we live in the illusion of a limited, small self. We think that it is all that we are. We exist in a state of mistaken identity. We have forgotten who we really are" (Grof, 1993, pp. 146–147). Thus, the Forgotten/Undiscovered pure Essence is nothing else than the Loss or the Never Had, it is the Absent Angel, one of the key characters in my existential drama therapy technique.

Addiction as Axis Mundi:
Re-centering Through Existential Drama Therapy

Clients who exhibit addictive behavior begin to organize their lives around the substance or practice they compulsively use or perform. The addiction becomes their axis mundi, the center of their world. Later, a fusion with this axis mundi occurs, and the addicted client is not able to distinguish anymore between self and the addiction, identifying with it. Some of the following existential drama therapy techniques have been described in detail elsewhere (Gheorghe, 2001, 2008). They are aimed at facilitating the deconstruction of the structure organized around addiction as axis mundi, the disidentification from addiction, and the reorganization around a different, meaningful axis mundi, which will facilitate the projection and the access to illo tempore.

Persona: Trapped In The Internal Cage Built Out Of Roles

A second warm-up technique that I use, somehow similar with the previous one, is Robert Landy's Role Cards (Landy, 2001, personal communication). After a careful selection, Landy came up with 70 roles that he believes are the most common in plays, movies, and stories. The client is asked to shuffle the cards where the roles are typed and place each card as quickly as possible in one of the following four groups that best describes how the client feels about himself or herself in that moment: This Is Who I Am, This Is Who I Am Not, I'm Not Sure If This Is Who I Am, and This Is Who I Want To Be.

Personification: Who Are You, My Dear?
Befriending the Addiction

A disidentification technique, which I elaborated during my work at Ohloff Outpatient Programs, implies a personification, and it uses dramatic projection (Johnson, 1998; Jones, 1996), role-taking and role-playing (Landy, 1994), improvisation and role reversal. The client is asked to think of his or her addiction in terms of a human being: Would it be a woman or man? What would be the age and the physical appearance of this person? But the expression of his/her face? What kind of clothes he/she wears? What is his or her behavior, voice and gestures? What his or her name would be?

The main goal of disidentification technique is to make the clients aware that they are not one with their addiction but they are a separate self that is fused with their addiction. Therefore, they are in relationship with their addiction. Consequently, they are able to act upon this relationship, to take a few steps back and contemplate both the addiction and their relationship with it/him/her. It is important to notice that these steps back and represent the way of achieving the aesthetic distance, which makes possible the contemplation of the ensemble (Gheorghe, 1994, 1996/2001). Disidentification is aimed to loosen (and eventually untie) the enmeshment (fusion) between the client and the substance ingested or the practice compulsively performed, preparing the client for the last step of this existential drama therapeutic technique, which involves the exploration of the relationship with the personified addiction.

I consider one's addiction as a representative form of one's shadow, in the Jungian sense. According to Lewis Hyde (1983), there are three ways of dealing with shadow figures. The first one is to declare that "everything on the dark side is 'not-God' and must be avoided or attacked." A second way of dealing with the shadow is to face it, address it, and have a dialog with it. "Such a dialog," Hyde says, "requires that the ego position be suspended for a moment, so that the shadow may actually speak." And finally, the third one would be to "switch allegiance and identify with the shadow itself" (Hyde, 1983, p. 255). It is not difficult to notice that denying/avoiding or attacking the addiction is the most frequent ways of how individuals and modern societies deal with substance abuse. The existential drama therapy that I developed focuses on the relationship created between the client and the addiction, exploring both its origin and its purpose, through role play and imaginary conversations: The personified addiction is faced in a non-confrontational manner and invited to dialog. When the client has reached a certain comfort and stability in terms of personal identity, role reversal can be used.

The achieving of aesthetic distance during the drama therapy session has a correspondent in the Rite of Passage Cycle. The precise moment when the client achieves aesthetic distance corresponds to the moment of understanding and accepting the new condition of being (Grainger, 1995) and it is situated between the stages of Transition and Incorporation. The aesthetic distance cannot exist before the transition ends and at the same time, it marks the beginning of the time when a new structure is incorporated. For those who are afraid of the Transition, existential drama therapy can initiate or create a Transition phase.

The Need for Transition

If we compare the first two cycles that form the operational frame of existential drama therapy, we notice an astonishing similarity: Both cycles share a Separation stage and Fusion is actually similar with Integration. What actually makes the difference between the two cycles is the presence of a third element, found exclusively within the Rite of Passage: the Transition. In fact, I can say that the Fusion-Individualization cycle is a primitive version of a Rite of Passage and when it becomes a vicious circle, it is part of the Forgetfulness of Being mode of existence. In fact, without the Transition stage, absolutely necessary for the change to take place, the Fusion-Individualization cycle becomes a vicious circle and is nothing more than a broken, incomplete Rite of Passage.

As it have been previously shown, the addictive behavior is characterized by (1) an urge and/or a need to follow an impulse, and great difficulty of not acting upon that impulse; and (2) a need to assuage the anxiety either by separation and loneliness, either by fusion and loss of individual identity. The addict, in his/her need to immediately act upon the impulse and in a state of forgetfulness of being fed back by the substance/practice abuse, viciously oscillates between fusion and separation, wanting and fearing them at the same time, without time and space allowed for Transition. In fact, the addict consciously or unconsciously avoids the Transition, which is actually a period of disorientation, and often implies discomfort and emotional pain. But, as Grainger writes, "before new life can be established, old life must have already died" (Grainger, 1995, p. 124). By not bypassing the difficulties of the Transition phase, the client introduces Transition into his initial Fusion-Separation cycle, breaking the vicious circle and transforming it into a Rite of Passage, which will result into conscious acceptance and Integration of the previously avoided material.

The vicious repetition of Fusion-Separation cycle is represented in my drama therapy technique by a mythological character, Sisyphus, condemned by gods for the rest of his life to carry a huge stone on the top of the mountain. Once there, the stone is dropped and Sisyphus has to go and bring it back, over and over again. In time, the addicts internalize this process and they identify themselves completely with their *Internalized Sisyphus.* I believe that the ceaseless reenactment of the addictive behavior is the result of a negative substitution: The anxious and fearful client replaces his/her Absent Angel (the essential Loss and/or Absence) with the Internalized/Internal Sisyphus.

During the drama therapy sessions, using dramatic projection, disidentification, personification, and reconstruction, the client achieves aesthetic distance. Consequently, the psychological and behavioral broken Rite of

Passage and its destructive effect (where the Transition is missing) is replaced by a complete Rite of Passage, which leads to Mindfulness of Being, understanding and acceptance Separation or Integration. Sisyphus' work is interrupted and the exploration of the Absent Angel begins.

Conclusion

This chapter is aimed at supporting or creating awareness about the need for multidisciplinary approach to addiction, in order to address the roots of this behavior, which are to be found in the social, cultural, and political environment of a given nation. It underlines that the deterioration of the current social relationships and of the public domain (extremely visible especially in the United States), is responsible for creating social loneliness and alienation. The consequences are: (1) lack of existential awareness and disconnection from the authentic sacred; (2) rejection and disregard of the so called "negative feelings" (sadness, yearning, nostalgia, etc.) and intolerance for discomfort; and (3) a tremendous increase of the basic level of the individual and collective anxiety, and consequently an increase (quantitatively and qualitatively) of the addictive behavior as a protection mechanism. The chapter also intends to draw attention to the natural, existential needs of human beings for togetherness and separation, and to the Rite of Passage which facilitates the reconnection of the society as a whole the paradigmatic, archetypal acts, from Illo tempore (the sacred time, the "place" and "time" where archetypes rest when they do not visit us).

References

APA. (2000). *Diagnostic and statistical manual of mental disorders*, fourth edition, text revision (DSM-IV-TR). Washington, DC: American Psychiatric Association.

Buber, M. (1965). *The knowledge of man.* New York: Harper & Row

Carrere, R. (2001). Personal communication.

Davis, J. (1999). *The diamond approach: The work of A. H. Almaas.* Boulder: Shamb'ala.

Eliade, M. (1991). *Eseuri: Mitul eternei reintoarceri. Mituri, vise si mistere.* Bucuresti: Editura Stiintifica.

Emunah, R. (1994). *Acting for real; Drama therapy process, technique and performance.* Levittown: Brunner/Mazel.

Gheorghe, C. (1994). *Persona: The internal cage.* Theater Play, Thespis Theater Timisoara, Romania.

Gheorghe, C. (1996). *Sophia.* Theater Play, Thespis Theater Timisoara, Romania.

Gheorghe, C. (2001). *The retrieval of the lost time: My three steps toward aesthetic distance.* Unpublished essay.

Gheorghe, C., & Rojas, P. (2005). *Individuality, individualism, individuation: The therapy and politics of separation.* Paper presented at the International Conference of Family Therapy, organized by American Association of Family Therapy (AFTA).

Gheorghe, C. (2008). The sacred and the profane food: Ritual and compulsion in dating disorders. In S. L. Brooke (Ed.), *The creative therapies and eating disorders* (pp. 194–208). Springfield, IL: Charles C Thomas Publishers, Ltd.

Grainger, R. (1995). *Drama and healing: The roots of drama therapy.* London: Jessica Kingsley Publishers.

Grof, C. (1993). *The thirst for wholeness: Attachment, addiction, and the spiritual path.* San Francisco: Harper.

Grof, S. (1985). *Beyond the brain: Birth, death and transcendence in psychotherapy.* New York: State University of New York Press.

Heidegger, M. (1962). *Being and time.* New York: Harper & Row.

Hyde, L. (1983). *The gift: Imagination and erotic life of property.* New York: Vintage Books, Random House.

Johnson, D. (1998). On the therapeutic action of the creative art therapies: The psychodynamic model. *The Arts in Psychotherapy, 25,* 85–99.

Jones, P. (1996). *Drama as therapy, theatre as living.* London: Routledge.

Landy, R. (1994). *Drama therapy: Concepts, theories and practices.* Springfield, IL: Charles C Thomas.

Lewis, P. (1988). The transformative process within the imaginal realm. *The Arts In Psychotherapy, 15,* 309–316.

May, R. (1977). *The meaning of anxiety.* New York: W.W. Norton & Company, Inc.

Peele, S. (1989). *Diseasing of America.* Boston: Houghton Mifflin Company.

Random House Webster's College Dictionary. (2000). New York: Random House.

Soros, G. (1998). *The crisis of global capitalism: Open society endangered.* New York: Public Affairs.

Yalom, I. D. (1980). *Existential psychotherapy.* Basic Books: Harper Collins Publishers.

Biography

Cosmin Gheorghe holds a Medical Degree in General Medicine, obtained at the University of Medicine and Pharmacy Timisoara, Romania, and he is a graduate of the Counseling Psychology program, concentration in Drama Therapy, from California Institute of Integral Studies in San Francisco. He is a Licensed Marriage and Family Therapist in California and New York. His 2008–2009 projects include the creation of a drama therapy certificate in Bogota, Colombia and a seminar in collaboration with Hôpital de la Chartreuse in Dijon, France. His writings include *The Sacred and the Profane Food: Ritual and Compulsion in Eating Disorders* and *Individuality, Individualism, Individuation: The Politics and Psychotherapy of Separation.* Together with Patricia Rojas, MFT, he founded in San Francisco "Synergis Counseling, Psychotherapy and Consulting," a private practice that reflects the idea of a systemic, multidisciplinary and meaningful approach to psychotherapy and life. Contact information: cosmin@SynergisCounseling.com or www.SynergisCounseling.com

Chapter 16

THE DARKEST ABYSS: POETRY THERAPY IN THE TREATMENT OF ADDICTIONS

Mari Alschuler

Poetry therapy (PT) involves the "intentional use of poetry and other literature to assist people with therapeutic and personal growth goals" (Alschuler, 2006, p. 253). PT had its roots in ancient Greece, but as an "organized treatment or adjunctive treatment modality" it began in "the early psychiatric hospital movement in the late 1800s," when inpatients wrote poems and published artwork in a hospital newsletter (p. 254). PT can be used in a variety of settings, including drug and alcohol treatment programs, schools, libraries, and in outpatient, inpatient, and residential settings.

PT uses the rhythms and images of written language "to access deeper aspects of the self" (Alschuler, 2006, p. 253). Three PT techniques are used frequently. First, the poetry therapist presents preexisting literature (poems, song lyrics) during a session. Second, the therapist provides writing exercises for clients to complete during or in between sessions. Third, within a family or group session, the members write a group or collaborative poem.

Clinically trained poetry therapists (PTR) or certified applied (developmental) poetry facilitators (CAPF) may use PT techniques with individuals, families, couples, and groups; PT is, however, primarily a group modality. The difference between a poetry therapy group and a creative writing or poetry workshop is its focus: "It is the significant difference between process and product" (Alschuler, 2006, p. 256). The PT group is about self-exploration and expression, while the writing workshop is about creating art to be published or performed. Clients should be informed that a PT group is not an English class and that spelling, grammar, syntax, whether they write in poetry or prose forms, use rhyme or not, are their choice. This helps to further differentiate between a writing workshop and a PT group. Literacy issues are of concern to poetry therapists, particularly in the choice of reading material selected to share with clients.

> Low literacy levels do not need to be barriers to the use of PT, however. Using a tape recorder, 'scribing' for an illiterate client, or assigning a peer to act as a writing surrogate for the client are all techniques that encourage the expression of language in all its forms. Clients who are not able to communicate in the therapist's language may also benefit from a peer transcribing their words, in addition to translating aloud to the group. Deaf or hard-of-hearing clients may also benefit from PT by utilizing signers to translate ASL. (Alschuler, 2006, p. 256)

Poems as a Confession–Poems as an Autobiography

Poetry by its nature is a product of condensation and compression, so it is natural that some facts get altered in the telling or writing. Andrew Hudgins (2001) has written about how poets may utilize various types of lies, or fictions: To him, some are "inevitable, others are merely convenient" (p. 183). He commented that some poets lie when they distill and collapse details like names, times, and places (the "lie of narrative cogency") to make "a coherent artistic product, the poem" (in Sontag & Graham, 2001, p. 183). Hudgins has suggested that even combining characters or incidents ("white lies"), which falsify the poem's background, are misrepresentations, even though the poet's intention is for "intensification and clarity" (p. 185). Another type of lie, according to Hudgins, is that of "texture," those imagistic details that accumulate in memory and paradox (p. 185).

Frost (2001) has asserted that:

> All poetry is autobiographical in its revelations of the motions a mind makes. The hesitancies, detours, innuendoes, spirals of lies and truths, as a person remembers or invents, are as essentially personal as the facts of that person's life. If readers look for event first, and take for granted the manner of telling, even so the texture, the syntax, the distribution of the literal and figurative, the timing of a writer's disclosures, false or true, are important in establishing, among other things, the authenticity of the work. . . . We doubt its authenticity in much the same way we may come to doubt a person's character. (in Sontag & Graham, 2001, p. 172)

Billy Collins (2001) has referred to Richard Hugo's suggestion of ways to free oneself from the bonds of memory and thus of direct autobiography. Hugo's "formula is that a poem as two subjects: a triggering subject that gets it going, and a generated subjected that the poem discovers along the way. The first subject is finally just a way of accessing the poem's true subject" (in Sontag & Graham, 2001, p. 85). Collins (2001) has reasoned that "we are, after all, the sum total of our own stories, our reiterated fictions" (p. 88). Thus, poets may choose to write through a mask or persona, or elect to "lie" about details, dates or facts, even when writing about the truths about their lives.

Facing Addiction–Entering Recovery

There are many poems across the centuries in which poets have described their first drink, drug, or experience of intoxication, from Rimbaud to Baudelaire to Joan Larkin, Jimmy Santiago Baca, and Raymond Carver, among others. In the introduction to **Last Call: Poems of Alcoholism, Addiction and Deliverance,** Skinner (1997) asserted that ". . . the alcoholic drinks, the drug addict shoots (or drops or smokes) to banish the self. It's not the world that's too much with the addict but the pressurized landscape within. . ." (p. xi). What first starts as a social lubricant feels at the time like "a revelation: a coping mechanism they never had, a buffer, a chemical pillow" (in Gorham & Skinner, p. xiii). When the coping mechanism becomes the problem, the addict/alcoholic often can no longer cope with life's ups and downs. As Jeffrey McDaniel (1997) noted, "Somewhere a junkie fixes the hole in his arm" ("Disasterology," in Gorham & Skinner, p. 62).

Tess Gallagher (1997), in "On Your Own," wrote about the addict's need to escape uncomfortable feeling states: ". . . I made out I was emotionally illiterate/so as not to feel a pain I deserved./ . . . I'm so scary some days/I'd run from myself" (in Gorham & Skinner, 1997, p. 92). In "The Heavens," Denis Johnson (1997) likened his struggles with addiction to those he imagined the stars experience: "From mind to mind/I am acquainted with the struggles/of these stars. The very same/chemistry wages itself minutely/in my person./It is all one intolerable war" (in Gorham & Skinner, p. 123).

In *A Season in Hell,* Rimbaud (1975) used violent imagery in poems such as "Drunken Morning":

> *The poison will stay in our veins even when, as the fanfares depart,*
> *We return to our former disharmony . . . little drunken vigil, blessed!*
> *If only for the mask that you have left us!*
> *. . . We have faith in poison.*
> *We will give our lives completely, every day.*
> *FOR THIS IS THE ASSASSINS' HOUR.* (p. 224)

In "The Drunken Boat," Rimbaud (1975) described his alcoholism as something he could not control "I drifted on a river I could not control,/No longer guided by the bargemen's ropes. . ." (p. 210). The image of a drifting, out of control boat continues: "Now I, a little lost boat in swirling debris, Tossed by the storm into the birdless upper air. . . could not fish up my body drunk with the sea" (p. 122). He was a "lost branch spinning" (p. 122). In "A Night in Hell," alcohol is "a terrific mouthful of poison that sets his guts "on fire. The power of the poison twists my arms and legs, cripples me, drives me to the ground" (p. 198). In "Second Delirium: The Alchemy of The Word," Rimbaud effectively used what now might be considered the technique of journaling to express his addiction:

> *It affected my health. Terror loomed ahead. I would fall again and again*
> *into a heavy sleep . . . and when I woke up, my sorrowful dreams continued.*
> *I was ripe for fatal harvest, and my weakness led me down dangerous roads to*
> *the edge of the world . . . I had been damned by the rainbow.* (p. 208)

Charles Baudelaire (1982) wrote poems about the internal torment of addiction. In "The Irreparable," he described "this long Remorse/which fattens on our heart/and fattens there like weevils in an oak/or vermin on a corpse" (p. 59). Only drugs or wine, he wrote, "is warranted to drown/this ancient enemy." Baudelaire also used personification in "The Soul of the Wine," in which the wine itself sings in its bottles, invoking people to break open the seal of the bottlecap so the wine can "bring you light and brotherhood!" Wine is a tempter, tempting people with false hope. Wine speaks: "Listen to my music . . . you will know happiness" (p. 113).

Jimmie Santiago Baca (1999) a Mexican-American poet, identified the period in his life and the feelings he was having when he first began using alcohol and drugs, in "The Lies Started":

> *I created a compartment*
> *where the liar existed, a small, dark cave where*
> *he cannibalized his heart and soul*
> *—kept away from others—*
> *isolating himself in a house of lies,*
> *going into the world only to drink and drug . . .*
> *. . . waking up in the morning remembering nothing,*
> *no words, no behavior, wallowing*
> *in murky, alcohol grogginess that padded the wounds,*
> *the hurts, the numbing pain of life . . .* (p. 18)

His addiction fueled crimes and led to incarcerations:

> *I lived for the drug, lived to get high,*
> *to lose myself in the darkest abyss of addiction.*
> *Parts of myself died, crawled away into holes . . .*
> *guttering away/into the sewer of addiction.* (p. 19)

Joan Larkin (1986) has written many poems about her struggles with addiction and recovery, most notably in the book, A Long Sound. In "Geneology," Larkin described the genetic factor:

I come from alcohol . . .
I was set down in it like a spark in gas . . .
My generations are of alcohol
And all that I could ever hope to bear. (p. 27)

Living "on the street," stoned on "seconal and wine," Larkin talked about how the substance

Wants more from you
It wants you
To drink
It doesn't mind if you die
I didn't mind. (p. 13)

In "Clifton," Larkin admitted she loved "booze and pills" and described how the pills let her drink,

The drink kept me from feeling
The Valium kept my hand from shaking. (p. 28)

Larkin (1986) finally stopped drinking and using. In "Goodbye," a farewell to the substances, she wrote: "You are saying good-bye to your last/drink. There is not lover/like her: bourbon, big gem/in your palm and steep/fiery blade in your throat,/deadeye down" (p. 31). The images of pain—the steep, fiery blade, the dead eye—intermingled with those of firm resolution—saying good-bye. When she stopped using, she felt it as an "unspeakable deprivation." Despite lingering memories and drug/booze-filled dreams, in sobriety Larkin experienced quiet moments, albeit mixed with doubt, in which her decision to live and survive girded her: "Often I am peaceful./I never imagined that" (p. 30).

Difficulties inherent in recovery—with its cycles of relapse, despair, and hope—are described in "Your Sister Life" in which Michael Burkard (1997) used personification to illustrate the desire to use. He compared the urge to use to having an "old sister" stop by and knock on the door to be let in—but in recovery he has the ability to say no to her, to keep her at arm's length. The recovering addict knows "she" is always present, and always a threat, but "You don't have to let her in" (in Gorham & Skinner, p. 148).

Instilling Hope

The element of hope is primary in poetry therapy. Poems are frequently selected for use in PT based on whether or not they have a hopeful tone, image, or ending. Recovery starts with "a shift in awareness, a turning away from materialism and obsession with the self, to trust in a benevolent creator—no matter the form or name" (Skinner, 1997, p. xxi). In recovery, the addict has a sense of wider understanding, connection to the world and its beauty, and is more able to open him or herself to connecting to others who suffer. The "redemptive understanding" of the recovering addict, like poetry, "accepts the double realm, the apparent fact of our suspension between the seen and the unseen" (p. xxii). Skinner ended the introduction with a hopeful note that "the news of poetry might call back a banished self, might literally save a life" (in Gorham & Skinner, 1997, pp. xxi–xxii).

Relapse is an expected part of the cycle of addiction. When Jimmie Santiago Baca (1999) relapsed, he watched himself fall down: "again I've been ensnared,/my soul filled with evil" (p. 26). There was still hope for another recovery as he recognized, in "The Day I Stopped":

> *I remember the last day*
> *when I ingested drugs, how the chilling filled*
> *my veins, my heart with corruption, venom,*
> *. . . all the work I'd done to stay clean*
> *. . . how that day . . . could be, would be, must be*
> *the day I stopped.* (p. 26)

Themes of hope continued to mark Baca's poems about recovery and release from prison, as in "I Have Roads in Me," which ended with an image about his drive to stay clean: "My heart restored,/I am guided/by stars/and a raging desire to live" (p. 28). In recovery, he memorialized those he had already lost to heroin, the streets, to prison, in "September" written in 1989, "Part of me died/with them. I am a cottonwood/lightning struck and scorched,/a black heart in the trunk. But part of me/still blossoms" (p. 110). In "I Will Remain," written while he was incarcerated, Baca (1990) envisioned release from prison:

> *a path that weaves through rock*
> *and swims through despair with fins of wisdom.*
> *A wisdom to see me through this nightmare,*
> *not by running from it; by staying to deal blow for blow.*
> *I will take the strength I need from me.* (p. 2)

Despite metaphors of blackened trees, heavy buckets that spill memories, ruins, abysses, gutters, in "Black Mesa" Baca (1989) believed "that whatever tragedy/happens in my life, I can stand on my feet/again and go on" (p. 120).

In the poem "In Western Massachusetts, Sixteen Months Sober," Larkin (1986) described how difficult it was in early recovery to write again: "To find words for this . . . /Words/I don't trust now" (p. 33). The poem ends with the hopeful image of "climbing this hill,/I'm picking up/this pen" (p. 33). A similar hopeful stance appeared at the end of "Addiction," by Cindy Goff (1999) in which she wrote about how the recovering addict has to relearn basic language: "Soon I will speak through ravens/but first I must gather my bones/and construct an alphabet" (in Gorham & Skinner, 1997, p. 105). When selecting poems for use in recovery-oriented therapy, the poetry therapist seeks writing that has a sense of hopefulness.

Stages of Change and Motivational Interviewing

The "stages of change model" in the treatment of addicts, utilizes a Transtheoretical Model (TTM) of behavioral change (Velasquez, Maurer, Crouch & DiClemente, 2001). The model has five distinct, cycling, and nonlinear stages of change. First is Precontemplation, in which clients do not yet accept or recognize they have a problem with addiction. Contemplation occurs when a client sees the problem and considers "whether to act" or not. The next stage, Preparation, occurs when a client begins to make actual, concrete plans to change. Action indicates that the client is actively doing something to change. Finally, Maintenance is a long-term process by which the client works to maintain the change.

People need a sense of mastery and ability to improve in order to succeed. Subjective states of mastery, efficacy, and purpose are important not just to our sense of self but to our sense of having the ability to make and sustain change. Motivational Interviewing (MI) is a technique for helping clients move through the stages of change as delineated by Miller and Rollnick (1991). Therapist skills are focused on the ability to:

- Express empathy
- Develop discrepancy
- Avoid argumentation
- Roll with resistance
- Support self-efficacy. (as cited in Velasquez et al., 2001, pp. 18–19)

MI strategies include asking open-ended questions, listening reflectively, remaining non-judgmental, providing affirmation, and summarizing client progress. Techniques may include psychoeducation, values clarification, problem solving, goal setting, relapse prevention planning, relaxation techniques, assertion training, role play, cognitive techniques, environmental restructuring, role clarification, reinforcement, social skills, and communication skills enhancement, needs clarification, assessment, and feedback (Velasquez et al., 2001, pp. 20–26). Many of these MI techniques involve writing, from lists to letters to journaling.

MI strategies and techniques may be modified in work with co-occurring disordered clients (mental illness with substance abuse). For example, clients dually diagnosed with addiction and mental illness can be given "modified 12-Step work" based on their cognitive and psychological level of functioning and presenting symptoms, according to Evans and Sullivan (2001). One example of modified step work might include journaling exercises, such as "give one example of someone who has been of help to you and explain how they were helpful" (p. 212). Another example could be to "describe a realistic, positive picture of your life in the future as you grow in your dual recovery" (p. 219) or to journal about "who or what is your Higher Power" (p. 226). Lists or list poems are also suggested, such as writing a list "of five specific things you like about yourself" (p. 239). Twelve-Step workbooks are used at some Anonymous meetings.

Linking Poetry Therapy to Addiction Treatment

Writing is an inherent component of the 12-Step model. Plasse (1995) believed that writing is a natural outlet within recovery programs: "The proliferation of inspirational literature attests to the importance of the written word in addiction recovery. People in recovery, even those with impoverished educations and lack of familiarity with books, quote sayings and recite parables" (p. 139). Knapp (1996), in describing her own experiences with alcoholism and recovery, wrote about attending 12-Step meetings: "When people talk [in meetings] . . . about their deepest pain, a stillness often falls over the room, a hush that's so deep and so deeply shared it feels like reverence. That stillness keeps me coming, and it helps keep me sober. . ." (p. 256). Knapp described the "language of 12-Step programs" as being repetitive: "Right from the start you hear the same clichés and catchphrases and slogans over and over and over. Don't drink, go to meetings, ask for help: the AA mantras. Keep It Simple. One Day at a Time. Let Go and Let God . . ." (p. 252).

The 12-Step model includes making amends to people the addicts/alcoholics have hurt in the past. Making a list of those who had been hurt leads the recovering person to make outreach to those people so identified. However, asking clients to write about other people in their lives, and events in their lives which involved other people, may lead to them writing about others without their permission, or write about or to others when the actuality of sending the writing to that person might have harmful consequences. Poetry therapists, therefore, may ask clients to write and then shred, flush, burn, or bury "unsent letters" in order to achieve the catharsis of self-expression while avoiding potential but unintentional injury to others.

By utilizing the techniques of MI, the therapist can implement poetry therapy techniques to assist in revealing and examining the client's typical ambivalence about getting and staying clean and sober (Springer, 2006, p. 72). During the first stage of change, precontemplation, the therapist can coach the client to examine a sense of ambivalence about their current substance use. It is also a good starting point for expressive writing. Springer (2006) suggested that the poetry therapist can examine and use the client's own written or spoken language, including symbol, image, and metaphor, to help understand "their state of mind" and to help the client move toward establishing "discrepancy between stated goals and actions. Talk of change can then begin with the client" (p. 72).

Skinner (1997) pointed out that using and recovering from using is a constant seesaw with parallels to the "contradiction and paradox" which are so "familiar" to poets (p. xx). This condition of spiritual submission, or readiness, is remarkably similar to the stance suggested by Alcoholics Anonymous for recovering addicts, who must "give up all our old ideas," and for whom "The result was nil until we let go absolutely" (in Gorham & Skinner, p. xx).

Metaphors, group writing exercises, and a non-judgmental therapeutic stance may open the recovering person to expressing "feelings that may not surface through other treatment modalities" (Howard, 1997, p. 85). Springer (2006) claimed that "images are the vehicle for expression of emotions, memories, desires, losses, trauma, and many kinds of psychic pain . . . Symbols are essential elements in therapeutic communication. . . . Working with the metaphor allows self-observation in the process of writing and the meaning one makes of the images chosen to express feeling" (p. 70). Techniques poetry therapists utilize with recovering addicts/alcoholics have included collaborative poetry, sentence stems, poems written to communicate with family members when it is too hard to have a direct conversation, journaling, poem writing, writing letters–sent and unsent–to parents or children, and creating "memorials" to help members grieve the end of a group (Alschuler, 2000; Gillispie, 2001; Morrow, 2002; Plasse, 1995).

Because institutions such as residential and inpatient drug treatment limit client choice (when to sleep, what group to attend, what to eat), the poetry therapist can have an important role in providing clients with choice, a first step toward self-efficacy and a sense of mastery and control. This writer (2000) always gave participants three choices in terms of participating in PT groups: "read what you wrote; read part of what you wrote; or pass" (p. 168).

Plasse (1995), in her work in a parenting group for recovering addicts, utilized journaling and poem writing. She found that group members were able to: Increase awareness of the damage done to [the addicts'] children through their drug addiction; move away from anomie and resistance and confront first their needs and then the needs of the children. She further emphasized that giving these parents the tools to express themselves in writing is a step toward preventing their return "back into the streets and the oblivion of drugs" (p. 137).

Writing, revising, and editing all contain the cognitive tools that portray mastery, self-efficacy, and control. Howard (1997) suggested that using metaphor and poetry can be helpful in relapse prevention, as elements of "control, perfection and isolation" are "essential to the disease" of addiction/alcoholism (p. 83). Group members recognize they are not alone, which helps to create a sense of universalization. This sense of belonging furthers group cohesion and is one of the primary healing aspects of group therapy, as well as for 12-Step meetings. The sharing of similar experience in a 12-Step meeting (the "qualification") provides a parallel experience.

Resistance can be countered through the use of the poem as transitional object, as well as through the therapist refocusing the client's attention on their own self-generated metaphors, symbols, and imagery. Poetry therapists can also instruct participants to use a persona (or mask) Examples of persona may include writing from the point of view of an archetypal or mythological character (Medusa, Helen of Troy, Cain), an animal, an inanimate object, a fictional character, or another real person.

Morrow (2002) acknowledged the frequent comings and goings of clients in substance abuse treatment; groups are always in the process of forming and reforming and clients are always leaving. Planned and unplanned termination are the grounds for helping the remaining group members deal with issues of abandonment, loss, and grief. Morrow utilized written group "memorials" which are compilations of selections of group members' writing previously produced during their PT group. Morrow stated that these memorials "make grieving-and thus remembering-possible" (p. 158). She introduced the memorial poems by first reading an excerpt to the group from Natalie Goldberg's book *Long Quiet Highway:*

> Whether we know it or not, we transmit the presence of everyone we have ever known in order to provide a sense of removal from direct revelation . . . and then we go on carrying that other person in our body, not unlike springtime when certain plants in fields we walk through attach their seeds in the form of small burrs to our socks, our pants, our caps, as if to say, 'Go on, take us with you, carry us to root in another place.' This is how we survive. . . . This is why it is important who we become, because we pass it on. (as cited in Morrow, 2002, p. 158)

Along with the group members, the therapist is also left to deal with these multiple losses, which may trigger some countertransferential feelings. This writer has suggested elsewhere (Alschuler, 2000) that the therapist could write poems at the end of sessions in lieu of process recordings or progress notes in order to "emotionally as well as intellectually process a session" (p. 167).

One of the primary goals of poetry therapy is self-expression as well as catharsis. Plasse (1995) described the recovering addict as housing poems inside of their struggles (p. 139). Dyer (1992) wrote that poetry is "a method of giving voice to what has been silenced" (p. 144). Dyer further suggested that utilizing all the creative therapies–poetry, art, movement, music, drama–"can transform pain and suffering into creation" (p. 149). Artistic images and metaphors "can give the client who suffers from silence a song of herself, an authentic reflection of all that is inside her" (p. 149).

Through reaching for authenticity and honesty, through the act of writing, personal truths may be uncovered, enacted, revealed, and released. At times, a writer may choose to use poetic techniques such as persona, metaphor, and symbol in order to address painful issues. The suffering addict or alcoholic can be assisted, through poetry therapy and similar techniques, to express their experiences, emotions, and hopes for the future.

References

Alschuler, M. (2000). Healing from addictions through poetry therapy. *Journal of Poetry Therapy, 5*(3), 143–151.

Alschuler, M. (2006). Poetry, the healing pen. In S. L. Brooke (Ed.), *Creative arts therapies manual: A guide to the history, theoretical approaches, assessment, and work with special populations of art, play, dance, music, drama, and poetry therapies* (pp. 253–262). Springfield, IL: Charles C Thomas.

Baca, J. S. (1989). *Black mesa poems.* NY: New Directions.

Baca, J. S. (1990). *Immigrants in our own land & selected early poems.* NY: New Directions.

Baca, J. S. (1999). *Set this book on fire!* Mena, AR: Cedar Hill.

Baudelaire, C. (1982). *Les fleurs du mal.* Trans. Richard Howard. Boston: Godine.

Burkard, M. (2001). Your sister life. In K. Sontag & D. Graham (Eds.), *After confession: Poetry as autobiography* (p. 148). St. Paul, MN: Graywolf.

Carver, R. (2001). Luck. In K. Sontag & D. Graham (Eds.), *After confession: Poetry as autobiography* (p. 175). St. Paul, MN: Graywolf.

Carver, R. (2001). Nyquil. In K. Sontag & D. Graham (Eds.), *After confession: Poetry as autobiography* (p. 173). St. Paul, MN: Graywolf.

Collins, B. (2001). My grandfather's tackle box: The limitations of memory-driven poetry. In K. Sontag & D. Graham (Eds.), *After confession: Poetry as autobiography* (pp. 81–94). St. Paul, MN: Graywolf.

Dyer, M. (1992). Poetry and children of alcoholics: Breaking the silence. *Journal of Poetry Therapy, 5*(3), 143–151.

Evans, K., & Sullivan, J. M. (Eds.) (2001). *Dual diagnosis: Counseling the mentally ill substance abuser.* 2nd ed. NY: Guilford.

Frost, C. (2001). Self-pity. After confession: Poetry as autobiography. In K. Sontag & D. Graham (Eds.), *After confession: Poetry as autobiography* (pp. 162–175). St. Paul, MN: Graywolf.

Gallagher, T. (1997). On your own. In S. Gorham & J. Skinner (Eds.), *Last call: Poems of alcoholism, addiction, and deliverance* (p. 92). Louisville, KY: Sarabande.

Gillispie, C. (2001). Recovery poetry 101: The use of collaborative poetry in a dual-diagnosed drug and alcohol treatment program. *Journal of Poetry Therapy, 15*(2), 83–92.

Goff, C. (1999). Addiction. In S. Gorham & J. Skinner (Eds.), *Last call: Poems of alcoholism, addiction, and deliverance* (p. 105). Louisville, KY: Sarabande.

Gorham, S., & Skinner, J. (Eds.) (1997). *Last call: Poems of alcoholism, addiction, and deliverance.* Louisville, KY: Sarabande.

Howard, A. A. (1997). The effects of music and poetry on the treatment of women and adolescents with chemical addictions. *Journal of Poetry Therapy, 11*(2), 81–102.

Hudgins, A. (2001). The glass anvil: The lies of the autobiographer. In K. Sontag & D. Graham (Eds.), *After confession: Poetry as autobiography* (pp. 182–196). St. Paul, MN: Graywolf.

Johnson, D. (1997). The heavens. In S. Gorham & J. Skinner (Eds.), *Last call: Poems of alcoholism, addiction, and deliverance* (p. 123). Louisville, KY: Sarabande.

Knapp, C. (1996). *Drinking: A love story.* NY: Delta.

Larkin, J. (1986). *A long sound.* Penobscot, ME: Granite Press.

Miller, W. & Rollnick, S. (1991). *Motivational interviewing: Preparing people to change addictive behavior.* NY: Guilford.

Morrow, D. (2002). A memorial: On recording the ending of a writing group at a recovery program for addiction. *Journal of Poetry Therapy, 15*(3), 157–161.

Plasse, B. (1995). Poetry therapy in a parenting group for recovering addicts. *Journal of Poetry Therapy, 8*(3), 135–142.

Rimbaud, A. (1975). *Complete works.* Trans. Schmidt, P. NY: Harper Colophon.

Skinner, J. (1997). Introduction. In S. Gorham & J. Skinner (Eds.), *Last call: Poems of alcoholism, addiction, and deliverance* (p. xi–xxiii). Louisville, KY: Sarabande.

Sontag, K. & Graham, D. (Eds.) (2001). *After confession: Poetry as autobiography.* St. Paul, MN: Graywolf.

Springer, W. (2006). Poetry in therapy: A way to heal for trauma survivors and clients in recovery from addiction. *Journal of Poetry Therapy, 19*(2), 69–82.

Velasquez, M., Maurer, G., Crouch, C., & Di Clemente, C. (2001). *Group therapy for substance abusers: A stages-of-change therapy manual.* NY: Guilford.

Biography

Mari Alschuler, LCSW, PTR, is a Licensed Clinical Social Worker in agency practice, and a Registered Poetry Therapist. She is the author of several professional journal articles and a book of poetry, *The Nightmare of Falling Teeth* (Pudding House Press, 1998). Ms. Alschuler holds a BA in Semiotics from Brown University, an MFA in Poetry from Columbia University, and masters' degrees in counseling psychology and organizational psychology (Teachers College/Columbia University), and social work (Fordham University). She is a Ph.D. student in Leadership and Education at Barry University, Miami Shores, Florida.

RAG DOLL

I can't shake
This image of a rag doll!
Please finally drop her
and stop the endless thrashing!

The utter fear
of not knowing
if this will stop in time.
Or if this will be
her last precious moment.

Looking up at you,
the same man
in the same position
whom she's looked up at before.
With trusting eyes,
with open heart,
with complete vulnerability.

And suddenly
"the original" that was painted
on her heart
disappears.
And she is just another rag doll.

Empty and alone
with black button eyes
that no longer sparkle.
And red frayed looped yarn hair
looking tattered and worn.

Unloved.
Completely and fully.
Unloved.

D. Desjardins (2004)

AUTHOR INDEX

271

SUBJECT INDEX

A

Adolescents, 8, 9, 51, 54, 62, 67, 69–79,
    101, 103, 105, 111, 117, 118, 121, 133,
    134, 136, 161, 177, 178, 267
Africa, 5–6
AIDS, 8, 10, 176, 202
Alcohol, 3, 4, 5, 6, 7, 9
Alexithymia, 63, 66, 104
Anxiety, 9, 16, 76, 86, 110, 124, 129, 130,
    137, 138, 141, 160, 162–174, 220, 221,
    241, 242, 243, 244, 245, 246, 247,
    248, 249, 253, 254, 255
Art Therapy, 3–105
Avatar, 86, 87, 101, 102
Australia, 9, 70, 78, 79, 166, 173

B

Brazil, 8
Butoh, 192, 199

C

Cannabis, 7, 10
Catharsis, 178, 184, 189, 195, 220, 227, 234,
    238, 249, 264, 266
Cocaine, 8, 10, 11, 121, 143, 144, 167, 195,
    196, 205, 241, 245
Chacian Technique, 167, 168, 173, 190, 192,
    197, 199, 200, 201
Child/Children, 9, 15, 19, 20, 34, 68, 98,
    100, 105, 106–119, 120–135, 138, 146,
    150, 160, 176, 181, 182, 204, 206, 214,
    224, 231, 232, 233, 247, 264, 265,
    266

China, 4

China, 4
Chinese 4, 11, 127, 135
Countertransference, 34, 116, 165, 173, 174,
    188

D

Dance/Movement Therapy, 162–174,
    186–203
Deaf/Hard of Hearing, 9, 11–36
Denial, 25, 62, 63, 81, 82, 83, 85, 95, 107,
    188, 199
Drama Therapy, 175–186, 204–255
DSM/DSM IV-TR, 14, 32, 158, 159, 245,
    254

E

Escapism, 140
Existential, 239–255

F

Fillial therapy, 9, 111, 112, 115, 117, 118,
    120, 122, 124, 125, 127, 129, 130, 132,
    133, 134, 135
Finitude, 81, 82, 84, 102

G

Global issues and substance abuse, 3–10
Greece, 7–8
Group therapy, 51, 65, 69, 71, 74, 75, 76, 77,
    78, 79, 83, 84, 102, 105, 191, 188,
    200, 265, 267

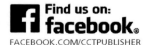